CHERYL DEGRAW, RN, M__
FLORENCE-DARLINGTON TECH__
FLORENCE, SOUTH CAR__

INSTRUCTOR'S RESOURCE MANUAL
FOR
MATERNAL-CHILD NURSING CARE

MARY ANN TOWLE • ELLISE ADAMS

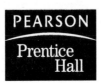

PEARSON
Prentice
Hall

Upper Saddle River, New Jersey 07458

Notice: Care has been taken to confirm the accuracy of the information presented in this book. The authors, editors, and the publisher, however, cannot accept any responsibility for errors or omissions or for consequences from application of the information in this book and make no warranty, express or implied, with respect to its contents.

The authors and the publisher have exerted every effort to ensure that drug selections and dosages set forth in this text are in accord with current recommendations and practice at time of publication. However, in view of ongoing research, changes to government regulation, and the constant flow of information relating to drug therapy and drug reactions, the reader is urged to check precautions. This is particularly important when the recommended agent is a new and/or infrequently employed drug.

The authors and publisher disclaim all responsibility for any liability, loss, injury, or damage incurred as a consequence, directly or indirectly, of the use and application of any of the contents of this volume.

All photography/illustrations not credited on page, under or adjacent to the piece, were photographed/rendered on assignment and are the property of Pearson Education/Prentice Hall Health.

Pearson Prentice Hall™ is a trademark of Pearson Education, Inc.
Pearson® is a registered trademark of Pearson plc
Prentice Hall® is a registered trademark of Pearson Education, Inc.

Pearson Education Ltd.
Pearson Education Singapore, Pte. Ltd.
Pearson Education Canada, Ltd.
Pearson Education—Japan
Pearson Education Australia PTY, Limited

Pearson Education North Asia Ltd.
Pearson Educación de Mexico, S.A. de C.V.
Pearson Education Malaysia, Pte. Ltd.
Pearson Education, Upper Saddle River, New Jersey

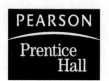

10 9 8 7 6 5 4 3 2 1
ISBN-10:   0-13-113673-9
ISBN-13: 978-0-13-113673-1

CONTENTS

PREFACE

Maternal-Child Nursing Care was written to provide the Practical/Vocational Nursing student with a foundation for providing safe, effective nursing care of mother and child within the community. This accompanying **Instructor's Resource Manual** is designed to support your teaching in this environment, and to reduce your preparation time for class. It will help you provide an optimal leaning experience for your students and their many leaning needs.

Each chapter in the Instructor's Resource Manual is thoroughly integrated with the corresponding chapter in the textbook *Maternal-Child Nursing Care*. Chapters are organized by learning outcomes, and the teaching unit flows from these outcomes. You will find the following features to support the objectives:

- The Concepts for Lecture in this manual may be used in their entirety for class presentation or they may be merged with the classroom activities for a mixture of teaching styles that will meet the needs of students with various learning styles.

- The Lecture Outlines can be found on your Instructor's Resource CD-ROM in PowerPoint. The number in the slide icon ● refers to the Concept for Lecture to which the slide correlates. Some lecture concepts have more than one slide, in which case the slide icon will contain a letter after the Concept for Lecture number.

- Suggestions for Classroom and Clinical Activities attempt to go beyond the traditional activities that have been the mainstay of nursing education for many years.

- The Resource Library identifies for you—the instructor—all the specific media resources and activities available for that chapter on the *Prentice Hall Nursing MediaLink CD-ROM,* Companion Website and Instructor's Resource CD-ROM. Chapter by chapter, the Resource Library helps you decide what resources from the CD-ROM, Companion Website, and Instructor's Resource CD-ROM to use to enhance your course and your students' ability to apply concepts from the book into practice.

This IRM also contains a new *Strategies for Success* module that includes discussion on learning theories, planning for instruction, how to use effective pedagogies, assessing learning, and more! There is also a guide on *Teaching Nursing to Students who Speak English as a Non-Native Language*. This tool is intended to guide you in reaching across cultural barriers to train nurses.

The following additional resources are also available to accompany this textbook. For more information or sample copies, please contact your Prentice Hall Sales Representative:

- **Study Guide ISBN 0-13-113727-1**—This workbook incorporates strategies for students to focus their study and increase comprehension of concepts of nursing care. It contains a variety of activities such as multiple choice, fill-in-the-blank, case studies, and more.

- **Prentice Hall Nursing MediaLink CD-ROM**—This CD-ROM is packaged with the textbook. It provides an interactive study program that allows students to practice answering NCLEX® style questions with rationales for right and wrong answers. It also contains an audio glossary, animations and video tutorials, and a link to the Companion Website (an Internet connection is required).

- **Companion Website www.prenhall.com/towle**—This online study guide is designed to help students apply the concepts presented in the book. Each chapter specific module features learning outcomes, NCLEX® review questions with rationales, chapter outlines for lecture notes, case studies, critical thinking questions, weblinks, an audio glossary, and more.

- **Instructor's Resource CD-ROM ISBN 0-13-113672-0**—This cross-platform CD-ROM provides text slides and illustrations in PowerPoint for use in classroom lectures. It also contains an electronic test bank, animations and video clips from the Prentice Hall Nursing MediaLink CD-Rom. This supplement is available to faculty upon adoption of the textbook.

- **Online Course Management Systems**—Also available are online companions for schools using course management systems. The OneKey Course Management solutions feature interactive assessment modules, electronic test bank, PowerPoint images, animations and video clips, and more. For more information about adopting an online course management system to accompany *Maternal-Child Nursing Care* please contact your Prentice Hall Sales Representative or go www.prenhall.com/nursing.

It is our hope that the information provided in this manual will decrease the time it takes you to prepare for class and will optimize the learning experience for your students.

TEACHING NURSING TO STUDENTS WHO SPEAK ENGLISH AS A NON-NATIVE LANGUAGE

We are fortunate to have so many multi-national and multi-lingual nursing students in the US in the 21st Century. As our classrooms become more diverse, there are additional challenges to communication, but we in the nursing education community are ready. Our goal is to educate competent and caring nurses to serve the health needs of our diverse communities.

We know that ENNL students experience higher attrition rates than their native English-speaking counterparts. This is a complex problem. However, there are teaching strategies that have helped many students be successful.

The first step toward developing success strategies is understanding language proficiency. Language proficiency has four interdependent components. Each component is pertinent to nursing education. Reading is the first aspect of language. Any nursing student will tell you that there are volumes to read in nursing education. Even native speakers of English find the reading load heavy. People tend to read more slowly in their non-native language. They also tend to recall less. Non-native speakers often spend inordinate amounts of time on reading assignments. These students also tend to take longer to process exam questions.

Listening is the second component of language. Learning from lectures can be challenging. Some students are more proficient at reading English than at listening to it. It is not uncommon for ENNL students to understand medical terminology, but to become confused by social references, slang, or idiomatic expressions used in class. The spoken language of the teacher may be different in accent or even vocabulary from that experienced by immigrant students in their language education. ENNL students may not even hear certain sounds that are not present in their native languages. Amoxicillin and Ampicillin may sound the same. Asian languages do not have gender-specific personal pronouns (he, she, him, her, etc.). Asian students may become confused when the teacher is describing a case study involving people of different genders.

Speaking is the third component of language proficiency. People who speak with an accent are often self-conscious about it. They may hesitate to voice their questions or to engage in discussion. Vicious cycles of self-defeating behavior can occur in which a student hesitates to speak, resulting in decreased speaking skills, which results in more hesitation to speak. Students may develop sufficient anxiety about speaking that their academic outcomes are affected. Students tend to form study groups with others who have common first languages. Opportunities to practice English are therefore reduced, and communication errors are perpetuated. When the teacher divides students into small groups for projects, ENNL students often do not participate as much as others. If these students are anxious about speaking, they may withdraw from classroom participation. ENNL students may feel rejected by other students in a small group situation when their input is not sought or understood.

The fourth aspect of language is writing. Spelling and syntax errors are common when writing a non-native language. Teachers often respond to student writing assignments with feedback that is too vague to provide a basis for correction or improvement by ENNL students. When it comes to writing lecture notes, these students are at risk of missing important details because they may not pick up the teacher's cues about what is important. They might miss information when they spend extra time translating a word or concept to understand it, or they might just take more time to write what is being said.

Another major issue faced by ENNL nursing students is the culture of the learning environment. International students were often educated in settings where students took a passive role in the classroom. They may have learned that faculty are to be respected, not questioned. Memorization of facts may have been emphasized. It may be a shock to them when the nursing faculty expect assertive students who ask questions and think critically. These expectations cannot be achieved unless students understand them.

Finally, the European-American culture, which forms the context for nursing practice, creates challenges. Because they are immersed in Euro-American culture and the culture of nursing, faculty may not see the potential sources of misunderstanding. For example, if a teacher writes a test question about what foods are allowed on a soft diet, a student who understands therapeutic diets may miss the question if s/he does not recognize the names of the food choices. Nursing issues with especially high culture connection are: food, behavior, law, ethics, parenting, games, or choosing the right thing to say. These topics are well represented in psychiatric nursing, which makes it a difficult subject for ENNL students.

MINIMIZING CULTURE BIAS ON NURSING EXAMS

Our goal is not really to eliminate culture from nursing or from nursing education. Nursing exists in a culture-dependent context. Our goal is to practice transcultural nursing and to teach nursing without undue culture bias.

Sometimes our nursing exam questions will relate to culture-based expectations for nursing action. The way to make these questions fair is to teach transcultural nursing and to clarify the cultural expectations of a nursing student in the Euro-American-dominated health care system.

Students must learn the cultural aspects of the profession before they can practice appropriately within it. Like other cultures, the professional culture of nursing has its own language (medical terminology and nursing diagnosis, of course). We have our own accepted way of dress, our own implements, skills, taboos, celebrations, and behavior. The values accepted by our culture are delineated in the ANA Code of Ethics, and are passed down to our young during nursing education.

It is usually clear to nursing educators that students are not initially aware of all the aspects of the professional culture, and that these must be taught. The social context of nursing seems more obvious to educators, and is often overlooked in nursing education. Some aspects of the social context of nursing were mentioned above (food, games, social activities, relationships, behavior, what to say in certain situations). Students must also learn these social behaviors and attitudes if they are to function fully in nursing. If they do not already know about American hospital foods, what to say when someone dies, how to communicate with an authority figure, or what game to play with a 5-year-old child, they must learn these things in nursing school.

Try for yourself the following test. It was written without teaching you the cultural expectations first.

CULTURE BIASED TEST

1. Following radiation therapy, an African American client has been told to avoid using her usual hair care product due to its petroleum content. Which product should the nurse recommend that she use instead?
   A. Royal Crown hair treatment
   B. Dax Wave and Curl
   C. Long Aid Curl Activator Gel
   D. Wave Pomade

2. A Jewish client is hospitalized for Pregnancy Induced Hypertension during Yom Kippur. How should the nurse help this client meet her religious needs based on the tradition of this holy day?
   A. Order meals without meat-milk combinations
   B. Ask a family member to bring a serving of *Marror* for the client
   C. Encourage her to fast from sunrise to sunset
   D. Remind her that she is exempt from fasting

3. Based on the Puerto Rican concept of *compadrazco*, who is considered part of the immediate family and responsible for care of children?
   A. Parents, grandparents, aunts, uncles, cousins, and godparents
   B. Mother and father, older siblings
   C. Mother, father, any blood relative
   D. Parents and chosen friends (*compadres*) who are given the honor of childcare responsibility

4. A 60-year-old Vietnamese immigrant client on a general diet is awake at 11 PM on a summer night. What is the best choice of food for the nurse to offer to this client?
   A. warm milk
   B. hot tea
   C. ice cream
   D. iced tea

5. Which of the following positions is contraindicated for a client recovering from a total hip replacement?
   A. Side-lying using an abductor pillow
   B. Standing
   C. Walking to the restroom using a walker
   D. Sitting in a low recliner

When you took this test, did it seem unfair? It was intended to test nursing behaviors that were based on culture-specific situations. Your immigrant and ENNL students are likely to face questions like these on every exam.

Item #1 is about hair care products for black hair. Option C is the only one that does not contain petroleum products. Students could know this, if they were given the information before the exam. Otherwise the item is culture-biased.

Item #2 is about the Jewish holiday Yom Kippur. To celebrate this holiday, it is customary to fast from sunrise to sunset, but people who are sick, such as the client in the question, are exempted from fasting. This is only unfair if students did not have access to the information.

Item #3 expects you to know about *compadrazco*, in which parents, grandparents, aunts, uncles, cousins, and godparents are all considered immediate family. This can be an important point if you are responsible for visiting policies in a pediatrics unit.

Item #4 tests knowledge about the preferred drink for an immigrant Vietnamese client. Many people in Asia feel comforted by hot drinks and find cold drinks to be unsettling.

Item #5 does not seem so biased. If you understand total hip precautions, it is a pretty simple question, unless you have never heard of a "low recliner". An ENNL student who missed this question, said, "I saw the chairs in clinical called 'geri chairs' and I know that the client cannot bend more than 90 degrees, but 'low recliner' was confusing to me. I imagined someone lying down (reclining) and I think this would not dislocate the prosthesis."

The best way to avoid culture bias on exams is to know what you are testing. It is acceptable to test about hip precautions, but not really fair to test about the names of furniture. The same is true of foods. Test about therapeutic diets, but not about the recipes (an African immigrant student advised us to say "egg-based food" instead of custard).

Behavior in social and professional situations is especially culture-bound. Behavior-based questions are common on nursing exams. Make behavior expectations explicit. Especially when a student is expected to act in a way that would be inappropriate in his or her social culture, these are very difficult questions. For example, we expect nurses to act assertively with physicians and clients. It is inappropriate for many Asian students to question their elders. When a client is their elder, these students will choose the option that preserves respect for the client over one that provides teaching. We must make our expectations very clear.

Finally, talk with your ENNL and immigrant students after your exams. They can provide a wealth of information about what confused them or what was ambiguous. Discuss your findings with your colleagues and improve your exams. Ultimately your exams will be clearer and more valid.

SUCCESS STRATEGIES

The following strategies were developed originally to help ENNL students. An interesting revelation is that they also help native English speakers who have learning styles that are not conducive to learning by lecture, or who read slowly, or have learning disabilities or other academic challenges.

STRATEGIES FOR PROMOTING ENNL STUDENT SUCCESS

1. You cannot decrease the reading assignment because some students read slowly, but you can help students prioritize the most important areas.

2. Allow adequate time for testing. The NCLEX is not a 1-minute-per-question test anymore. Usually 1.5 hours is adequate for a 50 item multiple-choice exam.

3. Allow students to tape lectures if they want to. You might have lectures audio-taped and put in the library for student access.

4. Speak clearly. Mumbling and rapid anxious speech are difficult to understand. If you have a problem with clarity, provide handouts containing the critical points. Provide the handouts anyway. You want to teach and test nursing knowledge, not note-taking skills.

5. Avoid slang and idiomatic expressions. This is harder than heck to do, but you can do it with practice. When you do use slang, explain it. This is especially important on exams. When in doubt about whether a word is confusing, think about what the dictionary definition would be, if there are two meanings, use another word.

6. Allow the use of translation dictionaries on exams. You can say that students must tell you what they are looking up, so they cannot find medical terminology that is part of the test.

7. Be aware of cultural issues when you are writing exams. Of course you will test on culture-specific issues, but be sure you are testing what you want to test (the student's knowledge of diets, not of recipes).

8. Feel free to use medical terminology, after all this is nursing school. However, when you use an important new term, write it on the board so students can spell it correctly in their notes.

9. In clinical, make the implied explicit. It seems obvious that safety is the priority, but if a student thinks the priority is respecting her elders, when a client with a new hip replacement demands to get out of bed there could be a disaster.

10. Hire a student who takes clear and accurate lecture notes to post his/her notes for use by ENNL and other students. The students will still attend class and take their own notes, but will have this resource to fill in the details that they miss.

11. SOA (spell out abbreviations).

12. Many international students learned to speak English in the British style. If something would be confusing to a British person, they will find it confusing.

13. Provide opportunities for students to discuss what they are learning with other students and faculty. A faculty member might hold a weekly discussion group where students bring questions. It can be interesting to find a student having no trouble tracing the path of a red cell from the heart to the portal vein, but having difficulty understanding what cream of wheat is ("I thought it was a stalk of grain in a bowl with cream poured on it").

14. Make it clear that questions are encouraged. When a student is not asking, and you think they may not understand, ask the student after class if s/he has questions. Make it easier for students to approach you by being approachable. Learn their names, and learn to pronounce them correctly. Hearing you try to pronounce their name might be humorous for them, and it will validate how difficult it is to speak other languages.

15. Take another look at basing grades on class participation. You may be putting inordinate demands on the ENNL students. Of course nurses must learn to work with others, but the nurse who talks most is not necessarily the best.

16. Be a role model for communication skills. You might even say in class when you talk about communication that if you respect a person who is trying to communicate with you, you will persist until you understand the message. Say, "Please repeat that," or "I think you said to put a chicken on my head, is that correct?" or "You want me to do what with the textbook?" It may be considered socially rude to ask people to repeat themselves repeatedly. Make it clear that this is not a social situation. In the professional role, we are responsible for effective communication. We cannot get away with smiling and nodding our heads.

17. In clinical, if a student has an accent that is difficult for the staff to understand, discuss clarification techniques (#16 above) to the student and staff member. Make it explicit that it is acceptable for the student to ask questions and for the staff to ask for clarification.

18. If your college has a writing center where students can receive feedback on grammar and style before submitting papers, have students use it. If you are not so fortunate, view papers as a rough draft instead of a final product. Give specific feedback about what to correct and allow students to resubmit.

19. Make any services available to ENNL students available to all students (such as group discussions and notes). These services may meet the learning needs of many students while preventing the attitude that "they are different and they get something I don't."

20. Faculty attitudes are the most important determinant of a successful program to promote the success of ENNL nursing students. Talk with other faculty about the controversial issues. Create an organized program with a consistent approach among the faculty. The rewards will be well worth the work.

STRATEGIES FOR SUCCESS

Sandra DeYoung, Ed.D., R.N.
William Paterson University
Wayne, New Jersey

IMPROVING OUR TEACHING

Every faculty member wants to be a good teacher and every teacher wants her or his students to learn. In particular, we want to achieve the student learning outcomes that our educational institutions say that we must achieve. How can we best meet both goals? We cannot just teach as we were taught. We have to learn a variety of teaching methods and investigate best practices in pedagogy. We also have to learn how to measure student learning outcomes in practical and efficient ways. The next few pages will introduce you to principles of good teaching and ways to evaluate learning. Keep in mind that this is only an introduction. For a more extensive study of these principles and pedagogies, you might consult the resources listed at the end of this introduction.

LEARNING THEORY

In order to improve our teaching, we must have some familiarity with learning theory. Nurses who come into educational roles without psychology of learning courses in their background should read at least an introductory level book on learning theories. You should, for example, know something about stages and types of learning; how information is stored in memory and how it is retrieved; and how knowledge is transferred from one situation to another.

BEHAVIORIST THEORIES

Behaviorist theories are not in as much favor today as they were 25 years ago, but they still help to explain simple learning. Conditioning and reinforcement are probably concepts with which most educators are familiar. Conditioning explains how we learn some simple movements and behaviors that result in desired outcomes, such as a nurse responding when an alarm sounds on a ventilator. Reinforcement refers to the fact that behavior which is rewarded or reinforced tends to reoccur. Therefore, reinforcement is a powerful tool in the hands of an educator.

COGNITIVE LEARNING THEORIES

Cognitive learning theories are much more sophisticated and deal with how we process information by perceiving, remembering, and storing information. All of these processes are a part of learning. One of the most useful concepts in cognitive theory is that of mental schemata.

Schemata (plural) are units of knowledge that are stored in memory. For example, nurses must develop a schema related to aseptic technique. Once a schema is stored in memory, related information can be built on it. For instance, changing a dressing is easier to learn if the learner already has a schema for asepsis.

Metacognition is another concept identified in cognitive theories. This concept refers to thinking about one's thinking. To help learners who are having difficulty mastering certain material, you might ask them to think about how they learn best and to help them evaluate whether they really understand the material.

Transfer of learning occurs when a learner takes information from the situation in which it is learned and applies it to a new situation. Transfer is most likely to occur if the information was learned well in the first place, if it can be retrieved from memory, and if the new situation is similar to the original learning situation. Educators can teach for transfer by pointing out to students how a concept is applied in several situations so that learners know that the concept is not an isolated one, and the students begin to look for similar patterns in new situations.

ADULT LEARNING THEORIES

Adult learning theories help to explain how learning takes place differently for adults than for children. Adults usually need to know the practical applications for the information they are given. They also want to see how it fits with their life experiences. When teaching young adults and adults, nurse educators need to keep in mind adult motivation for learning.

LEARNING STYLE THEORIES

Learning style theories abound. Research has shown that some learners are visually oriented, some are more auditory or tactile learners; some are individualistic and learn best alone, others learn best by collaboration; some deal well with abstract concepts and others learn better with concrete information. Measurement instruments that can determine preferred learning styles are readily available. Although not many educators actually measure their students' learning styles, they should at least keep learning styles in mind when they plan their instruction.

PLANNING FOR INSTRUCTION

With some background knowledge of how students learn, the nurse educator can begin to plan the learning experiences. Planning includes developing objectives, selecting content, choosing pedagogies, selecting assignments, and planning for assessment of learning. All nurse educators come to the teaching process already knowing how to write objectives. Objectives can be written in the cognitive, psychomotor, and affective domains of learning. In the cognitive domain, they can be written at the knowledge, comprehension, application, analysis, and synthesis levels of complexity. The critical aspect of objectives is that you need to keep referring to them as you plan your lesson or course. They will help you focus on the "need to know" versus the "nice to know" material. They will help you decide on which assignments will be most suitable, and they will guide your development of evaluation tools.

SELECTING ASSIGNMENTS

Selecting and developing out-of-class assignments calls for creativity. You may use instructor manuals such as this for ideas for assignments or you may also develop your own. To encourage learning through writing, you can assign short analysis papers, position papers or clinical journals, all of which promote critical thinking. Nursing care plans of various lengths and complexity may be assigned. You may create reading guides with questions to help students read their textbooks analytically. You might also ask students to interview people or observe people to achieve various objectives.

USING EFFECTIVE PEDAGOGIES

Selecting teaching methods or pedagogies takes considerable time. You must consider what you are trying to achieve. To teach facts, you may choose to lecture or assign a computer tutorial. To change attitudes or motivate learners, you may use discussion, role-playing, or gaming. Developing critical thinking may be done effectively using critical thinking exercises, concept maps, group projects, or problem-based learning. There are what I will call *traditional* pedagogies, *activity-based* pedagogies, and *technology-based* pedagogies.

TRADITIONAL PEDAGOGIES

Traditional pedagogies include lecture, discussion, and questioning. Lecturing is an efficient way to convey a great deal of information to large groups of people. However, the lecture creates passive learning. Learners just sit and listen (or not) and do not interact with the information or the lecturer. Research has shown that students learn more from active learning techniques, i.e. from being able to talk about, manipulate, reduce, or synthesize information. So, if you are going to lecture, it would be wise to intersperse lecture with discussion and questioning.

Discussion gives students an opportunity to analyze and think critically about information that they have read or were given in a lecture. By discussing key concepts and issues, they can learn the applicability of the concepts and see how they can transfer to varied situations. Discussions can be formal or informal, but they generally work best if they are planned. For a formal discussion, students must be held accountable for preparing for it. The teacher becomes a facilitator by giving an opening statement or question, guiding the discussion to keep it focused, giving everyone a chance to participate, and summarizing at the end.

Questioning is a skill that develops over time. The first principle to learn is that you have to give students time to answer. Most teachers wait only one second before either repeating the question or answering it themselves. You should wait at least three to five seconds before doing anything, to allow students time to think and prepare a thoughtful answer. Research has revealed that most instructor-posed questions are at a very low level (lower-order), eliciting recall of facts. But questioning can be used to develop critical thinking if it is planned. Higher-order questions are those that require students to interpret information, to apply it to different situations, to think about relationships between concepts, or to assess a situation. If you ask higher-order questions during your classes or clinical experiences, students will rise to the occasion and will be challenged to provide thoughtful answers.

ACTIVITY-BASED PEDAGOGIES

Activity-based teaching strategies include cooperative learning, simulations, games, problem-based learning, and self-learning modules, among others. Cooperative learning is an old pedagogy that has received more research support than any other method. This approach involves learners working together and being responsible for the learning of group members as well as their own learning. Cooperative learning groups can be informal, such as out-of-class study groups, or can be formally structured in-class groups. The groups may serve to solve problems, develop projects, or discuss previously taught content.

Simulations are exercises that can help students to learn in an environment that is low risk or risk free. Students can learn decision making, for example, in a setting where no one is hurt if the decision is the wrong one. Simulations in skill laboratories are frequently used to teach psychomotor skills. Simulations can be written (case studies), acted out (role playing), computer-based (clinical decision-making scenarios), or complex technology-based (active simulation mannequins).

Games can help motivate people to learn. Factual content that can depend on memorization such as medical terminology can be turned into word games such as crossword puzzles or word searches. More complex games can teach problem solving or can apply previously learned information; board games or simulation games can be used for these purposes.

Problem-Based Learning (PBL) provides students with real-life problems that they must research and analyze and then develop possible solutions. PBL is a group activity. The instructor presents the students with a brief problem statement. The student group makes lists of what they know and don't know about the problem. They decide what information they must collect in order to further understand the problem. As they collect the information and analyze it, they further refine the problem and begin to investigate possible solutions. The educator serves as a facilitator and resource during the learning process and helps keep the group focused.

Self-learning modules are a means of self-paced learning. They can be used to teach segments of a course or an entire course or curriculum. Modules should be built around a single concept. For example, you might design a module for a skill lab based on aseptic technique; or you could develop a module for a classroom course around the concept of airway impairment. Each module contains components such as an introduction, instructions on how to use the module, objectives, a pretest, learning activities, and a posttest. Learning activities within a module should address various learning styles. You should try to include activities that appeal to visual learners and tactile learners, conceptual learners and abstract learners, individual and collaborative learners, for example. Those activities could be readings, audiovisuals, computer programs, group discussion, or skills practice. The educator develops and tests the module and then acts as facilitator and evaluator as learners work through the module.

Technology-Based Pedagogies

Technology-based pedagogies include computer simulations and tutorials, Internet use, and distance learning applications. Computer simulations were discussed briefly above. They include decision-making software in which a clinical situation is enacted and students are asked to work through the nursing process to solve problems and achieve positive outcomes. They also include simulation games such as SimCity which can be a useful tool in teaching community health principles. Computer tutorials are useful for individual remedial work such as medication calculations or practice in taking multiple-choice test questions.

The Internet is a rich resource for classroom use and for out-of-class assignments. There are hundreds of websites that can be accessed for health-related information. Students need to be taught how to evaluate the worth of these websites. The criteria they should apply to this evaluation include identifying the intended audience, the currency of the information, the author's credentials or the affiliated organization, and content accuracy. Students may not know how to identify online journal sources compared to other websites. It is worth spending time, therefore, teaching students how to use the Internet before giving them such assignments. If your classroom is Internet access enabled, you can visually demonstrate how to identify and use appropriate Web sites. For example, if you want students to find relevant information for diabetic teaching, you can show them the differing value of information from official diabetes associations versus pharmaceutical sites versus chat rooms or public forums.

You may be using this instructor manual in a distance learning course. Distance learning takes the forms of interactive television classes, Webcasting, or online courses. In any form of distance learning, students are learning via the technology, but they are also learning about technology and becoming familiar with several computer applications. Those applications may include synchronous and asynchronous applications, streaming video and multimedia functions.

Assessing Learning

You can assess or evaluate learning in a number of ways. Your first decision is whether you are just trying to get informal, ungraded feedback on how well students are learning in your class, or whether you are evaluating the students for the purpose of assigning a grade. Following are a number of techniques that can be used for one or both purposes.

Classroom Assessment Techniques

Classroom Assessment Techniques (CATs) are short, quick, ungraded, in-class assessments used to gauge students' learning during or at the end of class. Getting frequent feedback on students' understanding helps educators to know if they are on the right track and if students are benefiting from the planned instruction. If you wait until you give a formal quiz or examination, you may have waited too long to help some students who are struggling with the material. The most popular CAT is probably the *Minute Paper*. This technique involves asking students to write down, in one or two minutes, usually at the end of class, what was the most important thing they learned that day or what point or points remain unclear. A related technique is the *Muddiest Point,* in which you ask the class to write down what the "muddiest" part of the class was for them. In nursing, *Application Cards* can be especially useful. After teaching about a particular concept or body of knowledge, and before you talk about the applications of the information, ask the students to fill out an index card with one possible clinical application of the information. This technique fosters application and critical thinking. Always leave class time during the following session to give feedback on the CAT results.

Another means of doing a quick assessment of learning in the classroom is the use of a *classroom (or student) response system,* sometimes called *clicker* technology. By the use of radio frequency technology, a laptop computer, projector, and student remote controls (the clickers), an instructor can pose a written question on the screen and ask students to use their clickers to select the correct answer. The answers are then tallied and can be projected as a graph of results on the screen. This technology permits quick assessment of student understanding of critical information and keeps students active during a lecture. Classroom response systems are often made available by publishers in conjunction with their textbooks.

Tests and Examinations

Tests and examinations are also used to assess or evaluate learning. Tests should be planned carefully to measure whether learning objectives have been met. You should form a test plan in which you decide the number of test items to include for each objective as well as the complexity of the items. Just as objectives can be written at the knowledge through synthesis levels of knowing, test items can be written at each level, too. Some types of items lend themselves to the lower levels of knowing, such as true-false and matching items, while multiple-choice and essay questions can be used to test higher levels.

TRUE-FALSE QUESTIONS

True-false questions are used simply to determine if the student can determine the correctness of a fact or principle. This type of question should be used sparingly, because the student has a 50% chance of guessing the correct answer. Well written true-false questions are clear and unambiguous. The entire statement should be totally true or totally false. An example of a question that is ambiguous is:

(T F) A routine urinanalyis specimen must be collected with clean technique and contain at least 100 ml.

The answer to this question is false because the specimen does not require 100 ml of volume. However the clean technique part of the question is true. Because part of the statement is true and part is false, the question is misleading. A better question is:

(T F) A routine urinalysis specimen must be collected with clean technique.

True-false questions can be made more difficult by requiring the student to explain why the statement is true or false.

MATCHING QUESTIONS

Matching questions also test a low level of learning—that of knowledge. They are most useful for determining if students have learned definitions or equivalents of some type. They should be formatted in two columns, with the premise words or statements on the left and the definitions or responses on the right. You should have more responses than premises so that matching cannot be done simply by process of elimination. Instructions should be given that indicate if responses can be used more than once or even not used at all. An example of a matching question is:

Match the definition on the right with the suffix on the left. Definitions can be used only once or not at all.

_____ 1. –itis   a. presence of

_____ 2. –stalsis   b. abnormal flow

_____ 3. – rrhage   c. inflammation

_____ 4. –iasis   d. discharge or flow

_____ 5. –ectomy   e. contraction

                          f. surgical removal of

MULTIPLE-CHOICE QUESTIONS

Multiple-choice questions can be written at the higher levels of knowing, from application through evaluation. At these higher levels they can test critical thinking. A multiple-choice question has two parts. The first part, the question, is also called the *stem*. The possible answers are called *options*. Among the options, the correct one is called the *answer,* while the incorrect options are termed *distractors*. You can word stems as questions or as incomplete statements that are completed by the options. For example, an item written as a question is:

WHAT IS A QUICK WAY TO ASSESS THE APPROXIMATE LITERACY LEVEL OF A PATIENT?

  a. Pay attention to her vocabulary as she speaks.

  b. Give her an instruction sheet to read.

  c. Administer a literacy test.

  d. Ask her whether she graduated from high school.

The same knowledge can be tested by a stem written as an incomplete statement:

A QUICK WAY TO ASSESS THE APPROXIMATE LITERACY LEVEL OF A PATIENT IS TO

  a. pay attention to her vocabulary as she speaks.

  b. give her an instruction sheet to read.

  c. administer a literacy test.

  d. ask her whether she graduated from high school.

Notice the differing formats of each item. When the stem is a question it is also a complete sentence, so each option should be capitalized because each is also a complete sentence and each ends with a period. When the stem is an incomplete statement, it does not end with a period, so the options which complete the statement do not begin with a capital letter but do end with a period. Stems should be kept as brief as possible to minimize reading time. Avoid negatively stated stems. For example, a poor stem would be, "Which of the following is not a good way to assess a patient's literacy level?" It is too easy for readers to miss the word "not" and therefore answer incorrectly. If you feel compelled to write negative stems occasionally, be sure to capitalize or underline the word "not", or use the word "except" as in the following example: "All of the following are good ways to assess a patient's literacy level EXCEPT." In this case, the reader is less likely to miss the negative word because of the sentence structure and also because the word "except" is capitalized.

Options usually vary from three to five in number. The more options you have, the more difficult the item. However, it is often difficult to write good distractors. Be sure that your options are grammatically consistent with the stem. Next is a test item in which all of the options do not fit grammatically with the stem:

The lecture method of teaching is best suited to

  a. when the audience already knows a lot about the topic.

  b. large audiences.

  c. times when you are in a hurry to cover your material and don't want to be interrupted.

  d. young children.

Not only are the options grammatically inconsistent, they are also of varied lengths. Attempt to keep the options about the same length. The following re-statement of the item corrects the problems with grammar and with length:

The lecture method of teaching is best suited to

a. an audience that already knows the topic.

b. an audience that is very large.

c. times when you must cover your material quickly.

d. an audience of young children.

Distractors that make no sense should never be used. Instead, try to develop distractors that reflect incorrect ideas that some students might hold about a topic.

ESSAY QUESTIONS

Essay-type questions include short answer (restricted response questions) and full essays (extended response questions). These types of items can be used to test higher-order thinking. Extended-response essays are especially suited to testing analysis, synthesis, and evaluation levels of thinking. An example of an essay that might test these higher order levels of thinking is: Explain how exogenous cortisone products mimic a person's normal cortisol functions and why long-term cortisone administration leads to complications. Also explain how nursing assessment and intervention can help to reduce those complications.

The educator must plan how the essay is going to be graded before the test is given. An outline of required facts and concepts can be developed and points given to each. Then a decision must be made as to whether it is appropriate to give points for writing style, grammar, spelling, and so on.

TEST ITEM ANALYSIS

After a test is given, an analysis of objective items can be conducted. Two common analyses are *item difficulty* and *item discrimination*. Most instructors want to develop questions that are of moderate difficulty with around half of the students selecting the correct answer. A mixture of fairly easy, moderate, and difficult questions can be used. The difficulty index can be easily calculated by dividing the number of students who answered the question correctly by the total number of students answering the question. The resulting fraction, converted to a percentage, gives an estimate of the difficulty, with lower percentages reflecting more difficult questions.

Item discrimination is an estimate of how well a particular item differentiates between students who generally know the material and those that don't. Another way of saying it is that a discriminating item is one that most of the students who got high scores on the rest of the examination got right and most of the students who got low scores got wrong. The discrimination index can be calculated by computer software or by hand using a formula that can be found in tests and measurement textbooks.

HELPFUL RESOURCES

These few pages are but an introduction to teaching techniques. To be fully prepared for the educator role, you will need to enroll in formal courses on curriculum and teaching or do more self-learning on educational topics. For more information, you might consult the following print and Web-based resources:

DeYoung, S. (2003). *Teaching Strategies for Nurse Educators*, Upper Saddle River, NJ: Prentice Hall.

Web sites:

www.crlt.umich.edu/tstrategies/teachings.html

www.gmu.edu/facstaff/part-time/strategy.html

www.ic.arizona.edu/ic/edtech/strategy.html

CHAPTER 1
THE LPN/LVN IN MATERNAL-CHILD, COMMUNITY-BASED NURSING

RESOURCE LIBRARY

 COMPANION WEBSITE

CDC mortality data

IMAGE LIBRARY

Figure 1-1 Nursing process model.
Figure 1-2 Interdisciplinary team with LPN/LVN.

Figure 1-3 Decision-making model.
Figure 1-4 Delegation model.

LEARNING OUTCOME 1

Describe the historical changes in maternity care and pediatrics.

CONCEPTS FOR LECTURE

1. Maternal-child nursing is the care of women through pregnancy, childbirth, and postpartum and care of children from birth through the teenage years.
2. From 1900 to the early 1940s childbirth shifted from care provided by untrained personnel to care provided by physicians, from the home to the hospital setting.
3. In the 1960s through the 1980s use of spinal block anesthesia led to the use of forceps for delivery and respiratory distress in the neonate, causing cesarean deliveries to increase.

    In the 1990s formal prenatal classes were formed, birthing suites were built, and epidural anesthesia was used for pain relief.
4. The Association of Women's Health, Obstetrics and Neonatal Nursing (AWHONN) was formed to improve the health of women and newborn infants after maternity nursing became a specialty.

    Today, couples are postponing childbirth to pursue a career, resulting in a greater risk of complications and fetal anomalies.
5. Pediatrics is medical science related to the diagnosis and treatment of childhood illness.

    Laws have been passed to protect children's rights, such as Aid to Families with Dependent Children, Child Health Assessment Program of Medicaid, and Women, Infants, Children (WIC) program. Aid is included in name of program and needs to be capitalized
6. Nursing has evolved from providing for the sick person's activities of daily living to a knowledge-based discipline requiring specialized education and professional judgment.

POWERPOINT LECTURE SLIDES

(NOTE: The number on each PPT Lecture Slide directly corresponds with the Concepts for Lecture.)

1 Maternal-Child Nursing Care
- Care of women through pregnancy, childbirth, and postpartum
- Care of children from birth through the teenage years

2 History of Maternity Nursing
- 1900–1940s
  ○ Childbirth care shifted to care by physicians
  ○ Health care moved from the home environment to the hospital setting
  ○ Improvements in anesthesia
  ○ AWHONN founded
  ○ Two- or three-day hospital stays

3 History of Maternity Nursing
- 1960s–1980s
  ○ Spinal block anesthesia use led to
    – Use of forcep deliveries
    – Respiratory distress in neonates
    – Increased number of cesarean deliveries
- 1990s
  ○ Formal prenatal classes developed
  ○ Birthing suites were built
  ○ Epidural anesthesia replaced spinal block

4 History of Maternity Nursing
- 2000s
  ○ Postponing childbirth to pursue career
    – Greater risk of complications
    – Increased fetal anomalies
  ○ Importance of client teaching

History of Pediatric Nursing
- Pediatrics
  - Diagnosis and treatment of childhood illness
- Middle Ages
  - Childhood lasted until 7 years of age
- Theorists developed childhood development theories
  - Erikson, Piaget
- Laws developed to protect children's rights

6 Changes in Nursing
- Providing for sick person's ADL and handmaiden to doctor
- Changed to knowledge-based discipline
- Four features of nursing practice (ANA)
  - Attend to full range of human responses to health and illness—holistic care
  - Integrate objective and subjective data
  - Apply scientific knowledge
  - Provide caring relationship

SUGGESTIONS FOR CLASSROOM ACTIVITIES	SUGGESTIONS FOR CLINICAL ACTIVITIES
• Have students review Table 1-1 and discuss events in Maternal-Child Nursing. • Have students look up the AWHONN organization to find the latest clinical updates and evidence-based practice guidelines.	• Have students research the requirements for participation in programs such as WIC and Medicaid.

LEARNING OUTCOME 2

Describe the steps of the nursing process.

CONCEPTS FOR LECTURE

1. The nursing process is a systematic approach that guides the care planning process.

   The steps of the nursing process are assessing, diagnosing, planning, implementing, and evaluating.

POWERPOINT LECTURE SLIDES

(NOTE: The number on each PPT Lecture Slide directly corresponds with the Concepts for Lecture.)

 Nursing Process
- Systematic approach when planning and implementing nursing care
  - Assessing
  - Diagnosing
  - Planning
  - Implementing
  - Evaluating

SUGGESTIONS FOR CLASSROOM ACTIVITIES	SUGGESTIONS FOR CLINICAL ACTIVITIES
• Have students review the nursing process care plan in the chapter and discuss the critical thinking questions.	• Have students develop a care plan using the nursing process for a client they are assigned to care for in the health care setting.

LEARNING OUTCOME 3

Describe the benefit of research for nursing practice.

CONCEPTS FOR LECTURE

1. Research gives direction to nursing practice through changes in current practice.
   Areas of research affecting nursing care are mortality, sudden infant death syndrome, and morbidity.

POWERPOINT LECTURE SLIDES

(NOTE: The number on each PPT Lecture Slide directly corresponds with the Concepts for Lecture.)

1 Research-Based Nursing Practice
- Research gives direction to nursing practice
- Areas of research
  - Mortality
  - Sudden Infant Death Syndrome
  - Morbidity
- Uses of research
  - Documentation quality of care
  - Revision of standards-of-practice policies

SUGGESTIONS FOR CLASSROOM ACTIVITIES

- Discuss factors that affect areas of research and the advantages of evidence-based nursing practice.
- Refer to mortality rates in Tables 1-2 and 1-3 when discussing importance of research.

SUGGESTIONS FOR CLINICAL ACTIVITIES

- Have students research the birthrates, mortality rates, and morbidity rate in the city or state they live in.

LEARNING OUTCOME 4

Describe community-based nursing practice.

CONCEPTS FOR LECTURE

1. Community-based nursing is nursing care provided to individuals, families, and groups in any setting they are in.
2. Effective community-based programs have the following characteristics: community participation, community assessment, measurable objectives, monitoring and evaluation processes, and interventions.
3. Community-based nursing encompasses primary, secondary, and tertiary levels of care.
4. Culturally proficient care includes awareness of the similarities and differences among cultures and a competence in caring for clients from other cultures.

POWERPOINT LECTURE SLIDES

(NOTE: The number on each PPT Lecture Slide directly corresponds with the Concepts for Lecture.)

1 Community-Based Practice
- Care provided to individuals, families, groups in any setting

2 Characteristics of Effective Community-Based Programs (*Healthy People 2010*)
- Community participation
- Community assessment
- Measurable objectives
- Monitoring and evaluation process
  - Interventions for change, cultural relevance

3 Community-Based Practice
- Levels of care
  - Primary care
    - Health prevention to maintain health and prevent illness
  - Secondary care
    - Treatment of illness to return client to health
  - Tertiary care
    - Management of chronic, terminal, complicated, long-term health care problems

4 Culturally Proficient Care
- Cultural awareness
  ○ Knowledge of similarities and differences among cultures
- Cultural competence
  ○ Skills, knowledge, attitudes of cultures
- Cultural proficiency
  ○ Using cultural competence to plan and provide nursing care

---

SUGGESTIONS FOR CLASSROOM ACTIVITIES

- Have students examine the *Healthy People 2010* document for initiatives in maternal-child nursing and community-based health care.
- Have students review Box 1-1 and discuss ways to provide culturally competent nursing care to clients from differing cultures.
- Assign students to list agencies where community-based nursing services are performed.

SUGGESTIONS FOR CLINICAL ACTIVITIES

- Have students provide nursing care to clients of a culture different from the student's culture.
- Schedule students to obtain clinical experiences in community agencies that provide services to women and children.

LEARNING OUTCOME 5

Describe LPN/LVN roles in maternal-child nursing.

CONCEPTS FOR LECTURE

1. Roles of the LPN/LVN include collaborating with the interdisciplinary team, utilizing the nursing process, problem solving using inductive and deductive reasoning, using critical thinking to solve problems, and utilizing critical thinking care maps to organize information and select relevant interventions.

   A major role of LPN/LVNs is health promotion teaching.

POWERPOINT LECTURE SLIDES

(NOTE: The number on each PPT Lecture Slide directly corresponds with the Concepts for Lecture.)

 Roles of the LPN/LVN
- Collaborating with the interdisciplinary team
- Utilizing the nursing process
- Using problem solving skills
  ○ Inductive reasoning
  ○ Deductive reasoning
- Using critical thinking
  ○ Critical thinking care maps
- Teaching health promotion

SUGGESTIONS FOR CLASSROOM ACTIVITIES

- Assist students in developing a critical thinking care map from a case study on a maternal client and a pediatric client.
- Discuss use of complementary and alternative therapies in Box 1-5.

SUGGESTIONS FOR CLINICAL ACTIVITIES

- Have students develop a critical thinking care map using a client cared for in the health care setting.

LEARNING OUTCOME 6

Describe decision making and prioritizing as they relate to nursing scope of practice.

CONCEPTS FOR LECTURE

1. LPNs/LVNs are held to a standard of reasonable and prudent care as designated by the Nurse Practice Act, the Board of Nursing Rules or Position Statements, and agency policies.

   The LPN/LVN needs to know what he/she is competent to perform to provide safe nursing care.

   The LPN/LVN needs to attend in-service programs to develop competence in new procedures or equipment.

2. Decision making is based on knowledge and competency about performing nursing care.

3. The LPN/LVN must establish priorities when planning and implementing nursing care to provide safe and effective care.

POWERPOINT LECTURE SLIDES

(NOTE: The number on each PPT Lecture Slide directly corresponds with the Concepts for Lecture.)

1 Decision Making
- Standards of reasonable and prudent care are designated by:
  - Nurse Practice Act
  - Board of Rules or Position Statements
  - Agency policies
- Maintenance of competence in practice
  - Attend in-service education

2 Decision Making

3 Prioritizing and Implementing
- Most critical aspects of care must be initiated first
  - Airway, breathing, circulation
- Next priority is client safety and comfort
- Plan and implement care for several clients at a time

SUGGESTIONS FOR CLASSROOM ACTIVITIES

- Have students contact the State Board of Nursing and review the standards of practice for an LPN/LVN.
- Discuss guidelines for decision making in Box 1-2.
- Discuss guidelines for priority setting in Table 1-4.

SUGGESTIONS FOR CLINICAL ACTIVITIES

- Have students review agency policies in the health care facility where they are having the clinical rotations.
- Discuss decisions made and how the students prioritized nursing care in the health care setting.

LEARNING OUTCOME 7

Describe the delegation process related to nursing scope of practice.

CONCEPTS FOR LECTURE

1. Delegation is transferring to a competent individual the authority or right to perform selected nursing tasks in a selected situation.

   The LPN/LVN retains accountability when delegating or assigning nursing care to unlicensed personnel. According to NCSBN, some states allow LPN/LVNs to delegate, other states allow LPN/LVNs to assign.

2. The five rules of delegation are right task, right circumstances, right person, right direction/communication, and right supervision.

3. The nursing task being delegated must be selected based on client assessment, the individual situation, and the skill of the individual being delegated to.

4. Redelegation: A delegated task may not be redelegated to another person.

POWERPOINT LECTURE SLIDES

(NOTE: The number on each PPT Lecture Slide directly corresponds with the Concepts for Lecture.)

1 Delegation
- Transfer authority or right to perform nursing task to competent individual in a selected situation
- Retain accountability for tasks delegated
- Base delegation on:
  - Client assessment
  - Individual situation
  - Skill of individual unlicensed person

2 Delegation
- Five rules of delegation
  - Right task
  - Right circumstances
  - Right person
  - Right direction/communication
  - Right supervision

Delegation
- Direction for delegation:
  - What is to be done
  - Expected outcome of task
  - Possible complications
  - What unlicensed person should do if complications happen

4 Delegation
- Unlicensed person accepting delegated task may not **redelegate** task to someone else
- Unlicensed person is not qualified to delegate nursing care

- Licensed nurse is accountable for outcome of task delegated or assigned
- Supervision is giving direction for and inspecting task performed

---

SUGGESTIONS FOR CLASSROOM ACTIVITIES

- Have students contact the State Board of Nursing to review the duties of unlicensed personnel.
- Review the National Council of State Boards of Nursing Premises for Delegating Tasks in Box 1-3.

SUGGESTIONS FOR CLINICAL ACTIVITIES

- Have students delegate or assign appropriate nursing tasks to unlicensed personnel in the clinical setting.

CHAPTER 2
LEGAL AND ETHICAL ISSUES IN MATERNAL-CHILD NURSING

RESOURCE LIBRARY

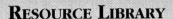 **COMPANION WEBSITE**

Healthy People 2010
State Policies for Minors

📖 IMAGE LIBRARY

Figure 2-1 *Healthy People 2010* identifies objectives for each indicator (USDHHS, 2000).

Figure 2-2 A sample power of attorney for health care plus organ donor form.

Figure 2-3 An incident report form.

Figure 2-4 Obtaining informed consent is the responsibility of the person performing the procedure. The nurse may be asked to witness the consent signature.

LEARNING OUTCOME 1

Describe federal initiatives to protect children.

CONCEPTS FOR LECTURE

1. The US government established programs to improve children's care, such as Medicaid's Early and Periodic Screening, Diagnosis and Treatment; Women, Infants, and Children's program; National School Lunch Program.
2. The U.S. Department of Health and Human Services released *Healthy People 2000* and *Healthy People 2010* to develop goals and objectives for health care.
3. The nurse should understand general guiding principles of legal and ethical issues affecting children and obtain legal advice for complex issues.

POWERPOINT LECTURE SLIDES

(NOTE: The number on each PPT Lecture Slide directly corresponds with the Concepts for Lecture.)

1 Federal Government Programs to Improve Children's Care
- Medicaid's Early and Periodic Screening, Diagnosis and Treatment (EPSDT)
- Women, Infants, and Children (WIC) program
- National School Lunch Program

2 U.S. Department of Health and Human Services
- *Healthy People 2000*
- *Healthy People 2010*

3 Legal and Ethical Issues Affecting Children
- Vary from state to state
- Need to understand general principles
- Obtain legal advice for complex issues

SUGGESTIONS FOR CLASSROOM ACTIVITIES

- Have students review the goals and objectives for *Healthy People 2010* at *http://www.healthypeople.gov* Discuss goals involving care of children.
- Have students research legal and ethical issues affecting the health care of children in the state in which they live. Discuss their research findings in class.
- Have students view state's regulations on sex education and sexually transmitted diseases.

SUGGESTIONS FOR CLINICAL ACTIVITIES

- None

LEARNING OUTCOME 2

Describe parents' rights as they relate to the care of children.

CONCEPTS FOR LECTURE

1. With few exceptions, parents have the authority to make decisions for their minor children regarding health care.

   The LPN/LVN must provide nursing care in an unbiased manner and report all concerns to the supervising RN.

POWERPOINT LECTURE SLIDES

(NOTE: The number on each PPT Lecture Slide directly corresponds with the Concepts for Lecture.)

1 Parents' Rights
- Authority to make decisions for minor children
- Right to give informed consent for procedures
- Right to have nursing care provided in an unbiased manner

1a Exceptions to Parents' Rights
- Parents are incapacitated and unable to make decision
- Actual or suspected child abuse or neglect
- Parents' choice does not permit life-saving procedures for child

SUGGESTIONS FOR CLASSROOM ACTIVITIES

- Review the steps and rationales for witnessing informed consent in Procedure 2-1.
- Discuss the legalities regarding who can sign an informed consent.

SUGGESTIONS FOR CLINICAL ACTIVITIES

- Have students review informed consents in assigned client's medical records when in the clinical setting.

LEARNING OUTCOME 3

Describe client rights as they relate to children.

CONCEPTS FOR LECTURE

1. Some states have a mature minor act that allows children to make decisions about their treatment.

   Emancipated minors are responsible for their own health care decisions and expenses.

   The Client's Bill of Rights needs to be explained in age-appropriate language.
2. Children need to be given as much control as possible by including them in decisions about their health care.

   It is the responsibility of the nurse to help the client and family understand how to participate in the client's care.
3. Children have the same rights to privacy and confidentiality as adults do.

POWERPOINT LECTURE SLIDES

(NOTE: The number on each PPT Lecture Slide directly corresponds with the Concepts for Lecture.)

1 Child's Rights
- Mature Minor Act
- Emancipated minors
- Client's Bill of Rights

2 Expectations of Parents and Children in Health Care
- Provide accurate and complete information about health issues
- Increase knowledge about diagnosis and treatment
- Be responsible for their own actions
- Report changes in client condition
- Keep appointments
- Meet financial obligations for health care

3 Privacy and Confidentiality
- Privacy: screening from view
- Confidentiality: keep secret any privileged information
- Parents may have right to access their dependent child's medical record

LEARNING OUTCOME 4

Name situations that the nurse must legally report to public agencies.

CONCEPTS FOR LECTURE

1. If a client's health problem puts the community at risk, or if child abuse or neglect is suspected, the nurse must notify the appropriate public health or law enforcement agency.

   The nurse who fails to report suspicions may be held liable by the courts.

   The nurse must record detailed information in the client's chart and complete report forms provided by investigating agencies.

2. The federal Patient Self-Determination Act requires health care institutions to inform clients of their rights to treatment, including advance directives or "living wills.

   The nurse needs to use effective therapeutic communication to help resolve conflict in regard to the rights to treatment or to withhold treatment.

POWERPOINT LECTURE SLIDES

(NOTE: The number on each PPT Lecture Slide directly corresponds with the Concepts for Lecture.)

1 Legally Reportable Situations
   • Communicable diseases
   • Child abuse or neglect
   • Threats to injure oneself
   • Suspicion of abuse

2 Patient Self-Determination Act

SUGGESTIONS FOR CLASSROOM ACTIVITIES	SUGGESTIONS FOR CLINICAL ACTIVITIES
• Have students discuss situations that are reportable to appropriate agencies. • Have students review the Client Self-Determination Act. • Arrange for a nurse or counselor from the Health Department or from an Abuse Prevention Center to speak with students about reportable situations.	• Role-play the use of therapeutic communication techniques for situations in need of resolving conflicts of treatment.

LEARNING OUTCOME 5

Describe the difference between legal and ethical issues.

CONCEPTS FOR LECTURE

1. Ethical issues are situations that require intervention based on a system of values and ideas that are shaped from a sense of right or wrong.

   Legal issues are situations that require intervention based on state or federal laws.

POWERPOINT LECTURE SLIDES

(NOTE: The number on each PPT Lecture Slide directly corresponds with the Concepts for Lecture.)

1 Legal and Ethical Issues
   • Ethical Issues
      ○ Intervention based on values and ideas
   • Legal issues
      ○ Intervention based on state or federal laws

SUGGESTIONS FOR CLASSROOM ACTIVITIES	SUGGESTIONS FOR CLINICAL ACTIVITIES
• Identify situations and discuss whether they are legal or ethical issues.	• None

LEARNING OUTCOME 6

Describe common legal and ethical issues that can affect the mother, child, and family.

CONCEPTS FOR LECTURE

1. The nurse must keep an open mind about legal and ethical situations and provide nonjudgmental nursing care to the mother, child, and family.

   The nurse must be familiar with the state and federal laws governing situations such as assisted reproduction, nontraditional parents, pregnancy after rape, and barrier-breaking technologies.

POWERPOINT LECTURE SLIDES

(NOTE: The number on each PPT Lecture Slide directly corresponds with the Concepts for Lecture.)

1. Legal and Ethical Issues
   - Assisted reproduction
   - Nontraditional parents
   - Pregnancy after rape
   - Barrier-breaking technologies

SUGGESTIONS FOR CLASSROOM ACTIVITIES

- Review steps in making ethical decisions (Box 2-2).
- Divide students into groups and have them discuss case studies of legal and ethical issues. Have them share their answers with the class.

SUGGESTIONS FOR CLINICAL ACTIVITIES

- None

LEARNING OUTCOME 7

Describe the practical and vocational nurse's role in legal/ethical issues.

CONCEPTS FOR LECTURE

1. The LVN/LPN's nursing practice is guided by the nurse's Code of Ethics and the Scope and Standards of Practice.
2. When providing nursing care to a client who has legal or ethical issues, the priorities are therapeutic listening, critical thinking, and awareness of the law.
3. Nursing interventions for clients with legal and ethical issues are based on the situation in which they occur.

POWERPOINT LECTURE SLIDES

(NOTE: The number on each PPT Lecture Slide directly corresponds with the Concepts for Lecture.)

1. LPN/LVN's Role in Legal and Ethical Issues
   - Follow Scope and Standards of Practice
   - Provide testimony
   - Do no harm
   - Participate in ethics committees
   - Refer to support groups

2. Priorities in Nursing Care
   - Therapeutic listening
     ○ Reflecting, open-ended questions, silence
   - Critical thinking
   - Awareness of the law

3. Nursing Interventions in Legal or Ethical Situations
   - Practice within limits of state nurse practice act
   - Know laws of state practicing in
   - Never advise client based on your values
   - Uphold client confidentiality

3a. Nursing Interventions in Legal or Ethical Situations
   - Collaborate with other health care members
   - Practice culturally sensitive nursing care
   - Provide quality nursing care
   - Report incidents promptly and accurately

SUGGESTIONS FOR CLASSROOM ACTIVITIES

- Review the nurse's Code of Ethics (Box 2-3).
- Assign students to research other cultures and discuss how to provide culturally sensitive nursing care (Box 2-5).

SUGGESTIONS FOR CLINICAL ACTIVITIES

- Assign students to provide nursing care to clients from differing cultures. In postconference, have students discuss any problems encountered in caring for these clients and families.

CHAPTER 3
NURSING CARE OF THE FAMILY

RESOURCE LIBRARY

 CD-ROM

Defining families

📖 **IMAGE LIBRARY**

Figure 3-1 (A) Families come in many different sizes, racial or gender mixtures, and types. (B) Evidence indicates that children raised in a homosexual family are at no greater developmental or dysfunctional risk than children raised in a heterosexual family.

🌐 **COMPANION WEBSITE**

Premature labor & birth

Figure 3-2 Blended families are a regular part of U.S. culture in the 21st century.
Figure 3-3 Genogram.
Figure 3-4 Ecomap.
Figure 3-5 Home assessment.
Figure 3-6 Neighborhood or community assessment.

LEARNING OUTCOME 1
Describe family assessment techniques such as genogram and ecomap.

CONCEPTS FOR LECTURE

1. A family is defined as two or more people related by blood or marriage who reside together or two or more individuals who come together for the purpose of nurturing.
2. A family assessment is an ongoing process of examining the relationships and functioning of members of a family.
3. A genogram is a diagram of relationships of members of the family.
4. An ecomap is a diagram of interactions of family members with the immediate environment.
   While keeping an open mind and a nonjudgmental attitude, the LPN/LVN assists the RN with family and environmental assessments to facilitate a move toward healthy relationships.

POWERPOINT LECTURE SLIDES

(NOTE: The number on each PPT Lecture Slide directly corresponds with the Concepts for Lecture.)

1 Family
  - Two or more people related by blood or marriage who reside together
  - Two or more individuals who come together for the purpose of nurturing

2 Family Assessment
  - Process of examining relationships and functioning of members
    ○ Genogram
    ○ Ecomap

3 Genogram

4 Ecomap

SUGGESTIONS FOR CLASSROOM ACTIVITIES

- Have students draw a genogram of their own families to identify family relationships.

SUGGESTIONS FOR CLINICAL ACTIVITIES

- Have students develop a genogram of a family to whom they are providing nursing care.

LEARNING OUTCOME 2

Describe the effect of cultural and religious beliefs on family functioning.

CONCEPTS FOR LECTURE

1. Family-centered care is treatment to a designated client with recognition that the family system or unit may also need intervention.
2. Culture is a style of behavior patterns, beliefs, and products of human works within a given community or population.
3. Culture theory describes factors of culture that should be considered when working with families.
4. Religion is a belief in a superhuman power recognized as a creator or governor of the universe.

   Ethnicity is identity based on common ancestry, race, religion, and culture.

   The LPN/LVN must not stereotype members of different cultures and must be able to provide care by identifying specific aspects of the family's cultural and religious beliefs.

POWERPOINT LECTURE SLIDES

(NOTE: The number on each PPT Lecture Slide directly corresponds with the Concepts for Lecture.)

1 Family-Centered Care
  - Treatment to client includes treatment of family system

2 Culture
  - Style of behavior patterns
  - Beliefs
  - Products of human works
  - Within a given community or population

3 Culture Theory
  - Cultural factors considered when working with families
    ○ Communication
    ○ Space
    ○ Time
    ○ Role

3a Four Main Cultural Groups in U.S.
  - Rasa Latina
  - Asian Pacific
  - American Black
  - Caucasian

4 Religion/Ethnicity
  - Religion
    ○ Belief in a superhuman power
  - Ethnicity
    ○ Identity based on common ancestry, race, religion, culture
    ○ Race is biological deviations

SUGGESTIONS FOR CLASSROOM ACTIVITIES

- Have students research different types of cultures and discuss nursing care that needs to be considered for these groups (Box 3-1).
- Arrange for people from different cultures to speak to students about their cultural beliefs in health care.

SUGGESTIONS FOR CLINICAL ACTIVITIES

- Have students interview clients from a different culture. Have students observe the roles of each family member. Develop a nursing care plan based on the cultural beliefs and religion of that client.

LEARNING OUTCOME 3

Describe the characteristics of family systems.

CONCEPTS FOR LECTURE

1. There are many types of family units such as the nuclear family, extended family, single-parent family, blended family, foster family, interracial family, communal family, and cult family.

POWERPOINT LECTURE SLIDES

(NOTE: The number on each PPT Lecture Slide directly corresponds with the Concepts for Lecture.)

1 Types of Family Units
  - Nuclear family
  - Extended family
  - Single-parent family
  - Blended family

2. Family systems theory states that the family system maintains a flexible boundary that can adjust or adapt to the needs of its members.
3. The LPN/LVN must have a basic understanding of how a family functions and how to assess that functioning.

1a Types of Family Units
- Foster family
- Interracial family
- Communal family
- Cult family

2 Family Systems Theory
- Adaptability

3 Functions of the Family
- Provide economic support
- Satisfy emotional needs for love and security
- Provide sense of place and position in society

SUGGESTIONS FOR CLASSROOM ACTIVITIES

- Discuss types of family units and how family functioning affects health care.

SUGGESTIONS FOR CLINICAL ACTIVITIES

- Have students interview families to determine the type of family unit and how the family perceives their health care.

LEARNING OUTCOME 4

Describe the normal changes a family undergoes over time.

CONCEPTS FOR LECTURE

1. Family development theory describes changes that occur through predictable stages the family undergoes over time.
   Family Development Theory has predictable *stages* the family undergoes over time.

POWERPOINT LECTURE SLIDES

(NOTE: The number on each PPT Lecture Slide directly corresponds with the Concepts for Lecture.)

1 Family Development Theory
- Predictable stages of a family life cycle

SUGGESTIONS FOR CLASSROOM ACTIVITIES

- Review stages of the family life cycle in the family development theory (Table 3-1).

SUGGESTIONS FOR CLINICAL ACTIVITIES

- None

LEARNING OUTCOME 5

Describe the characteristics of a family under stress.

CONCEPTS FOR LECTURE

1. The LPN/LVN must be able to identify characteristics of families under stress and understand when to seek assistance and guidance from the supervising Registered Nurse.

POWERPOINT LECTURE SLIDES

(NOTE: The number on each PPT Lecture Slide directly corresponds with the Concepts for Lecture.)

1 Characteristics of Family Under Stress
- Become defensive
- Blame others for their problems
- Use ineffective communication and problem solving
- Cause individuals to feel unwanted, unloved, worthless
- Block communication, leading to additional stress

SUGGESTIONS FOR CLASSROOM ACTIVITIES	**SUGGESTIONS FOR CLINICAL ACTIVITIES**
• Compare the differences in stress and coping between healthy families and unhealthy families (Box 3-3).	• Have students assess for signs of abuse when completing client assessments. Review Box 3-2.

LEARNING OUTCOME 6

Identify the role of the Practical/Vocational Nurse in family assessment and care.

CONCEPTS FOR LECTURE

1. The LPN/LVN's role is to assist with data collection, report findings, and implement the written plan of care.

POWERPOINT LECTURE SLIDES

(NOTE: The number on each PPT Lecture Slide directly corresponds with the Concepts for Lecture.)

 Role of LPN/LVN in Family Assessment and Care
- Data collection
- Report findings
- Implement written plan of care

SUGGESTIONS FOR CLASSROOM ACTIVITIES	**SUGGESTIONS FOR CLINICAL ACTIVITIES**
• Have students contact the State Board of Nursing to obtain information on the scope of practice of the LPN/LVN. Discuss their findings in class.	• Assign students to assist an RN with completing a family assessment and in implementing a plan of care for a family.

LEARNING OUTCOME 7

Apply the nursing process to care of the family.

CONCEPTS FOR LECTURE

1. The LPN/LVN utilizes the steps of the nursing process when planning and implementing nursing care to clients and families.

POWERPOINT LECTURE SLIDES

(NOTE: The number on each PPT Lecture Slide directly corresponds with the Concepts for Lecture.)

 Nursing Process When Caring for the Family
- Collect data on family
- Identify appropriate nursing diagnoses
- Plan and implement interventions for nursing care
- Evaluate nursing care

SUGGESTIONS FOR CLASSROOM ACTIVITIES	**SUGGESTIONS FOR CLINICAL ACTIVITIES**
• Review steps of the nursing process when discussing nursing care of a client or family.	• Utilizing the steps of the nursing process, have students complete a nursing care plan or concept map on an assigned client and family.

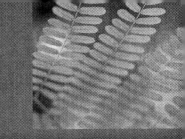

CHAPTER 4
REPRODUCTIVE ANATOMY AND PHYSIOLOGY

RESOURCE LIBRARY

 CD-ROM

Spermatogenesis
Oogenesis
Conception
Human Genome Project

IMAGE LIBRARY

Figure 4-1 Gametogenesis involves meiosis within the ovaries and testicles.

Figure 4-2 (A) Normal female sets of genes (karyotype). (B) Normal male karyotype. (C) Karyotype of a male who has trisomy 21, Down syndrome. Note that position 21 has one extra chromosome.

Figure 4-3 Expanding view from DNA strand to chromosome.

Figure 4-4 Transmission of traits. Children manifest physical characteristics related to their racial or ethnic groups.

Figure 4-5 Example of transmission of disease.

Figure 4-6 The testes.

Figure 4-7 Self-examination of the testes should be done monthly to check for the possibility of testicular cancer. Young men are at higher risk for this than other groups.

Figure 4-8 Structure of a mature sperm cell.

Figure 4-9 Male reproductive organs.

Figure 4-10 Fallopian tubes and ovaries.

Figure 4-11 Various stages of development of the ovarian follicles.

Figure 4-12 Structures of the uterus.

Figure 4-13 (A) Internal female reproductive organs. (B) Uterine ligaments that support reproduction structures.

Figure 4-14 Variations in uterine position.

Figure 4-15 External female reproductive organs (adult parous woman).

Figure 4-16 Structures of the breast.

Figure 4-17 Relationship between the pituitary gland and milk production.

Figure 4-18 Some positions for inspection of the breast.

Figure 4-19 (A) Check each breast using the pads of the fingers, feeling all parts of the breast. (B) While holding one hand behind your head, palpate your breast.

Figure 4-20 Squeeze the nipple and look for any drainage.

Figure 4-21 Female reproductive cycle showing interrelationships of hormones, phases of the ovarian cycle, and phases of the uterine cycle.

Figure 4-22 (A) Stages of male pubic hair and external genital development. (B) Stages of female pubic hair development.

LEARNING OUTCOME 1

Explain the developmental steps of spermatogenesis and oogenesis.

CONCEPTS FOR LECTURE

1. Gametogenesis is the formation of sex cells in males and females.
2. Spermatogenesis or sperm production begins at puberty and continues until death.

    Shortly before puberty, spermatogonia (sperm precursor cells) increase in number by the process of mitosis, resulting in two cells containing 46 chromosomes including the Y chromosome.
3. Oogenesis is the development of the female gamete or ovum.

POWERPOINT LECTURE SLIDES

(NOTE: The number on each PPT Lecture Slide directly corresponds with the Concepts for Lecture.)

1 Gametogenesis
- Sex cell formation
- Meiosis within the ovaries and testicles

1a Gametogenesis

2 Spermatogenesis
- Sperm production begins at puberty, continues to death

Oogenesis occurs during fetal development from the process of meiosis, which results in an ovum with 23 chromosomes, one of which is an X chromosome.

- Spermatogonia increase in number by mitosis
- Results in 2 cells containing 46 chromosomes
- Cells split into 2 cells with 23 chromosomes in each
- Contains Y chromosome

3 Oogenesis
- Development of female gamete or ovum
- Occurs during fetal development by meiosis
- Results in ovum with 23 chromosomes
- Contains X chromosome

SUGGESTIONS FOR CLASSROOM ACTIVITIES

- Compare development of sperm in the male with development of ovum in the female.

SUGGESTIONS FOR CLINICAL ACTIVITIES

- None

LEARNING OUTCOME 2

Describe basic information about genes in relation to reproduction.

CONCEPTS FOR LECTURE

1. The unique combination of traits a person has results from that person's genetic makeup.

   Genetic coding is determined by a person's chromosomes, which are structures of DNA and protein.

   In humans, there are 22 sets of chromosomes (autosomes) and two sex chromosomes in each set.

   Genetic information is contained in DNA's pairs of chemical components, which are the proteins adenine, thymine, guanine, and cytosine.

   The human genome (complete set of DNA) contains 3 billion base pairs.

POWERPOINT LECTURE SLIDES

(NOTE: The number on each PPT Lecture Slide directly corresponds with the Concepts for Lecture.)

1 Chromosomes
- Structures of DNA and protein
- Governs development of organism
- Determines genetic coding
- 23 sets with 2 sex chromosomes
- 3 billion base pairs composed of proteins

1a Chromosomes (Figure 4-2 A and B)

1b Chromosomes (Figure 4-3)

SUGGESTIONS FOR CLASSROOM ACTIVITIES

- Have students develop a genogram of their own family.

SUGGESTIONS FOR CLINICAL ACTIVITIES

- None

LEARNING OUTCOME 3

List the essential and accessory organs of the male and female reproductive systems.

CONCEPTS FOR LECTURE

1. The essential organs of the male reproductive system are the pair of gonads or testes.

   The tunica vaginalis testis covers the front and sides of the testes and epididymis.

   The tunica albuginea covers the outside of the testes and forms the septum between the lobules.

   Seminiferous tubules are composed of long narrow coiled tubes in the lobules.

POWERPOINT LECTURE SLIDES

(NOTE: The number on each PPT Lecture Slide directly corresponds with the Concepts for Lecture.)

1 Male Reproductive Organs
- Testes
- Tunica vaginalis testis
- Tunica albuginea
- Seminiferous tubules

1a Male Reproductive Organs (Figure 4-6)

2. The male and female accessory organs are the reproductive ducts, supportive glands, and external genitalia.
3. The essential organs of the female reproductive system are the ovaries, which contain about 1 million ovarian follicles.

The corpus luteum is a glandular structure that forms from a ruptured follicle.

 Male Accessory Organs
- Reproductive ducts
  ○ Epididymis
  ○ Spermatic cord (vas deferens)
  ○ Ejaculatory duct
  ○ Urethra

 Male Accessory Organs
- Reproductive glands
  ○ Seminal vesicles
  ○ Prostate gland
  ○ Bulbourethral or Cowper's gland

 Male Accessory Organs (Figure 4-9)

Male Accessory Organs
- External Genitalia
  ○ Penis
  ○ Glans
  ○ Prepuce or foreskin
  ○ Scrotum

Functions of Male Organs
- Testes
  ○ Produce testosterone
  ○ Sperm production
- Epididymis
  ○ Where sperm mature
  ○ Sperm develop ability to move

Functions of Male Organs
- Seminal vesicles
  ○ Produce thick yellowish fluid to nourish sperm
- Prostate gland
  ○ Produces thin milky fluid to activate sperm
- Bulbourethral or Cowper's gland
  ○ Secretes mucus-like fluid

Functions of Male Organs
- Penis
  ○ Organ of copulation
- Scrotum
  ○ Covers testes, epididymis, vas deferens

Male Sex Hormones
- Follicle-stimulating hormone
  ○ Spermatognesis
- Testosterone
  ○ Development of male accessory organs
  ○ Greater muscle mass and strength
  ○ Masculine characteristics

 Female Reproductive Organs
- Ovaries
  ○ Contain 1 million ovarian follicles
  ○ Corpus luteum

 Female Reproductive Organs (Figure 4-13)

3b Female Accessory Organs
- Reproductive Ducts
  - Fallopian tubes
  - Uterus
  - Vagina
- Reproductive Glands
  - Bartholin's gland
  - Breasts

3c Female Accessory Organs (Figure 4-16)

3d Female Accessory Organs
- External Genitalia
  - Mons pubis
  - Labia majora and minora
  - Clitoris

3e Female Accessory Organs (Figure 4-15)

SUGGESTIONS FOR CLASSROOM ACTIVITIES	**SUGGESTIONS FOR CLINICAL ACTIVITIES**
• Have students view the videos on the male and female reproductive systems. • Have students label diagrams of the anatomy of the male and female reproductive system to review the structures.	• Perform physical assessments on the male and female reproductive systems. • Teach the male client to perform testicular self-examination. • Teach the female client to perform breast self-examination.

LEARNING OUTCOME 4

Describe the general function of each organ of the male and female reproductive systems.

CONCEPTS FOR LECTURE

1. The testes are responsible for production of testosterone in the cells between the septum and seminiferous tubules and of sperm in the walls of the seminiferous tubules.

   The epididymis is where the sperm mature and develop the ability to move.

2. Seminal vesicles produce a thick, yellowish fluid rich in fructose to provide energy for the sperm.

   The prostate gland produces a thin milky fluid that helps to activate sperm and to maintain their motility.

   The bulbourethral or Cowper's gland secretes a mucus-like fluid to neutralize the acid environment of the urethra and lubricate the end of the penis.

3. The penis is the organ of copulation.

   The scrotum covers the testes, epididymis, and lower end of vas deferens.

POWERPOINT LECTURE SLIDES

(NOTE: The number on each PPT Lecture Slide directly corresponds with the Concepts for Lecture.)

 1 Functions of Male Organs
- Testes
  - Produce testosterone
  - Sperm production
- Epididymis
  - Where sperm mature
  - Sperm develop ability to move

 2 Functions of Male Organs
- Seminal vesicles
  - Produce thick yellowish fluid to nourish sperm
- Prostate gland
  - Produces thin milky fluid to activate sperm
- Bulbourethral or Cowper's gland
  - Secretes mucus-like fluid

4. The ovaries contain ovarian follicles, which develop into Graafian follicles (mature follicles) and release a ripened ovum (egg).

   The fallopian tubes transport the ovum from the ovary toward the uterus and are the site of fertilization.

   The uterus is the organ where implantation takes place.

   The vagina connects the cervix to the vaginal opening. It is the site of deposition of sperm and the passageway for the delivery of the infant.

   The clitoris, located behind the junction of the labia majora and labia minora, is for sexual arousal and pleasure.

   The Bartholin's gland secretes a thin, mucus-like substance that produces lubrication during sexual intercourse.

   The breasts contain milk-secreting glandular cells for nourishment of the newborn.

3 Functions of Male Organs
- Penis
  - Organ of copulation
- Scrotum
  - Covers testes, epididymis, vas deferens

4 Functions of Female Organs
- Ovaries
  - Contain ovarian follicles
- Fallopian tubes
  - Transport ovum
  - Site of fertilization
- Uterus
  - Organ of implantation

4a Functions of Female Organs
- Vagina
  - Site of deposition of sperm
  - Passageway for delivery of infant
- Clitoris
  - Site for sexual arousal and pleasure
- Bartholin's gland
  - Secretes thin mucus-like substance for lubrication

4b Functions of Female Organs
- Breasts
  - Contain milk-secreting cells for nourishment of newborn

4c Breast Self-Examination (Figure 4-18)

4d Breast Self-Examination (Figure 4-19)

4e Breast Self-Examination (Figure 4-20)

SUGGESTIONS FOR CLASSROOM ACTIVITIES

- Develop a matching quiz with the organs on the left and the organ function on the right.

SUGGESTIONS FOR CLINICAL ACTIVITIES

- Have students practice breast self-examination on breast models
- Have students teach breast self-examinations to assigned clients.
- Have students demonstrate breast self-examination at a Health Fair.

LEARNING OUTCOME 5

Discuss the primary functions of the sex hormones.

CONCEPTS FOR LECTURE

1. The anterior pituitary gland releases follicle-stimulating hormone when the male enters puberty. Follicle-stimulating hormone stimulates spermatogenesis to occur.

   Testosterone causes development of male accessory organs, greater muscle mass and strength, and masculine characteristics.

POWERPOINT LECTURE SLIDES

(NOTE: The number on each PPT Lecture Slide directly corresponds with the Concepts for Lecture.)

1 Male Sex Hormones
- Follicle-stimulating hormone
  - Spermatognesis

2. The anterior pituitary gland releases follicle-stimulating hormone causing a follicle to enlarge and move closer to the surface of the ovary until the follicle ruptures and releases the ovum.

   The ovary produces estrogen and progesterone. Estrogen is responsible for the development and maintenance of the secondary sex characteristics and growth of the endometrium. Progesterone stimulates thickening and vascularization of the endometrium. Decrease in progesterone results in menses as the endometrium sloughs off.

   Pitocin released from the pituitary stimulates milk production and stimulates contraction of the uterus.

- Testosterone
  - Development of male accessory organs
  - Greater muscle mass and strength
  - Masculine characteristics

2 Female Sex Hormones
- Follicle-stimulating hormone
  - Follicle maturation
- Estrogen
  - Development and maturation of secondary sex characteristics

3 Female Sex Hormones
- Progesterone
  - Stimulates thickening and vascularization of endometrium
- Oxytocin (Pitocin)
  - Stimulates milk production
  - Stimulates uterine contractions

SUGGESTIONS FOR CLASSROOM ACTIVITIES

- Develop a matching quiz with the hormone on the left and the function on the right

SUGGESTIONS FOR CLINICAL ACTIVITIES

- None

LEARNING OUTCOME 6

Discuss the phases of the menstrual cycle and correlate each with physical changes during a 28-day cycle.

CONCEPTS FOR LECTURE

1. The menstrual cycle occurs with regularity from their onset (menarche) until the cycle ends (menopause).
   The average length of the menstrual cycle is 28 days.
   The menstrual cycle is divided into three phases: menses, proliferative phase, and secretory phase.
2. The phases of sexual response are excitement, plateau, orgasm, and resolution.
   The nurse must be able to explain the phases of the menstrual cycle and correlate each with physical changes during the 28-day cycle.
   The nurse uses knowledge of the sexual response when teaching clients about their own and their partner's sexual responses and when identifying sexual dysfunction.

POWERPOINT LECTURE SLIDES

(NOTE: The number on each PPT Lecture Slide directly corresponds with the Concepts for Lecture.)

1 Menstrual Cycle
- Occurs from onset (menarche) to cycle end (menopause)
- Average 28-day cycle
- Three phases
  - Menses
  - Proliferative phase
  - Secretory phase

2 Sexual Response
- Four phases
  - Excitement
  - Plateau
  - Orgasm
  - Resolution

SUGGESTIONS FOR CLASSROOM ACTIVITIES

- Explain the phases of the menstrual cycle, including the hormone changes.
- Discuss physiologic changes in the sexual response cycle—see Table 4-1.

SUGGESTIONS FOR CLINICAL ACTIVITIES

- None

LEARNING OUTCOME 7

Explain the process of lactation.

CONCEPTS FOR LECTURE

1. Lactogenesis or milk production begins in pregnancy due to sustained levels of estrogen and progesterone.

   Colostrum is a translucent, yellow fluid rich in protein, antibodies, and other substances to meet the needs of the newborn.

   Stimulation of the nipple causes the pituitary gland to secrete oxytocin.

   Pitocin causes milk-ejecting cells in the lactiferous sinus to contract, forcing colostrum and then milk from the nipple.

   A week after delivery, estrogen and progesterone decrease causing the mammary glands to change from producing colostrum to producing mature milk.

   The nurse uses knowledge of the process of lactation when helping the new mother with breastfeeding techniques.

POWERPOINT LECTURE SLIDES

(NOTE: The number on each PPT Lecture Slide directly corresponds with the Concepts for Lecture.)

[1] Process of Lactation (Lactogenesis)
- Colostrum rich in protein, antibodies
- Nipple stimulation causes secretion of oxytocin
- Oxytocin (Pitocin) causes milk ejection from nipple

[1a] Lactation (Figure 4-17)

SUGGESTIONS FOR CLASSROOM ACTIVITIES

- Use diagrams to explain the process of lactogenesis.
- Have a Lactation Consultant speak to the students about breastfeeding and what to teach the client about breastfeeding.

SUGGESTIONS FOR CLINICAL ACTIVITIES

- Have students observe breastfeeding mothers and perform a breast assessment.

CHAPTER 5
REPRODUCTIVE ISSUES

RESOURCE LIBRARY

CD-ROM

Breast cancer
Erectile dysfunction
Conception
H.I.V.
Spermatogenesis

COMPANION WEBSITE

Contraception
Teen pregnancy

IMAGE LIBRARY

Figure 5-1 Left, orange peel; right, peau d'orange cancerous changes in a breast.

Figure 5-2 Postmastectomy exercises.

Figure 5-3 The multisystem effects of premenstrual syndrome.

Figure 5-4 Sites of uterine fibroid tumors.

Figure 5-5 Conization: removal of a cone-shaped section of the cervix.

Figure 5-6 Common sites for endometriosis.

Figure 5-7 Rape evidence collection kit contains a step-by-step system to gather samples for evidence.

Figure 5-8 Types of penile implants.

Figure 5-9 TURP.

Figure 5-10 Some sexually transmitted infections.

Figure 5-11 Methods of contraception (*from top right*): Mirena intrauterine device (IUD), applicator for female condom, delivery catheter, Norplant subcutaneous contraceptive, vaginal ring, male condom, "the pill," diaphragm, and contraceptive patch.

Figure 5-12 (A) Basal body temperature chart with ovulation indicated. (B) Determining elasticity of cervical mucus (spinnbarkeit) to predict day of ovulation.

Figure 5-13 The male condom.

Figure 5-14 The female condom.

Figure 5-15 Application of spermicide and placement of vaginal diaphragm.

Figure 5-16 Longer-term contraceptive devices include Norplant and the vaginal ring.

Figure 5-17 Permanent sterilization.

Figure 5-18 (A) Formation of identical (monozygotic) twins. (B) Formation of fraternal (dizygotic) twins.

Figure 5-19 Adolescents require age-appropriate teaching about sexuality and sexually transmitted infections.

Figure 5-20 Spontaneous abortion (or miscarriage).

LEARNING OUTCOME 1

Define key terms.

CONCEPTS FOR LECTURE

1. Reproductive issues involve physical disorders that can have an impact on psychological health.

POWERPOINT LECTURE SLIDES

(NOTE: The number on each PPT Lecture Slide directly corresponds with the Concepts for Lecture.)

 Woman's Reproductive Health Issues
- Breast disorders
  - Malignant vs. Nonmalignant
- Uterine disorders
- Ovarian disorders
- Pelvic floor disorders
- Rape trauma syndrome

1a Men's Reproductive Health Issues
- Testicular and epididymus disorders
- Erectile dysfunction
- Prostate disorders

1b Family Planning Issues
- Infections
  ○ Sexually transmitted infections
- Contraception
- Genetic testing
  ○ Infertility
  ○ Chromosomal abnormalities

1c Family Planning Issues
- Adolescent sexuality and teenage pregnancy
- Unintended pregnancy
- Abortion
- Adoption
- Pregnancy after 35

SUGGESTIONS FOR CLASSROOM ACTIVITIES

- Define reproductive health disorders and discuss the psychological impact on the client.
- Have students do key terms exercise on companion website.

SUGGESTIONS FOR CLINICAL ACTIVITIES

- Have students teach assigned clients how to do breast self-examination.
- Arrange for students to observe a nurse working at a mammogram clinic at an outpatient center.

LEARNING OUTCOME 2

Describe possible causes of reproductive issues.

CONCEPTS FOR LECTURE

1. Breast disorders may be detected by the woman during a monthly breast self-exam, during a physical examination by the primary care provider, or by mammography.
2. Breast cancer is the second leading cause of cancer-related deaths among women.
3. Most women experience minor discomforts just prior to and during menstruation related to hormone changes.

    Menopause is the cessation of menstruation that occurs between 35 and 58 years of age due to stopped functioning of ovaries.
4. Fibroid tumors are common among women of all ages, probably due to estrogen secretion.

    Endometrial cancer is a common, slow-growing tumor that affects women between 50 and 70 years of age.

    Most cervical cancers result from infection by the human papillomavirus.

    Endometriosis occurs when endometrial tissue grows outside the uterine cavity and may lead to infertility.
5. Cysts may become large and rupture, causing bleeding; thus a surgical emergency could occur.

    Ovarian cancer is the most lethal of female reproductive cancers.
6. Relaxation or damage of pelvic muscles may result in prolapse or displacement of the pelvic organs.

POWERPOINT LECTURE SLIDES

(NOTE: The number on each PPT Lecture Slide directly corresponds with the Concepts for Lecture.)

1 Breast Disorders
- Nonmalignant Breast Disorders
  ○ Caffeine intake
  ○ Increased estrogen
- Malignant Breast Disorders
  ○ Estrogen related

2 Breast Disorders (Figure 5-1)

3 Uterine Disorders
- Premenstrual syndrome
  ○ Imbalance of estrogen and progesterone
  ○ Increased prolactin and aldosterone
- Menopause
  ○ Cessation of ovary functioning

3a Premenstrual Syndrome (Figure 5-3)

4 Uterine Tumors
- Nonmalignant fibroids
- Endometrial cancer
- Cervical cancer
- Endometriosis
  ○ May be related to estrogen secretion

7. With rape or incest, the psychological trauma is as great as or greater than the physical trauma.
8. Testicular cancer, which is the most common cancer of men between 15 and 35 years of age, has a greater than 90% cure rate.

    Infections of the male reproductive system are often caused by sexually transmitted diseases and could result in infertility and sexual dysfunction.
9. Erectile dysfunction is caused by any disorder that impairs circulation, interrupts nerve or hormone intervention, or by trauma that results in scar tissue.
10. Benign prostatic hyperplasia is a growth of the prostate gland, which most commonly affects men over the age of 50.

    Prostate cancer is a leading type of cancer in men, which has a 5-year cure rate of 100% when diagnosed early and confined to the prostate. It is a testosteronerelated condition.
11. The most common sexually transmitted diseases are chlamydia, genital herpes, gonorrhea, genital warts, trichomoniasis, and syphilis.

4a Uterine Tumors (Figure 5-4)

5 Ovarian Disorders
- Polycystic ovary syndrome
  ○ Related to increased LH, estrogen, androgen, decreased FSH
- Ovarian cancer
  ○ Most lethal reproductive cancer

6 Pelvic Floor Disorders
- Cystocele
- Rectocele
- Uterine prolapse
  ○ Ligaments stretched, thinned with aging, damaged during delivery

7 Rape Trauma Syndrome
- Rape
- Incest
  ○ Psychological trauma and physical trauma

8 Testicular and Epididymus Disorders
- Testicular cancer
- Epididymitis, Orchitis, Prostatitis
  ○ Caused by sexually transmitted diseases

9 Erectile Dysfunction (Figure 5-8)

10 Prostate Disorders
- Benign prostatic hyperplasia
  ○ Testosterone and estrogen related
- Prostate cancer
  ○ Testosterone related

11 Infections
- Sexually transmitted diseases
- Human immunodeficiency virus and acquired immunodeficiency syndrome
- Candidiasis

SUGGESTIONS FOR CLASSROOM ACTIVITIES

- Assign students to research a sexually transmitted disease and present the findings to the class.
- Divide students into groups and have them answer questions on a case study involving reproductive health issues. Have them share the answers with the class.

SUGGESTIONS FOR CLINICAL ACTIVITIES

- Have students teach male clients how to perform testicular self-exam.
- Have students go to a drugstore to see how many types of birth control they can find. Have them discuss the effectiveness of the different birth control methods they find.

LEARNING OUTCOME 3

Discuss the medical and surgical interventions used to treat the client with reproductive issues.

CONCEPTS FOR LECTURE

1. Physical disorders, including infection, hormonal imbalance, and structural defects, may be treated medically or, at times, surgically.

    Some disorders cannot be treated, and they result in infertility.

POWERPOINT LECTURE SLIDES

(NOTE: The number on each PPT Lecture Slide directly corresponds with the Concepts for Lecture.)

1 Treatment of Breast Disorders
- Surgery
  ○ Lumpectomy, Mastectomy
  ○ Mammoplasty

- Radiation
- Chemotherapy
- Pharmacologic treatment

1a Treatment of Uterine Disorders
- Diet
- Exercise
- Relaxation techniques
- Hormone replacement therapy

1b Treatment of Uterine Tumors
- Surgery
  - Myomectomy
  - Hysterectomy with or without salpingo-oophorectomy
  - Cervical laser, conization
- Pharmacologic treatment

1c Treatment of Ovarian Disorders
- Laparoscopic surgery
- Pharmacologic treatment
- Abdominal hysterectomy with bilateral salpingo-oophorectomy
- Radiation

1d Treatment of Pelvic Floor Disorders
- Kegel exercises
- Hysterectomy
- Vaginal pessary

1e Treatment of Rape Trauma Syndrome (Figure 5-7)

1f Treatment of Testicular and Epididymus Disorders
- Surgery
- Radiation
- Pharmacologic treatment

1g Treatment of Erectile Dysfunction
- Pharmacologic treatment
- Penile implants

1h Treatment of Prostate Disorders (Figure 5-9)

1i Treatment of Infections
- Pharmacologic treatment

SUGGESTIONS FOR CLASSROOM ACTIVITIES

- Discuss the use of markers to identify risk for cancers in males and females.
- Review medications used for reproductive disorders. Discuss administration, adverse effects, and nursing concerns.
- Review manifestations and treatment of sexually transmitted diseases in Table 5-8.

SUGGESTIONS FOR CLINICAL ACTIVITIES

- Arrange for students to observe reproductive surgeries, if possible, or to do preoperative and/or postoperative nursing care.

LEARNING OUTCOME 4

Identify nursing diagnosis and nursing interventions to assist the couple with reproductive issues.

CONCEPTS FOR LECTURE

1. Nursing diagnoses for reproductive issues include: Risk for Disturbed Body Image, Sexual Dysfunction, Deficient Knowledge.

2. Couples wishing to postpone pregnancy need information about contraception. The nurse should encourage the client to speak with the health care provider for the appropriate type of contraception. Some methods may not be recommended with certain physical disorders.

3. The nurse's responsibility in managing clients with infertility is to provide emotional support and teaching. Other methods may be used to become pregnant, but there is an increased risk of a multifetal pregnancy.

4. Multifetal pregnancies, other than twins, occur most commonly from the use of fertility drugs or in vitro fertilization. The nurse needs to monitor for complications of a multifetal pregnancy, such as preterm labor, pregnancy-induced hypertension, gestational diabetes, or uterine rupture.

5. Adolescent girls, women over 30, and couples who have a family history of genetic anomalies are at a higher risk for developing a fetus with chromosomal abnormalities than other couples. Chromosomal defects result in a variety of physical anomalies, including malformations and underdeveloped structures or body systems. The nurse needs to be knowledgeable about genetics to communicate information to the client.

   A combination of peer pressure, feelings of invincibility, elevation of sex hormones and sex drive may lead the adolescent to engage in premarital sexual intercourse, resulting in pregnancy and/or sexually transmitted diseases.

   The nurse must encourage early and continued prenatal care to help the pregnant adolescent have a good pregnancy outcome.

6. Abortion is the termination of a pregnancy before the fetus is viable. This may be caused by a genetic abnormality or hormonal problem in embryo, infection, drug problem, systemic disorder or abnormality in mother. After an abortion, the entire family needs support and grief counseling.

7. Pregnancies after the age of 35 years need assistance with the lifestyle changes required by raising an infant.

POWERPOINT LECTURE SLIDES

(NOTE: The number on each PPT Lecture Slide directly corresponds with the Concepts for Lecture.)

1 Nursing Diagnoses for Reproductive Issues
- Risk for Disturbed Body Image
- Sexual Dysfunction
- Deficient Knowledge

2 Contraception (Figure 5-11)

3 Infertility
- Provide emotional support and teaching
- Recommend counseling when needed
- Clarify medical and surgical options
- Assist with exploring financial resources

3a Infertility (Figure 5-17)

4 Multiple Pregnancy
- Monitor for complications
  - Preterm labor
  - Pregnancy-induced hypertension
  - Gestational diabetes
  - Uterine rupture

4a Dizygotic Twins (Figure 5-18)

5 Chromosomal Abnormalities (Figure 4-2)

5a Adolescent Sexuality and Teenage Pregnancy
- Encourage early and continued prenatal care
- Refer to appropriate social services
- Teach issues related to sexuality
- Encourage open lines of communication between parents and children
- Develop programs to provide accurate information

6 Abortion (Figure 5-21)

6a Adoption
- Assist mother in decision-making
- Make appropriate referrals
- Provide emotional support

7 Pregnancy after 35
- Provide emotional support and teaching
- Allow client to express feelings
- Assist client to develop coping skills
- Refer to social services

SUGGESTIONS FOR CLASSROOM ACTIVITIES

- Have students brainstorm nursing diagnoses that are appropriate to use with reproductive issues.
- Discuss a case study of a client with a reproductive issue.

SUGGESTIONS FOR CLINICAL ACTIVITIES

- Have students develop a plan of care or a concept map for a client with a reproductive issue.

LEARNING OUTCOME 5

Provide appropriate care for the couple with reproductive issues.

CONCEPTS FOR LECTURE

1. The couple experiencing psychological and emotional problems about reproductive issues may require long-term support and professional counseling.

   When discussing sexual relations with the couple, the nurse needs to express compassion, be understanding, and be open-minded and nonjudgmental.

POWERPOINT LECTURE SLIDES

(NOTE: The number on each PPT Lecture Slide directly corresponds with the Concepts for Lecture.)

1 Nursing Care
- Identify nature of disorder
- Provide emotional support
- Teach self-care
- Prevent complications

1a Nursing Care
- Use nonjudgmental attitude
- Use open communication
- Use matter-of-fact approach
- Assure confidentiality
- Evaluate effectiveness

SUGGESTIONS FOR CLASSROOM ACTIVITIES

- Role-play a situation of a couple with reproductive issues to demonstrate how to communicate and provide emotional support to the couple.

SUGGESTIONS FOR CLINICAL ACTIVITIES

- Have students discuss and demonstrate how to use therapeutic communication with clients with reproductive issues.

RESOURCE LIBRARY

 COMPANION WEBSITE

Prenatal care by race
Herbs in pregnancy
Vegetarian pregnancy
Pre-eclampsia

IMAGE LIBRARY

Figure 6-1 Highly sensitive periods during the embryonic stage.

Figure 6-2 At fertilization, the following sequence (called an *acrosome reaction*) occurs.

Figure 6-3 Ovulation, fertilization, and implantation.

Figure 6-4 Sequence of development of the embryo from primary germ layers.

Figure 6-5 Placenta.

Figure 6-6 (A) Human prenatal development from conception to 10 weeks. (B) Human fetal development: 12 weeks, 20 weeks, 24 weeks, and 30 weeks.

Figure 6-7 Fetal circulation.

Figure 6-8 The embryo at 7 weeks.

Figure 6-9 Development of the external reproductive structures.

Figure 6-10 The embryo at 8 weeks.

Figure 6-11 (A) Hegar's sign. (B) Goodell's and Chadwick's signs.

Figure 6-12 Increase in oxygen consumption among body organs during pregnancy.

Figure 6-13 Supine hypotensive syndrome.

Figure 6-14 Linea nigra.

Figure 6-15 (A) Amniocentesis. (B) Umbilical blood sample.

Figure 6-16 Data on the fetal heart rate is collected regularly throughout the woman's pregnancy.

Figure 6-17 U.S. infant mortality rate by race and ethnicity, 1995–2002.

Figure 6-18 The gestational wheel can be used to calculate the EDB (estimated date of birth).

Figure 6-19 Prenatal exercises.

Figure 6-20 Kegel exercises are often taught during pregnancy.

Figure 6-21 Providing prenatal classes specifically for teens can improve the learning environment for young mothers.

Figure 6-22 Weight gain form shows the typical pattern of weight gain in pregnancy.

Figure 6-23 (A) Height of the fundus during second trimester at 16, 20, and 24 weeks. (B) The height of the fundus is measured at prenatal visits during the third trimester.

LEARNING OUTCOME 1

Define key terms.

CONCEPTS FOR LECTURE

1. Preconception is care given to help the couple identify their pregnancy risk and prepare for conception.
2. Fertilization or conception is the process of uniting two sex cells into one.
3. Embryonic development begins with the fertilized egg called the zygote and develops into the morula, and then the blastocyst within 5 days.
4. Implantation is the embedding of the blastocyst into the endometrium of the uterus.

     The trophoblast develops villi, which secrete human chorionic gonadotropin by 8 to 10 days after fertilization. Chorionic villi develop into the placenta.

POWERPOINT LECTURE SLIDES

(NOTE: The number on each PPT Lecture Slide directly corresponds with the Concepts for Lecture.)

1 Preconception
 • Identify pregnancy risks
 • Prepare for conception

2 Fertilization (Figure 6-2)

2a Fertilization (Figure 6-3)

3 Embryonic Development (Figure 6-4)

4 Implantation
 • Blastocyte embeds into endometrium
 • Villi produces human chorionic gonadotropin (HCG)

Corpus luteum is maintained by human chorionic gonadotropin and continues to produce estrogen and progesterone until the placenta takes over by 11–12 weeks after implantation.

5. Amniotic fluid, which is reabsorbed and replaced every 3 days, has many important functions for the developing fetus.

6. The placenta is a highly vascular organ connecting the mother to the fetus. Functions of the placenta are transport, hormone production, and production of fatty acids, glycogen, and cholesterol for fetal use.

- HCG maintains corpus luteum
- HCG stimulates corpus luteum to produce estrogen and progesterone
- Placenta takes over production of estrogen and progesterone by 11–12 weeks

5 Amniotic Fluid
  - Reabsorbed and replaced every 3 days
  - Important functions for the developing fetus

6 Placenta (Figure 6-5)

SUGGESTIONS FOR CLASSROOM ACTIVITIES

- Show a video on fertilization and implantation to assist with understanding the process of conception.

SUGGESTIONS FOR CLINICAL ACTIVITIES

- None

LEARNING OUTCOME 2

Describe factors that influence prenatal development.

CONCEPTS FOR LECTURE

1. A healthy pregnancy begins before conception with good health habits.
2. Because production of sperm is a continuous process, men can decrease risks of fetal anomalies by avoiding smoking and industrial chemicals for 3 to 4 months prior to conception.

    Maternal behaviors can have negative effects on the fetus.

    The role of the nurse in caring for the pregnant woman involves a great deal of client education and emotional support.

POWERPOINT LECTURE SLIDES

(NOTE: The number on each PPT Lecture Slide directly corresponds with the Concepts for Lecture.)

1 Preconception
  - Good eating patterns
  - Regular exercise
  - Weight control
  - Male contribution
    ○ Smoking
    ○ Industrial chemical exposure

2 Maternal Negative Effects
  - Smoking
  - Alcohol
  - Illicit drugs
  - Medications, chemicals
  - Nutrition deficiencies
  - Infectious diseases

SUGGESTIONS FOR CLASSROOM ACTIVITIES

- Review medications that are pregnancy category X and explain the consequences of taking these medications.
- Discuss the effects of smoking on the fetus.
- Examine the consequences of having an infectious disease such as rubella or CMV while pregnant.

SUGGESTIONS FOR CLINICAL ACTIVITIES

- Have students develop an education program promoting healthy behaviors while pregnant.

LEARNING OUTCOME 3

Describe fetal development.

CONCEPTS FOR LECTURE

1. Fetal development is very systematic, occurring cephalocaudal, proximal to distal and from general to specific.

POWERPOINT LECTURE SLIDES

(NOTE: The number on each PPT Lecture Slide directly corresponds with the Concepts for Lecture.)

1 Fetal Development (Figure 6-6)

During fetal development, all body systems are formed in the first 8 weeks.

2. The cardiovascular system develops from a series of tubes, with the heart beginning to beat on day 21.
3. The respiratory system begins to develop during week 6 and is developed by week 23. Surfactant begins to develop between weeks 20-23 and continues to mature to week 35.
4. The central nervous system is present by week 6. The peripheral nervous system continues to develop for 7-10 years.
5. The gastrointestinal system begins to develop by week 4. The fetus swallows and produces bile by week 12 and produces meconium by week 16.
6. The renal system develops in stages, and the kidneys ascend to their normal location. The fetus produces urine in the 10th week and urinates in week 11.
7. Sex of the fetus is determined at conception and can be identified in week 12.
8. A primitive skeleton covered by muscles is formed by week 6. Fetal movement can be seen on ultrasound by week 7. Fetal movement is felt by the mother between weeks 16-20.
9. In the integumentary system, fat develops in last 4-6 weeks gestation. Lanugo disappears in week 28. Fingernails and toenails reach end of digit by 36th week. Skin color is determined at conception.

2 Cardiovascular System
- Series of tubes develops into heart
- Heart begins to beat on day 21
- Most heart anomalies occur during weeks 6-8

2a Fetal Circulation (Figure 6-7)

3 Respiratory System
- Lung buds form during week 6
- Developed by week 23
- Surfactant develops from weeks 20-35

4 Nervous System
- Entire central nervous system is formed by week 6
- Peripheral nervous system continues to develop for 7-10 years

4a Special Senses (Figure 6-8)

5 Gastrointestinal System
- Begins formation in week 4
- Swallows amniotic fluid and makes bile by week 12
- Meconium is made by week 16

6 Renal System
- Kidneys develop in stages
- Ascends to normal location
- Produces urine by week 10
- Urinates by week 11

7 Reproductive System (Figure 6-9)

8 Musculoskeletal System
- Primitive skeleton covered by muscles by week 6
- Fetal movement on ultrasound by week 7
- Fetal movement felt by mother between weeks 16-20

9 Integumentary System
- Fat develops in last 4-6 weeks.
- Lanugo disappears in week 28
- Fingernails and toenails develop by end of 36th week
- Skin color is determined at conception

SUGGESTIONS FOR CLASSROOM ACTIVITIES

- Have students label a diagram of fetal circulation comparing differences between fetal and neonatal circulation.
- Show a video of fetal development to help students understand how the major organs are formed.

SUGGESTIONS FOR CLINICAL ACTIVITIES

- Have students develop a poster explaining fetal development.

Identify signs of pregnancy and maternal changes throughout pregnancy.

CONCEPTS FOR LECTURE

1. Presumptive signs of pregnancy are indicators, not diagnostic of pregnancy.
2. Probable signs of pregnancy could indicate pregnancy but are not diagnostic of pregnancy.
3. Positive signs of pregnancy are diagnostic of a pregnancy.
4. Most pregnancies progress as planned. The LPN/LVN is responsible for collecting data and for recognizing and reporting symptoms of complications.
5. The key to a healthy pregnancy is regular prenatal care, including client teaching and early detection of complications.

POWERPOINT LECTURE SLIDES

(NOTE: The number on each PPT Lecture Slide directly corresponds with the Concepts for Lecture.)

1 Presumptive Signs of Pregnancy
- Amenorrhea, breast changes
- Nausea and vomiting
- Urinary frequency, fatigue
- Abdominal enlargement, quickening

2 Probable Signs of Pregnancy
- Positive pregnancy test
- Ballottement
- Uterine changes

3 Positive Signs of Pregnancy
- Hearing fetal heart tones
- Visualization of fetus
- Fetal movement felt by examiner

4 Reproductive System
- Uterine growth 1cm/week
- Braxton Hicks contractions
- Breasts enlarge and secrete colostrum

5 Cardiovascular System
- Pulse rate increases by 10–15 beats per minute
- Cardiac output increases
- Increased blood flow to uterus and kidneys
- Increased blood volume resulting in physiologic anemia

5a Supine Hypotensive Syndrome (Figure 6-13)

5b Respiratory System
- Chest increases as enlarged uterus displaces diaphragm
- Decreased airway resistance allows more oxygen into lungs
- Swelling of nasal mucosa

5c Renal System
- Urinary frequency
- Glomerular infiltration increases
- Tubular reabsorption increases

5d Gastrointestinal System
- Morning sickness begins week 6 and ends week 12
- Gastric reflux due to relaxation of cardiac sphincter
- Constipation due to decreased peristalsis

5e Musculoskeletal System
- Altered center of gravity
- Increased lumbar curve
- Relaxed pelvic joints
- Muscle cramps

5f Integumentary System (Figure 6-14)

5g Endocrine System
- Prolactin stimulates milk production
- Oxytocin stimulates uterine contractions, let-down reflex
- Gestational diabetes

Suggestions for Classroom Activities	Suggestions for Clinical Activities
• Compare the presumptive, probable, and positive signs of pregnancy. • Assign groups of students a body system and have them present to the other groups the changes that the maternal body undergoes during pregnancy.	• Arrange for students to observe in an antepartum office and write a paper about the observation.

LEARNING OUTCOME 5

Discuss nutritional requirements during pregnancy.

CONCEPTS FOR LECTURE

1. During pregnancy, the woman should add 300 kcalories per day to the diet.

   When breastfeeding, add 500 kcalories per day to the diet.

   Add 2 milk servings and 1 meat serving to meet the additional calories needed during pregnancy.

   The pregnant woman should drink 1.5 to 2 liters of fluids per day to maintain adequate fluid intake.

POWERPOINT LECTURE SLIDES

(NOTE: The number on each PPT Lecture Slide directly corresponds with the Concepts for Lecture.)

 Nutrition
- Add 300 kcalories a day to diet
- Add 500 kcalories a day when breastfeeding
- Add 2 milk servings and 1 meat serving
- Drink 1.5 to 2 liters fluids per day

Suggestions for Classroom Activities	Suggestions for Clinical Activities
• Review the food pyramid and discuss a well-balanced diet for the pregnant woman. Examine an appropriate diet for a vegetarian. Discuss the need for folic acid before becoming pregnant. See Box 6-1. • Arrange for a dietician or nutritionist to speak to students about an appropriate diet for a pregnant woman. • Examine the use of herbs during pregnancy. See Box 6-4.	• Have students develop a teaching plan for a well-balanced diet for the pregnant woman that includes the additional calories and examples of meal plans.

LEARNING OUTCOME 6

Discuss common maternal discomforts during pregnancy and their treatment.

CONCEPTS FOR LECTURE

1. Numerous discomforts occur in a woman's body during pregnancy. Many discomforts are due to changes in hormone levels.

POWERPOINT LECTURE SLIDES

(NOTE: The number on each PPT Lecture Slide directly corresponds with the Concepts for Lecture.)

 Maternal Discomforts during Pregnancy (Table 6-4)

Suggestions for Classroom Activities	Suggestions for Clinical Activities
• Have students complete a case study of a newly pregnant woman who is experiencing many discomforts of pregnancy. Have them discuss the treatment for each discomfort.	• Arrange to students to observe a midwife or nurse practitioner do antepartum physicals and teaching in an OB/GYN office.

LEARNING OUTCOME 7

Discuss prenatal care and client teaching related to prenatal care.

CONCEPTS FOR LECTURE

1. Goals of prenatal care are a healthy and prepared mother who has minimal discomforts, safe delivery of fetus, and prepared family.
2. Naegele's rule is used to determine the estimated date of birth.
3. Routine office visits are scheduled to monitor the pregnant woman and fetus.
4. Nurses have a responsibility to teach good health practices, including nutrition, exercise, and eliminating risky behaviors.

POWERPOINT LECTURE SLIDES

(NOTE: The number on each PPT Lecture Slide directly corresponds with the Concepts for Lecture.)

1 Goals of Prenatal Care
- Healthy, prepared mother who has minimal discomforts
- Safe delivery of fetus
- Prepared family

1a Prenatal Terminology
- Gravida—number of pregnancies
- Para—number of deliveries after 24 weeks gestation
- Abortion—loss of pregnancy before 24 weeks 20 weeks gestation
- Preterm delivery—delivery after 24 weeks but before 38 weeks
- Term delivery—delivery between 38–42 weeks
- Postterm—delivery after 42 weeks gestation

2 Naegele's Rule (Figure 6-18)

3 Prenatal Office Visits
- Every 4 weeks for first 28 weeks
- Every 2 weeks during weeks 29 to 36
- Every week after 36 weeks until delivery

4 Teach Healthy Behaviors
- Good nutrition
- Exercise
- Avoid hyperthermia
- Home safety

4a Prenatal Teaching/Classes
- Self-care
- Labor process
- Signs of complications
- Infant care
- Follow-up care

SUGGESTIONS FOR CLASSROOM ACTIVITIES

- Review client teaching topics for health promotion during pregnancy. See Box 6-5.
- Discuss warning signs of pregnancy—Table 6-6.

SUGGESTIONS FOR CLINICAL ACTIVITIES

- Have students attend a childbirth education class and report on what they learned from the class.

CHAPTER 7
LABOR AND DELIVERY

RESOURCE LIBRARY

CD-ROM

Breech birth
Second stage of labor
Delivery of Infant
Placenta cord blood
Applying umbilical cord alarm system
Leopold's maneuvers
Video: *First Stage of Labor*
Video: *Second Stage of Labor*
Video: *Transition*
Video: *Cesarean Delivery*

IMAGE LIBRARY

Figure 7-1 Birthing room in a women and babies hospital.
Figure 7-2 Flowsheet showing hormone theory of how labor begins.
Figure 7-3 Cervical effacement and dilatation of the cervix in a primigravida woman.
Figure 7-4 Female pelvis.
Figure 7-5 Measuring the station of the fetal head while it is descending.
Figure 7-6 Fetal attitude.
Figure 7-7 Fetal lie.
Figure 7-8 Cephalic presentations.
Figure 7-9 Breech presentations.
Figure 7-10 ROA.
Figure 7-11 Palpating the sutures in the skull to determine position of the fetus.
Figure 7-12 Effects of labor on the fetal head.
Figure 7-13 Contraction patterns in first, second, and third stages of labor.
Figure 7-14 (A) The nurse helps the client in labor assume a side-lying position to promote efficiency of contractions and maternal comfort. (B) Birthing ball facilitates fetal descent and fetal rotation, and helps increase the diameter of the pelvis. (C) Birthing bar.
Figure 7-15 Massage techniques for back labor.
Figure 7-16 Distribution of pain in labor.
Figure 7-17 (A) Paracervical block (sensory pathways and site of interruption in relation to fetus). (B) Pudendal block. (C) Placement of epidural and spinal anesthetics. (D) Illustrates the epidural space, located between the dura and the vertebra.
Figure 7-18 Technique of local injection prior to episiotomy.

COMPANION WEBSITE

Birthplan

Figure 7-19 Cervical dilatation (actual sizes).
Figure 7-20 Amniotomy is a very common procedure performed during labor.
Figure 7-21 Crowning of the fetus.
Figure 7-22 Two most common episiotomy incisions.
Figure 7-23 Mechanisms of labor: left anterior occiput position.
Figure 7-24 Birthing sequence.
Figure 7-25 Hollister cord clamp.
Figure 7-26 Placental separation.
Figure 7-27 Neonatal measurements taken immediately after birth.
Figure 7-28 (A) Identification band on infant. (B) Umbilical alarm attached to newborn infant. (C) Nurse takes footprint of baby.
Figure 7-29 Performing Leopold's maneuvers to determine fetal lie.
Figure 7-30 (*Left*) Location of FHR when fetus is in LOA position. (*Right*) Other transducer placements.
Figure 7-31 (A) External electronic fetal monitoring device showing graph readout. (B) Beltless tocodynamometer system features remote telemetry that allows the laboring mother more mobility.
Figure 7-32 (A) Nurse provides massage to sacral area. (B) Direction of abdominal effleurage for the latent and active phases of the first stages of labor.
Figure 7-33 Some birthing positions.
Figure 7-34 Birthing sequence with mother in supine position.
Figure 7-35 A newborn infant being suctioned with a DeLee mucus trap to remove excess secretions from the mouth and nares.

LEARNING OUTCOME 1

Define key terms.

CONCEPTS FOR LECTURE

1. Theories have been developed to answer why labor begins: the overdistention theory and the hormonal theory.
2. Labor progresses in an identifiable sequence of events.

POWERPOINT LECTURE SLIDES

(NOTE: The number on each PPT Lecture Slide directly corresponds with the Concepts for Lecture.)

1 Beginning of Labor Theories
- Overdistention Theory
  - Hollow organs empty themselves when over-distended
- Hormonal Theory
  - Fetal cortisol, progesterone
  - Estrogen, oxytocin

1a Hormonal Theory (Figure 7-2)

2 Signs of Impending Labor
- Lightening
- Braxton Hicks contractions
- Bloody show
- Ruptured membranes
  - Spontaneous, premature
- Sudden increase in energy

2a True vs. False Labor (Table 7-1)

SUGGESTIONS FOR CLASSROOM ACTIVITIES

- Discuss the differences between false labor and true labor. Have two students role-play a nurse explaining to a pregnant client that she is in false labor and how to determine when she is in true labor. Have the observers discuss the emotional status of the pregnant woman being sent home.

SUGGESTIONS FOR CLINICAL ACTIVITIES

- Arrange for students to observe in a labor triage unit and write a short paper on the types of clients seen and the outcome of their nursing care.

LEARNING OUTCOME 2

Discuss appropriate nursing actions for women who present for admission when in labor.

CONCEPTS FOR LECTURE

1. Upon admission, the most important concerns are the stage of labor, the condition of the mother, and the condition of the fetus.

POWERPOINT LECTURE SLIDES

(NOTE: The number on each PPT Lecture Slide directly corresponds with the Concepts for Lecture.)

1 Assessing the Client on Admission
- When did the contraction begin?
- How far apart are the contractions and how long do they last?
- Have the membranes ruptured? (Has the water broken?)
- Is this your first pregnancy? How long were previous labors?

1a Client Assessment
- Maternal vital signs
- Urine dipstick for glucose and protein
- Fetal heart rate
- Contractions
- Vaginal examination

1b Cervical Changes (Figure 7-3)

1c Client Assessment
- Nitrazine test of vaginal secretions
- Signs of pregnancy-induced hypertension
  ○ Edema
  ○ Altered reflexes
  ○ Clonus

SUGGESTIONS FOR CLASSROOM ACTIVITIES

- Present a case study of a labor client in class. Have students discuss what information is necessary to know about the medical history, the obstetric history, and the presenting assessment.

SUGGESTIONS FOR CLINICAL ACTIVITIES

- Arrange for a labor and delivery nurse to explain to the students the procedure for admission of a laboring client. Have students assist with an admission of a labor client.
- Have students review a client chart for the admission data collected by the labor and delivery nurse. Discuss the importance of knowing the client's medical history.

LEARNING OUTCOME 3

Describe variables affecting labor and delivery.

CONCEPTS FOR LECTURE

1. Variables affecting labor include the 5Ps: passage, passenger, powers, position, and psyche.

   The passage consists of the size and shape of the maternal pelvis to accommodate the fetus. In cephalopelvic disproportion, the maternal pelvis is smaller than the fetal head, making vaginal delivery impossible.

   The station refers to the relationship between the fetus and the maternal ischial spines. The fetus is fully engaged when at 0 station.

   The passenger refers to the size of the fetus and the relationship of fetal parts to the maternal uterus and pelvis.

   The attitude is the relationship of fetal parts to one another. Flexion of the head and extremities makes for an easier labor.

   The fetal lie is the relationship of the fetal position to the maternal pelvis. Ideally, the fetus should be in a longitudinal lie in relation to the long axis of the maternal pelvis.

   The fetal presentation is the body part of the fetus that is closest to the cervix, such as in vertex presentation the occiput is closest to the cervix. Breech position is the buttocks closest to the cervix.

   Fetal position is the relationship of the presenting part to the four quadrants of the maternal pelvis, such as left or right, anterior or posterior.

   The largest part of the fetus is the head, which will accommodate to fit through the maternal pelvis.

2. The primary power is the involuntary muscle contraction of the myometrium in response to oxytocin.

POWERPOINT LECTURE SLIDES

(NOTE: The number on each PPT Lecture Slide directly corresponds with the Concepts for Lecture.)

1 Passage (Figure 7-4)

1a Passage (Figure 7-5)

1b Passenger (Figure 7-6)

1c Passenger (Figure 7-7)

1d Passenger (Figure 7-8)

1e Passenger (Figure 7-9)

2 Power
- Contractions
  ○ Frequency
  ○ Duration
  ○ Intensity
- Ferguson's reflex

2a Power (Figure 7-13)

3 Position (Figure 7-14)

4 Psyche
- Emotional status
  ○ Past experiences
  ○ Expectations
  ○ Culture
  ○ Ideas about behavior
- Fear and anxiety

The secondary power is Ferguson's reflex, or the spontaneous urge to push the fetus through the birth canal.

3. The position of the mother relieves muscle tension, supports areas of the body, and provides distraction. The side-lying position prevents supine hypotension syndrome.

4. The psyche is the emotional status of the mother. The fear and anxiety of the labor process stimulates the sympathetic nervous system.

SUGGESTIONS FOR CLASSROOM ACTIVITIES

- Have students identify the correct terminology for fetal positions. See Table 7-2 and Figure 7-10.
- Discuss positioning of the labor client and the influence on the fetus of different positions.
- Have students research cultural practices of the different cultures that live in the area where they will have clinical rotations. Refer to Box 7-1 and search the Web for cultural practices.

SUGGESTIONS FOR CLINICAL ACTIVITIES

- On a pregnant model, demonstrate the mechanisms that occur to allow the fetal head to progress through the pelvis during delivery. Refer to Figures 7-11 and 7-12.

LEARNING OUTCOME 4

Identify various methods of pain relief used during labor.

CONCEPTS FOR LECTURE

1. Pain in labor may begin as a mild ache and progresses to a great intensity, which is relieved on delivery of the fetus.

2. Nonpharmacologic and pharmacologic methods may be used for pain relief during labor.

POWERPOINT LECTURE SLIDES

(NOTE: The number on each PPT Lecture Slide directly corresponds with the Concepts for Lecture.)

1 Pain in Labor (Figure 7-16)

2 Nonpharmacologic Pain Relief
- Light activity
- Relaxation techniques
- Counterpressure
- Natural childbirth
  ○ Breathing and relaxation

2a Pharmacologic Pain Relief (Figure 7-17)

2b Pharmacologic Pain Relief (Figure 7-18)

SUGGESTIONS FOR CLASSROOM ACTIVITIES

- Discuss methods of nonpharmacologic support of the laboring client. Refer to Box 7-5.
- Discuss medications used for pain relief and the adverse effects on the mother and fetus. Refer to Table 7-3.

SUGGESTIONS FOR CLINICAL ACTIVITIES

- Have students attend a childbirth education class where alternative pain relief methods are taught to the pregnant woman and support person.
- Have students observe placement of an epidural catheter and nursing care during epidural administration.

LEARNING OUTCOME 5

Differentiate the stages of labor.

CONCEPTS FOR LECTURE

1. In order to determine whether labor is progressing in a normal pattern, the nurse must understand the stages of labor and the mechanism by which the infant maneuvers its way through the birth canal.
2. To stimulate and shorten labor, an amniotomy or artificial rupture of fetal membranes may be performed.

   To prevent tearing of the perineal and anal tissue and to aid in delivery, an episiotomy or cutting of the perineal tissue may be performed.

POWERPOINT LECTURE SLIDES

(NOTE: The number on each PPT Lecture Slide directly corresponds with the Concepts for Lecture.)

1 Stages of Labor
- First Stage
  - Latent, active, transition
- Second Stage
  - Clamping of the umbilical cord
  - Collecting cord blood
- Third Stage
  - Schultze mechanism
  - Duncan mechanism
- Fourth Stage

1a Transition Stage of Labor (Figure 7-19)

2 Amniotomy (Figure 7-20)

SUGGESTIONS FOR CLASSROOM ACTIVITIES

- Have students view videos on the stages of labor and compare the nursing care for each stage.
- Show students an amnihook and explain nursing care of the client when the membranes are artificially ruptured.
- Have students research cord blood banking, uses of the cord blood, and cost of storage.

SUGGESTIONS FOR CLINICAL ACTIVITIES

- Have students teach a newly delivered client how to care for an episiotomy, including administering perineal care and setting up a sitz bath.
- Examine a placenta to demonstrate the fetal side and the maternal side.

LEARNING OUTCOME 6

Discuss the mechanisms of labor.

CONCEPTS FOR LECTURE

1. The mechanisms of labor are the cardinal movements the fetus makes as the fetus moves through the pelvis to delivery.

POWERPOINT LECTURE SLIDES

(NOTE: The number on each PPT Lecture Slide directly corresponds with the Concepts for Lecture.)

1 Mechanisms of Labor (Figure 7-23)

SUGGESTIONS FOR CLASSROOM ACTIVITIES

- With a pelvis and a doll, demonstrate the cardinal movements the fetus makes to descend through the pelvis.

SUGGESTIONS FOR CLINICAL ACTIVITIES

- None

LEARNING OUTCOME 7

Identify nursing diagnoses and nursing interventions to assist in the labor process.

CONCEPTS FOR LECTURE

1. The LNP/LVN uses nursing diagnoses in the planning of nursing care for the laboring client.
2. The goals of nursing interventions are to assist the client and support persons through the labor process.
3. Nursing care during labor involves providing non-pharmacologic and pharmacologic comfort measures for the mother and monitoring the well-being of the infant.

POWERPOINT LECTURE SLIDES

(NOTE: The number on each PPT Lecture Slide directly corresponds with the Concepts for Lecture.)

[1] Nursing Diagnoses during Labor
- Pain related to the labor process
- Anxiety
- Deficient Knowledge
- Risk for Ineffective Individual Coping related to fatigue and the birth process

[1a] Nursing Diagnoses during Labor
- Altered Urinary Elimination
- Deficient Fluid Volume
- Risk for Infection

[2] Nursing Interventions during Labor
- Maintain standards of practice
- Review prenatal records for presence of complications
- Provide encouragement and emotional support by using therapeutic communication
- Assess comfort level and ability to cope
- Evaluate effectiveness of comfort measures
- Listen to and respect needs of client

[3] Nursing Interventions during Labor
- Provide ice chips and oral care
- Encourage muscle relaxation, massage, effleurage
- Promote breathing techniques
- Assist with epidural placement and monitor complications
- Administer Pitocin (oxytocin) to augment labor, as ordered.
- Prepare for delivery

SUGGESTIONS FOR CLASSROOM ACTIVITIES

- Have students calculate an IV Pitocin solution to determine the mL/hr to infuse. Discuss nursing considerations for the administration of Pitocin.
- Have students practice breathing and relaxation techniques. Refer to Table 7-4 for breathing techniques.

SUGGESTIONS FOR CLINICAL ACTIVITIES

- Assign student to assist a labor and delivery nurse with a laboring client.

LEARNING OUTCOME 8

Provide appropriate care for a client during labor and delivery.

CONCEPTS FOR LECTURE

1. The first priority in nursing care during labor and delivery is to assess maternal and fetal well-being with the progression of labor and delivery.

   The nurse must be constantly on the alert to see whether labor is progressing normally. If it is not, the care provider must be notified at once.

POWERPOINT LECTURE SLIDES

(NOTE: The number on each PPT Lecture Slide directly corresponds with the Concepts for Lecture.)

[1] Nursing Interventions during Labor
- Monitor the client and fetus
- Perform ongoing data collection

2. To deliver culturally competent care, the nurse must be alert to verbal and nonverbal expressions of the client and family.
3. Nursing care during and after delivery involves positioning the client, cleansing the perineum, encouraging the client to push, administering medications, and comforting the client.

- Perform Leopold's maneuver
- Apply the external fetal monitor
- Teach to change positions frequently
  - Side-lying, upright

1a External Fetal Monitor (Figure 7-31)

1b Vaginal Examinations
- Assess progression
  - Cervical effacement and dilatation
  - Fetal station
  - Fetal position

2 Culturally Competent Care (Box 7-4)

3 Nursing Care during Delivery
- Position client in lithotomy position or left side
- Cleanse perineum with antiseptic soap
- Encourage client to push

3a Delivery (Figure 7-34)

3b Nursing Care after Delivery
- Administer Pitocin after delivery of placenta.
- Take vital signs every 15 minutes for one hour
- Provide blankets for warmth
- Check fundus and vaginal flow
- Inspect the episiotomy and/or lacerations
- Encourage bonding with newborn

3c Episiotomy (Figure 7-22)

SUGGESTIONS FOR CLASSROOM ACTIVITIES

- Using a pregnant model, demonstrate Leopold's maneuver.
- Have students suck on a LifeSavers® candy to demonstrate cervical dilatation and effacement.

SUGGESTIONS FOR CLINICAL ACTIVITIES

- Have students assist with external fetal monitor placement and determining fetal tracing.

LEARNING OUTCOME 9

Describe important aspects of nursing care of the neonate immediately after birth.

CONCEPTS FOR LECTURE

1. The LPN/LVN needs to understand the care of the neonate that must be met immediately after delivery.
2. The Apgar score is performed at 1 minute and 5 minutes after delivery to evaluate the neonate's adaptation to extrauterine life.
3. For safety issues, proper identification must be made in the delivery room before the mother and infant are separated. Each time the infant is brought to the mother, the identification bands must be compared. Upon discharge the mother signs the identifying document that she has received her infant.

POWERPOINT LECTURE SLIDES

(NOTE: The number on each PPT Lecture Slide directly corresponds with the Concepts for Lecture.)

1 Delivery Room Care of Neonate
- Airway—suction
- Breathing—stimulate to breathe
- Circulation—administer oxygen if indicated
- Temperature—dry with warm blankets
- Examine umbilical cord—two arteries and one vein

2 Apgar Score (Table 7-5)

2a Measurements of the Neonate (Figure 7-27)

3 Identification of Neonate (Figure 7-28)

SUGGESTIONS FOR CLASSROOM ACTIVITIES

- Explain the temperature change for a newborn by comparing the delivery with the example of an adult taking a very warm shower and opening the shower curtain while wet before drying with a towel.
- Create newborn assessment scenarios in which students assign Apgar scores.

SUGGESTIONS FOR CLINICAL ACTIVITIES

- Have students assist with nursing care of a newborn after delivery.
- Have students check the newborn's identification band with the mother's identification band when transporting the newborn to the mother's room. Discuss any alarm system that may be used to prevent infant abduction.

CHAPTER 8
MATERNAL HIGH RISK NURSING CARE

RESOURCE LIBRARY

🔵 CD-ROM

Ectopic pregnancy
Pre-eclampsia
Evaluate deep tendon reflexes
Breech birth
Postpartum assessment

COMPANION WEBSITE

HIV/AIDS
Mental health in pregnancy

📖 IMAGE LIBRARY

Figure 8-1 Early pregnancy risk identification, showing the likely referral for each condition.

Figure 8-2 (A) Normal findings of a reactive nonstress test (NST). (B) Examples of a nonreactive NST.

Figure 8-3 A cerclage or purse-string suture is inserted into the cervix to prevent cervical dilation and pregnancy loss.

Figure 8-4 Implantation sites of ectopic pregnancy in order of frequency.

Figure 8-5 Placenta previa.

Figure 8-6 Abruptio placentae.

Figure 8-7 When a woman with heart disease begins labor, the caregivers must monitor her closely for signs of congestive heart failure.

Figure 8-8 (A) In a normal pregnancy, the passive quality of the spiral arteries permits increased blood flow to the placenta. (B) In pre-eclampsia, vasoconstriction of the myometrial segment of the spiral arteries occurs.

Figure 8-9 To elicit clonus, the nurse sharply dorsiflexes the foot.

Figure 8-10 Pre-eclampsia edema.

Figure 8-11 (A) Pregnant woman learning to do serum glucose monitoring. (B) Macrosomia.

Figure 8-12 Rh isoimmunization sequence.

Figure 8-13 Examples of twin presentation.

Figure 8-14 Nuchal cord.

Figure 8-15 Clamp and cut cord, leaving about 1 inch (2.5 cm) between the baby and the first clamp.

Figure 8-16 Prolapse of the umbilical cord.

Figure 8-17 (A) Technique of inserting a uterine catheter. (B) INTRAN Plus intrauterine pressure catheter.

Figure 8-18 Technique for internal direct fetal monitoring.

Figure 8-19 Fetal heart rate variability.

Figure 8-20 Types and characteristics of early, late, and variable decelerations.

Figure 8-21 Technique of obtaining fetal blood from the scalp during labor.

Figure 8-22 (A) Shoulder dystocia. (B) This position with pressure against the mother's knees may be helpful in clients with shoulder dystocia.

Figure 8-23 Vacuum extractor traction.

Figure 8-24 Forceps are composed of a blade, shank, and handle, and may have a cephalic and pelvic curve.

Figure 8-25 Pressure marks from forceps used during delivery may appear on the newborn's cheeks and jaws.

Figure 8-26 Anesthesia levels for a vaginal and cesarean birth.

Figure 8-27 The uterine incisions for cesarean birth.

Figure 8-28 Cesarean delivery.

Figure 8-29 Comprehensive checklist for perinatal loss.

Figure 8-30 Mastitis.

Figure 8-31 Peritonitis may develop with the spread of uterine infection via lymphatics.

LEARNING OUTCOME 1

Define key terms.

CONCEPTS FOR LECTURE

1. Complications can occur at any time during pregnancy, labor, delivery, and postpartum that can put the mother and fetus at high risk.

   Diagnostic studies can be performed to determine the status of the mother and/or the fetus.

POWERPOINT LECTURE SLIDES

(NOTE: The number on each PPT Lecture Slide directly corresponds with the Concepts for Lecture.)

 Key Terms
- High Risk Pregnancy, Labor and Delivery, Postpartum
  - Risk factors create high risk
  - Complications with bleeding
  - Other complications
- Maternal or Fetal Demise or Death
- Postpartum Depression and Postpartum Psychosis

1a Key Terms
- Fetal Well-being
  - Diagnostic tests performed to determine status of the fetus
- Maternal Well-being
  - Blood tests performed to determine the possibility of complications of the mother and/or fetus

SUGGESTIONS FOR CLASSROOM ACTIVITIES

- Develop a matching quiz with terms on the left side and definitions on the right side. Divide students in to groups and have them complete the quiz.

SUGGESTIONS FOR CLINICAL ACTIVITIES

- Assign students to clients in an antepartum unit or triage unit to observe monitoring and assessing clients with problem pregnancies. Discuss the physician's orders and nursing interventions in postconference.

LEARNING OUTCOME 2

Describe factors that put a woman at risk for complications of pregnancy.

CONCEPTS FOR LECTURE

1. Factors associated with high-risk childbearing are grouped according to the threat to health and the outcome of the pregnancy.

   The LPN/LVN may help collect data about risk factors.

POWERPOINT LECTURE SLIDES

(NOTE: The number on each PPT Lecture Slide directly corresponds with the Concepts for Lecture.)

 Risk Factors for Complications
- Risk-taking behaviors
  - Alcohol or other substance intake
  - Unguarded sexual intercourse
  - Multiple partners
  - Smoking
  - Poor nutritional habits or fad diets

1a Risk Factors (Figure 8-1)

SUGGESTIONS FOR CLASSROOM ACTIVITIES

- Have students identify risk factors and discuss the possible consequences to the fetus.
- Discuss signs and symptoms to assess for during a routine prenatal exam that would identify risk factors.

SUGGESTIONS FOR CLINICAL ACTIVITIES

- Have students review client's prenatal record to identify risk factors. Discuss how to counsel a pregnant client after risk factors are identified.

LEARNING OUTCOME 3

Describe diagnostic tests commonly used during pregnancy.

CONCEPTS FOR LECTURE

1. If signs of complications are detected, a variety of tests are used to assess fetal well-being.

   Prenatal care must include an assessment of maternal well-being. Routine prenatal maternal assessment includes vital signs, weight, and urine analysis for glucose and protein. If complications are detected, further diagnostic studies are indicated.

POWERPOINT LECTURE SLIDES

(NOTE: The number on each PPT Lecture Slide directly corresponds with the Concepts for Lecture.)

1 Diagnostic Tests for Fetal Well-being
- Ultrasound
- Amniocentesis
- Nonstress test
- Biophysical profile

1a Nonstress Test (Figure 8-2)

1b Diagnostic Tests for Maternal Well-being
- Maternal hemoglobin
- Indirect Coombs' test
- Multiple marker screen
- 1-hour glucose screen
- Vaginal culture

SUGGESTIONS FOR CLASSROOM ACTIVITIES

- Discuss the client preparation needed for diagnostic studies.
- Have students develop a client education sheet explaining the reason for the diagnostic studies and the preparation the client needs to do prior to the study being conducted.

SUGGESTIONS FOR CLINICAL ACTIVITIES

- Review client charts for results of diagnostic studies and blood studies. Compare normal with abnormal results and discuss what interventions were done.

LEARNING OUTCOME 4

Describe common complications of pregnancy, including symptoms, medical treatment, and nursing care.

CONCEPTS FOR LECTURE

1. Complications can be identified early through assessment and monitoring.

   Bleeding during pregnancy is always a potentially life-threatening condition for the mother and the fetus.

   Pregnancy puts additional workload on the client's damaged heart, resulting in congestive heart failure.

   Hypertensive disorders can lead to serious complications, resulting in death of the fetus or the mother.

   The client with diabetes prior to pregnancy has the same risks to the pregnancy as the client who develops gestational diabetes.

   The fetus has some protection from infection with intact membranes. Once the membranes rupture, the fetus is exposed to the infection.

   Most medication used to treat AIDS is safe to administer during pregnancy, decreasing the chance for the infant developing the disease.

   The nurse is responsible for early detection of complications, assisting with medical treatments, and providing emotional support.

POWERPOINT LECTURE SLIDES

(NOTE: The number on each PPT Lecture Slide directly corresponds with the Concepts for Lecture.)

1 High-Risk Pregnancy
- Menstruation
  - No treatment indicated
- Spontaneous abortion
  - Bleeding and cramping occur
  - Bedrest for several days
  - If bleeding stops, instruct to avoid strenuous activity, fatigue, sexual intercourse
  - If bleeding continues, physician performs D&C

1a Complications with Bleeding
- Habitual abortion
  - Causes by incompetent cervix
    - Cervix dilates in second trimester, expelling fetus
  - Circlage (Shirodkar procedure) is performed

1b Circlage (Figure 8-3)

1c Complications with Bleeding
- Ectopic pregnancy
  - Implantation of blastocyte outside uterine cavity
  - Ruptures causing bleeding in abdominal cavity, vaginal bleeding, shock
  - Immediate surgery
  - Embryo usually does not survive

1d Ectopic pregnancy (Figure 8-4)

1e Complications with Bleeding
- Placenta previa
  - Placenta lies near or covers cervical opening
  - Painless bleeding occurs as cervix begins to dilate and efface
  - Vaginal exams are contraindicated
  - Cesarean section is performed

1f Placenta Previa (Figure 8-5)

1g Complications with Bleeding
- Abruptio placenta
  - Premature separation of placenta
  - If small abruption, induce labor and allow vaginal delivery
  - If moderate or severe separation, perform cesarean section
  - Evaluate fetus for anemia and hypoxia
  - Evaluate mother for rigid and painful uterus, vaginal bleeding and hypovolemia

1h Abruptio placenta (Figure 8-6)

1i Hyperemesis Gravidarium
- Excessive vomiting leading to dehydration and electrolyte imbalance
  - Tachycardia, hypovolemia, hypotension, increase in BUN
  - Poor skin turgor, dry mucous membranes, urine output <30 mL/hr, protein and vitamin deficiency
- Treatment
  - Anti-emetics, oral or intravenous fluids, correct electrolyte imbalance

1j Cardiac Disorders
- Heart defect or cardiac damage due to disease or drug abuse increases workload on heart
- Signs of congestive heart failure
- Treatment
  - Constant heart monitoring during labor
  - Cesarean section delivery

1k Hypertensive Disorders
- Gestational hypertension
  - Increased blood pressure of 140/90 or higher

- No proteinuria
- Blood pressure return to normal within 12 weeks after delivery

11 Hypertensive Disorders
- Chronic hypertension
  - Blood pressure 140/90 or higher before pregnancy
  - High blood pressure continues more than 12 weeks after delivery

1m Hypertensive Disorders
- Pre-eclampsia and eclampsia
  - Progressive hypertension and proteinuria
  - Vasoconstriction decreases circulation to uterus, placenta, and kidneys
  - Fluid overload leads to cerebral edema, headache, visual disturbances, hyperactive deep tendon reflexes
  - Liver enlargement with epigastric pain and damage

1n Pre-eclampsia and Eclampsia (Figure 8-8)

1o Pre-eclampsia vs. Eclampsia
- Preeclampsia:
  - BP 30 mmHg systolic or 15 mm HG diastolic above normal
  - Weight gain of > I lb per week
  - 1+ protein in urine
  - Hyperreflexes
  - Headache, blurred vision, scotoma, irritability, epigastric pain
- Eclampsia:
  - BP 160/110 or higher
  - Generalized edema
  - Weight gain 2 or more lbs in few days to week
  - 2+ protein in urine
  - Reduced urine output
  - Grand mal seizures
  - Coma
  - Initiation of contractions
  - Death

1p Hypertensive Disorders
- Eclampsia
  - Pre-eclampsia progressing to grand mal seizures and coma
- HELLP syndrome
  - Pre-eclampsia with liver damage
  - Hemolysis, elevated liver enzymes, low platelet count
  - Results in ischemia and tissue damage

1q Hypertensive Disorders
- Treatment
  - Bedrest on left side
  - Well-balanced diet—high protein, moderate sodium
  - Antihypertensive drugs, diuretics, sedatives

- ○ CNS depressants—magnesium sulfate
- ○ Labor induction or cesarean delivery

1r Hypertensive Disorders
- Nursing Considerations
  - ○ Monitor blood pressure, urine output, proteinuria
  - ○ Monitor deep tendon reflexes
  - ○ Teach diet, activity, medications
  - ○ Perform fetal and maternal monitoring
  - ○ Prepare for labor induction or cesarean section delivery

1s Gestational Diabetes Mellitus
- Abnormal glucose metabolism caused by additional requirement for insulin
  - ○ Fetus may develop macrosomia, hypoglycemia
  - ○ Mother at risk for pre-eclampsia and ketoacidosis
  - ○ Treatment
    - – Monitor blood sugar, administer insulin
    - – Instruct in diet and activity

1t Infections
- Sexually transmitted diseases
- TORCH infections
- Treatment
  - ○ Maternal and fetal antibiotics or antivirals
  - ○ Cesarean section if active herpes lesions

1u Acquired Immunodeficiency Syndrome (AIDS)
- Caused by the human immunodeficiency virus (HIV)
- Treatment
  - ○ Zidovudine (ZDV) or azidothyamidine (AZT) therapy for mother and infant
  - ○ Cesarean delivery, no breastfeeding

1v Hemolytic Disorders
- Rh Incompatibility
  - ○ Mother is Rh negative and fetus is Rh positive
  - ○ Mother produces antibodies against Rh positive fetus
  - ○ Treatment: Rh immune globulin (RhoGAM) at 28 weeks gestation and within 72 hours of delivery

1w Hemolytic Disorders (Figure 8-12)

1x Hemolytic Disorders
- ABO Incompatibility
  - ○ Mother is type O and fetus is type A, B, or AB
  - ○ Mother's blood contains anti-A and anti-B antibodies which attack fetal blood

1y Multiple Pregnancy
- Carrying more than one fetus
- Risk for pre-eclampsia, gestational diabetes, preterm labor
- Type of delivery depends on presentation of fetuses

1z Multiple Pregnancy (Figure 8-13)

1aa Nursing Care with Complications of Pregnancy
- Assessment of mother and fetus with monitoring
- Administer intravenous infusions, blood transfusions if indicated
- Maintain bedrest with bathroom privileges
- Administer tocolytic medications, antihypertensive medications
- Provide emotional support and education

SUGGESTIONS FOR CLASSROOM ACTIVITIES

- Compare pre-eclampsia with eclampsia. See Box 8-4. Discuss differences in nursing care for both conditions.
- Develop case studies of clients with complications of pregnancies. Divide the students into groups and have them present the assigned case study and lead a discussion of the nursing care for the client.

SUGGESTIONS FOR CLINICAL ACTIVITIES

- Assign students to the antenatal unit to provide nursing care for a client with complications of pregnancy. Have the student present the client in postconference.
- Arrange for students to accompany a public health nurse on an antepartum visit. Have the students report on the assessment and teaching that was done by the public health nurse.

LEARNING OUTCOME 5

Describe common complications during labor and delivery, including the symptoms, medical interventions, and nursing care.

CONCEPTS FOR LECTURE

1. Most pregnancies end with a normal labor and delivery, but the possibility of anticipated and unanticipated complications exists.

    Preterm labor is contractions and cervical changes between the 20th and 37th weeks of gestation.
2. Induction of labor may be necessary if the risk to the mother or infant of continuing the pregnancy is greater than the risk of delivery.
3. Precipitous labor and/or delivery increase the risk of ruptured uterus, cervical and vaginal lacerations, hemorrhage, fetal distress, and fetal cerebral trauma.
4. A prolapsed umbilical cord compresses the umbilical cord against the cervix and the pelvis, resulting in fetal hypoxia and maybe death.
5. Dystocia is a difficult delivery that could occur due to fetal malposition or malpresentation, large fetus, ineffective uterine contractions, or small maternal pelvis.
6. In the absence of cephalopelvic disproportion, the delivery may be assisted with a vacuum or forceps.
7. A cesarean section may be a planned event or an emergency procedure to save the mother and/or fetus.
8. A vaginal birth may be attempted after a cesarean section, depending on the reason for the cesarean section, condition of the scar tissue, and the size of the fetus.
9. The nurse provides emotional support for the grieving family after fetal death, as well as monitors the progress of labor and prepares for delivery.

POWERPOINT LECTURE SLIDES

(NOTE: The number on each PPT Lecture Slide directly corresponds with the Concepts for Lecture.)

1 High-Risk Labor and Delivery
- Preterm labor
  - Onset of regular contractions and cervical changes between 20 and 37 weeks gestation
- Treatment
  - Hospitalization, tocolytic medications, corticosteroids
  - If contractions continue, labor continues to delivery

2 Induction of Labor
- Induction of labor is performed if risk of continuing pregnancy is greater than risk of delivery
- Methods of induction
  - Administer prostaglandin (PGE_1), artificial rupture of membranes (AROM), administer Pitocin infusion

3 Precipitous Delivery
- Rapid, unexpected delivery without attention of physician or nurse midwife
- Precipitous labor
  - Labor lasting less than three hours
- Increases risk of ruptured uterus, cervical and vaginal lacerations, hemorrhage, fetal distress, fetal cerebral trauma

10. The LPN/LVN must be prepared to assist the registered nurse with delegated tasks in providing care for the labor and delivery client.

4 Prolapsed Umbilical Cord
- Umbilical cord emerges through cervix before presenting part
- Treatment:
    - Vaginal exam to apply upward pressure to relieve pressure on cord
    - Turn to knee-chest position
    - Cover cord with wet towels
    - Emergency cesarean section

4a Prolapsed Umbilical Cord (Figure 8-16)

5 Dystocia
- Long, difficult, or abnormal labor pattern
- External or internal fetal monitoring is performed to obtain continuous tracing of fetal heart rate and uterine contractions
- Fetal blood sample may be drawn for blood gases
- Pressure may be applied above mother's pubis for difficult shoulder delivery

5a Dystocia (Figure 8-20)

6 Assisted Delivery (Figure 8-23)

6a Assisted Delivery (Figure 8-24)

7 Surgical Delivery or Cesarean Section
- Sign surgical consent
- Insert foley catheter
- Start intravenous infusion
- Shave prep
- Prepare for anesthesia
- Assist with delivery

7a Anesthesia (Figure 8-26)

7b Cesarean Delivery (Figure 8-28)

8 Vaginal Birth after Cesarean Section (VBAC)
- Vaginal birth depends upon:
    - Reason for cesarean section
    - Condition of scar tissue
    - Size of fetus
- Uterine stimulant is used with caution
- Frequent monitoring may be needed
- Prepare for emergency cesarean, if indicated

9 Fetal Demise or Fetal Death (Figure 8-29)

10 Nursing Care with Complications of Labor and Delivery
- Assess mother and fetus with frequent monitoring
- Assist with application of monitoring equipment
- Recognize normal and abnormal patterns and report to supervising nurse
- Administer intravenous fluids, medications, oxygen
- Prepare for delivery

LEARNING OUTCOME 6

Describe common complications during the postpartum period, including the symptoms, medical interventions, and nursing care.

CONCEPTS FOR LECTURE

1. The postpartum period usually progresses without problems, but complications may continue from before delivery or develop after delivery.

   Preeclampsia usually begins during pregnancy but can become worse in the first 24 to 48 hours after delivery.

2. Postpartum hemorrhage is most common within the first hour after delivery.

3. Infections may be prevented through good hygiene practices, such as daily bathing and handwashing.

4. Maternal death is rare during childbirth. It takes an emotional toll on the family, nurses, and medical staff.

5. The nurse must be prepared to refer the mother and family for counseling and follow-up care as appropriate.

POWERPOINT LECTURE SLIDES

(NOTE: The number on each PPT Lecture Slide directly corresponds with the Concepts for Lecture.)

1 High-Risk Postpartum
  • Pre-eclampsia (Figure 8-9)

2 Complications with Bleeding
  • Retained placenta
    ○ Treatment
      – Physician performs D&C to remove placental parts
  • Uterine atony
    ○ Uterus does not fully contract
    ○ Treatment
      – Fundal massage, administration of Pitocin or Methergine

2a Complications with Bleeding
  • Lacerations
    ○ Treatment
      – Physician sutures lacerations, administer intravenous fluids or blood transfusions, if needed

2b Complications with Bleeding
  • Disseminated Intravascular Coagulation (DIC)
    ○ Overactivation of blood clotting mechanism resulting in depletion of clotting factors and platelets
    ○ Treatment
      – Administer intravenous fluids, blood transfusions, oxygen, anticoagulants

2c Nursing Care with Bleeding Problems
  • Assess vital signs
  • Stop bleeding
  • Monitor intake and output
  • Administer medical treatment
  • Support client and family
  • Contact other resources

3 Postpartum Infections
- Mastitis
  - Infection of the breast
  - Treatment
    - Antibiotics, moist heat applications, analgesics, emptying the breast with frequent breastfeeding
- Wound infection
  - Redness, swelling, pain, purulent drainage of incision or laceration
  - Treatment
    - Antibiotics, wound care

3a Mastitis (Figure 8-30)

3b Postpartum Infections
- Puerperal infection
  - Infection of the uterus, can lead to septicemia
  - Fever 100.4°F or higher, chills, pelvic and abdominal pain, foul-smelling lochia
  - Treatment
    - Antibiotics

3c Puerperal Infections (Figure 8-31)

4 Maternal Death
- Listen to family's questions and respond appropriately
- Provide reassurance that everything possible is being done
- Review the situation and learn if anything could be done differently
- Debriefing helps to cope with feelings and emotions

5 Postpartum Depression
- Depression appears 4 weeks after delivery and upon weaning from the breast
  - Sadness, frequent crying, insomnia or excessive sleeping, appetite change, difficulty concentrating, feelings of worthlessness, lack of interest in usual activities, lack of concern for appearance

5a Postpartum Psychosis
- Major psychiatric disorder evident in first three months after delivery
  - Agitation, hyperactivity, insomnia, mood lability, confusion, irrational thoughts and behaviors, difficulty remembering or concentrating, poor judgment, delusions, hallucinations
  - Considered an emergency because of risk of suicide and infanticide

5b Postpartum Depression and Postpartum Psychosis
- Treatment
  - Medication
  - Individual and group counseling
  - Assistance meeting childcare and family needs
  - Referral to mental health professional

Nursing Care with Depression and Psychosis
- Teach signs and symptoms to client and family
- Assist in monitoring symptoms
- Monitor for side effects of medications
- Be supportive to family

SUGGESTIONS FOR CLASSROOM ACTIVITIES	SUGGESTIONS FOR CLINICAL ACTIVITIES
• Compare the responsibilities of the LPN/LVN with the responsibilities of the RN on a postpartum unit. • Have students identify risk factors postpartum depression and postpartum psychosis. Arrange for a mental health nurse to discuss nursing interventions for postpartum depression and postpartum psychosis. • Role-play how to communicate with a family when a maternal death has occurred. Discuss what measures can be taken to help the family grieve the loss of a mother and/or fetus.	• Assign student to provide nursing care for clients in a postpartum unit. • Have students develop a client education sheet on the complications that can occur in the postpartum period. Have them use this education sheet when educating the client for discharge.

CHAPTER 9
HEALTH PROMOTION OF THE NEWBORN

RESOURCE LIBRARY

CD-ROM

Circumcision
Breastfeeding & first foods

COMPANION WEBSITE

Umbilical cord alarm system
Circumcision bioethics
Infant massage

IMAGE LIBRARY

LEARNING OUTCOME 1

Define key terms.

CONCEPTS FOR LECTURE

1. The newborn is the infant from delivery through the first month of life.

   An understanding of the physiologic adaptation to extrauterine life guides the nurse's actions when setting priorities in the care of the newborn.

   The newborn's adaptation to extrauterine life is evaluated using the Apgar score.

2. Gestational age assessment is used to determine the accurate gestational age in weeks. It is determined from the last menstrual period.

   Reflexes are signs of neurologic integrity. Absent or slowed reflexes may indicate prematurity of the newborn.

   Disorders or congenital anomalies place the infant at high risk for conditions that may be life-threatening.

POWERPOINT LECTURE SLIDES

(NOTE: The number on each PPT Lecture Slide directly corresponds with the Concepts for Lecture.)

1. Key Terms
   - Newborn
     ○ Infant from delivery through the first month of life
   - Physiologic adaptation
     ○ Adapting to life outside the uterus
   - APGAR score
     ○ Evaluation of adaptation to life outside uterus

2. Key Terms
   - Gestational age
     ○ Accurate age in weeks from last menstrual period
   - Reflexes
     ○ Signs of neurologic integrity
   - High-risk newborn
     ○ Conditions of the newborn that may be life-threatening

SUGGESTIONS FOR CLASSROOM ACTIVITIES

- Develop a matching quiz with key terms on the left and definitions on the right. Have students complete the quiz for extra credit.

SUGGESTIONS FOR CLINICAL ACTIVITIES

- None

LEARNING OUTCOME 2

Discuss physiologic adaptation of the newborn.

CONCEPTS FOR LECTURE

1. An understanding of the physiologic adaptation to life outside the uterus guides the nurse's actions when setting priorities in the care of the newborn.

   The first priority of respiratory adaptation is to assist the newborn to establish respirations.

2. After clamping the umbilical cord, the fetal circulation contains structures that close due to the increase and decrease of thoracic pressures with respirations.

3. Upon delivery, body heat is lost by evaporation, convection, conduction, and radiation.

4. Newborns are not able to shiver to produce heat; therefore, cold stress may occur when excessive heat is lost.

POWERPOINT LECTURE SLIDES

(NOTE: The number on each PPT Lecture Slide directly corresponds with the Concepts for Lecture.)

1. Physiologic Adaptation of the Newborn
   - Respiratory adaptation
     ○ Spontaneous respirations
     ○ Stimulation by rubbing skin or tapping feet
     ○ Oxygen by mask to prevent hypoxia

1a. Respiratory Adaptation (Figure 9-1)

2. Physiologic Adaptation of the Newborn
   - Cardiovascular adaptation
     ○ Blood no longer flows through the umbilical arteries and veins
     ○ Thoracic pressure increases and decreases cause the closure of the foramen ovale and the ductus arteriosus

2a. Cardiovascular Adaptation (Figure 9-2)

3 Physiologic Adaptation of the Newborn
- Thermoregulatory adaptation
  - Upon delivery, body heat is lost by evaporation, convection, conduction and radiation
- Nursing interventions
  - Dry with warm blankets
  - Place infant on mother's warm skin
  - Cover with dry warm blankets and warm hat
  - Place under radiant warmer

3a Thermoregulatory Adaptation (Figure 9-3)

3b Thermoregulatory Adaptation
- Cold stress
  - Nonshivering thermogenesis
  - Increased metabolism burns stored brown fat resulting in
    - Respiratory distress
    - Hypoxia
    - Depletion of stores of glycogen

4 Cold Stress (Figure 9-4)

SUGGESTIONS FOR CLASSROOM ACTIVITIES

- Trace fetal circulation on a diagram of the fetal circulatory system. Have students identify changes that take place after delivery.
- Have students identify how heat loss occurs through evaporation, conduction, convection, and radiation.
- Explain brown fat and how the newborn maintains body heat. Have students identify ways to prevent cold stress.

SUGGESTIONS FOR CLINICAL ACTIVITIES

- Have students assist the nurse with newborn care at a delivery. Have students discuss their observations in postconference.

LEARNING OUTCOME 3

Discuss Apgar score.

CONCEPTS FOR LECTURE

1. The evaluation of the newborn's adaptation to extrauterine life is the Apgar score, which is assigned at 1 and 5 minutes after birth.

   A narcotic antagonist can be administered for respiratory depression if mother received a narcotic during labor.

2. The nurse performing CPR on the newborn must be qualified in the Neonatal Resuscitation Program (NRP).

POWERPOINT LECTURE SLIDES

(NOTE: The number on each PPT Lecture Slide directly corresponds with the Concepts for Lecture.)

1 APGAR Score
- Completed at 1 and 5 minutes after birth
- Score of 8–10 requires no intervention
- Score of 4–7 requires stimulation and oxygen
- Score of 0–3 requires immediate resuscitation
- Narcan is administered for narcotic-induced respiratory depression

1a APGAR Score (Table 7-5)

1b Neonatal Resuscitation Program (NRP) (Figure 9-5)

- Develop case studies of newborns in which students calculate the Apgar score.
- Review the steps of neonatal resuscitation.

- Have students assist the nurse with calculating the Apgar score after delivery of the newborn.

LEARNING OUTCOME 4

Describe physical characteristics of the newborn.

CONCEPTS FOR LECTURE

1. Within the first 1 to 2 hours after birth, the nurse completes an in-depth assessment to evaluate the newborn's adaptation to extrauterine life and to identify any complications or abnormalities.

    The LNP/LVN must understand the normal appearance and reflexes of the newborn and to identify and report deviations to the supervising nurse or physician.

POWERPOINT LECTURE SLIDES

(NOTE: The number on each PPT Lecture Slide directly corresponds with the Concepts for Lecture.)

1 Newborn Vital Signs
- Temperature—97.7–99.4°F (36.5–37.5°C)
- Pulse rate—110–160 bpm (brachial and femoral pulses)
- Respiratory rate—30–60 breaths per minute
- Blood pressure—60-80/40-45 at birth, 100/50 at day 10

1a Pain (Box 9-1)

1b Gestational Age
- Complete within 4 hours of birth
- Neuromuscular Maturity
- Physical Maturity

1c Gestational Age Assessment (Figure 9-9)

1d Characteristics of the Newborn
- General appearance (Figure 9-15)

1e Characteristics of the Newborn
- Head (Figure 9-16)

1f Characteristics of the Newborn (Figure 9-17)

1g Characteristics of the Newborn
- Chest
    - 12 inches to 13 inches in circumference
    - Nipples may secrete whitish fluid (witches' milk)
    - Heart murmurs may be normal
    - Diaphragmatic breathing pattern
    - Respirations are irregular with brief periods of apnea

1h Characteristics of the Newborn
- Abdomen
    - Soft, rounded without palpable masses
    - Umbilical cord should have 3 vessels
    - Bowel sounds present in all 4 quadrants
    - Meconium stools for 2–3 days
    - Voids 5–8 times a day

1i Characteristics of the Newborn
- Genitalia (Figure 9-19)

POWERPOINT LECTURE SLIDES *continued*

Characteristics of the Newborn
- Extremities
  - Symmetrical bilaterally
  - Each extremity ends with 5 digits
  - Strong muscle tone
  - Full range of motion
  - No hip displacement

SUGGESTIONS FOR CLASSROOM ACTIVITIES

- Have students view a video on the assessment of a newborn. Review normal and abnormal findings.

SUGGESTIONS FOR CLINICAL ACTIVITIES

- Have students practice newborn assessments on infant models in the laboratory and then assist with newborn assessments in the nursery.
- Have students complete a gestational age assessment and graph weight, height, and head circumference to determine whether or not the newborn is appropriate for gestational age, small for gestational age or large for gestational age.
- Have students use a noncognitive pain scale to determine the pain level of the newborn.

LEARNING OUTCOME 5

Describe neonatal reflexes.

CONCEPTS FOR LECTURE

1. Reflexes are signs of neurologic integrity. Some reflexes remain throughout life. Others disappear within 2 years.
2. Absent or slowed reflexes may indicate prematurity of the newborn.
3. Lingering reflexes may indicate neurologic lesions.

POWERPOINT LECTURE SLIDES

(NOTE: The number on each PPT Lecture Slide directly corresponds with the Concepts for Lecture.)

 Neonatal Reflexes
- Rooting reflex, sucking reflex
- Palmar grasp reflex, plantar grasp reflex
- Babinski reflex, stepping reflex
- Tonic neck reflex
- Moro reflex or startle reflex

SUGGESTIONS FOR CLASSROOM ACTIVITIES

- Demonstrate neonatal reflexes and discuss at what age reflexes disappear.

SUGGESTIONS FOR CLINICAL ACTIVITIES

- Have students practice demonstrating neonatal reflexes on infant models in the laboratory and then assist with performing neonatal reflexes on infants in the nursery.

LEARNING OUTCOME 6

Describe nursery care for the newborn.

CONCEPTS FOR LECTURE

1. Most infants are born without complications and only require routine nursing care.

POWERPOINT LECTURE SLIDES

(NOTE: The number on each PPT Lecture Slide directly corresponds with the Concepts for Lecture.)

 Nursery Care for the Newborn
- Airway maintenance
- Eye care
- Vitamin K administration
- Umbilical cord care
- Bathing
- Safety

SUGGESTIONS FOR CLASSROOM ACTIVITIES

- Arrange for a nursery nurse to discuss routine nursing care on the newborn in the nursery.

SUGGESTIONS FOR CLINICAL ACTIVITIES

- Assign students to perform newborn care in the nursery and develop a concept map or care plan on the newborn.

LEARNING OUTCOME 7

Discuss common procedures and screening tests for the newborn.

CONCEPTS FOR LECTURE

1. Newborn screening tests are performed to detect abnormalities in the newborn, allowing treatment to begin before further complications occur.
2. The most common procedures performed on the newborn are circumcisions and immunizations.

POWERPOINT LECTURE SLIDES

(NOTE: The number on each PPT Lecture Slide directly corresponds with the Concepts for Lecture.)

1 Newborn Screening Tests
- Hypoglycemia
- Phenylketonuria
- Bilirubin

1a Newborn Screening Tests (Figure 9-27)

2 Newborn Procedures
- Circumcision
- Immunizations

2a Newborn Procedures (Figure 9-28)

SUGGESTIONS FOR CLASSROOM ACTIVITIES

- Discuss the procedure for drawing blood from the newborn.
- Have students discuss the implications of performing newborn screening tests and the treatment for abnormal results.
- Assign students to research the pros and cons of having a circumcision performed. Have them discuss their findings in class.

SUGGESTIONS FOR CLINICAL ACTIVITIES

- Have students perform heel sticks for blood screening tests.
- Allow students to administer immunizations to newborns in the nursery.
- Arrange for students to observe circumcisions being performed and to monitor for bleeding after the procedure.

LEARNING OUTCOME 8

Discuss the newborn's nutritional needs and how they can be met.

CONCEPTS FOR LECTURE

1. A full-term infant needs 50 to 55 kcal/lb (110 to 120 kcal/kg), which equals 20 oz (600 mL) of breast milk or formula per day.

   The newborn's stomach holds approximately 20 to 30 mL in the first few days of life. The stomach capacity increases to 60-90 mL within the first week after birth. 60 to 90 mL.
2. The American Academy of Pediatrics recommends breast milk for the first year of life.

   Colostrum, a thin, yellow fluid containing protein, calories, and immune globulins, protects the infant from intestinal infections and assists with passage of meconium.

POWERPOINT LECTURE SLIDES

(NOTE: The number on each PPT Lecture Slide directly corresponds with the Concepts for Lecture.)

1 Newborn Nutrition
- 50 to 55 kcal/lb (110 to 120 kal/kg) or 20 oz (600 mL) of breast milk or formula per day
- At birth, newborn's stomach holds about 20 mL
- End of first week, newborn's stomach holds 60–90 mL
- Feed every 2–4 hours to meet nutritional needs

2 Breastfeeding
- AAP recommends breastfeeding for first year of life
- Colostrum contains protein, calories, immune globulins

3. When feeding, the mother should be instructed to hold the infant's head higher than the stomach to prevent aspiration of stomach contents.

- Breastfeeding
  - 10 to 30 minutes a side per feeding
  - 8–12 times a day.

2a Breastfeeding (Figure 9-30)

2b Breastfeeding (Figure 9-31)

3 Bottlefeeding
- Feed 15mL first few days, then increase gradually
- Position head higher than stomach
- Burp when half of feeding consumed

3a Bottlefeeding (Figure 9-32)

SUGGESTIONS FOR CLASSROOM ACTIVITIES

- Arrange for a Lactation Consultant to talk to the class about breastfeeding and techniques to use when teaching a client how to breastfeed.
- Have students research different types of formula. Have them discuss when to use each formula.

SUGGESTIONS FOR CLINICAL ACTIVITIES

- Have students make rounds with the lactation consultant to observe how to assist the client and infant with breastfeeding.
- Have students attend a prenatal class in which newborn nutrition is taught. Have them write a paper on the pros and cons of breastfeeding versus bottle-feeding.

LEARNING OUTCOME 9

Discuss parent teaching related to care of the newborn.

CONCEPTS FOR LECTURE

1. The LPN/LVN reviews discharge instructions with the parents to evaluate their understanding of infant care.
2. Diapers should be checked and changed frequently to monitor the amount of output and to maintain skin integrity of the diaper area.
3. Infants are cleansed with a warm, moist washcloth until the umbilical cord falls off. Once the umbilical cord falls off, tub baths may be given.
4. The newborn likes the security and warmth of being swaddled and may sleep 20 to 22 hours a day when swaddled.
5. Safety issues need to be stressed to the parents to avoid injury to the newborn.

POWERPOINT LECTURE SLIDES

(NOTE: The number on each PPT Lecture Slide directly corresponds with the Concepts for Lecture.)

1 Discharge Teaching
- Elimination
  - Voids 8–10 times a day
  - Pass meconium within 24 hours after delivery
  - Transitional stools passed after several feedings
  - Formed brown stools pass after solid food is eaten
  - Diapers should be checked and changed frequently

2 Diapering (Figure 9-33)

3 Hygiene
- Bathing
- Umbilical cord care
- Perineal care
- Circumcision care

3a Hygiene (Figure 9-34)

4 Sleep (Figure 9-35)
- Swaddling
- Sleeps 20–22 hours a day

5 Safety
- Car seat safety
- Falls
- Head support

SUGGESTIONS FOR CLASSROOM ACTIVITIES	SUGGESTIONS FOR CLINICAL ACTIVITIES
• Have students develop a discharge teaching sheet for newborn care at home. Have them use the discharge sheet in the clinical setting.	• Have students attend a discharge teaching class or observe the nurse giving discharge instructions to the parents of the newborn.

LEARNING OUTCOME 10

Describe signs of respiratory distress in the newborn.

CONCEPTS FOR LECTURE

1. The newborn should be observed frequently for signs of respiratory distress. Subtle changes may indicate difficulty maintaining gas exchange.

POWERPOINT LECTURE SLIDES

(NOTE: The number on each PPT Lecture Slide directly corresponds with the Concepts for Lecture.)

1 Signs of Respiratory Distress
- Tachypnea, orthopnea
- Grunting
- Flaring nostrils
- Retractions
- Fluid retention

1a Respiratory Distress (Figure 9-18)

SUGGESTIONS FOR CLASSROOM ACTIVITIES	SUGGESTIONS FOR CLINICAL ACTIVITIES
• Discuss signs of respiratory distress and list the priorities of treatment. • Have students view a video on respiratory distress and treatment.	• Have students practice neonatal resuscitation on an infant simulation model.

LEARNING OUTCOME 11

Discuss conditions and treatment of the high-risk newborn.

CONCEPTS FOR LECTURE

1. The role of the LPN is one of assisting the RN with data collection, meeting the basic needs of the newborn, and documenting nursing care administered.

   Newborns with congenital heart defects need to be assessed for heart murmurs and monitored for signs and symptoms of congestive heart failure.

   The most common type of hemorrhage is intraventricular hemorrhage, which can occur in premature infants who deliver vaginally.
2. The most common cause of hyperbilirubinemia is physiologic jaundice from the normal breakdown of red blood cells. The most common cause of pathologic jaundice is Rh incompatibility. Treatment for hyperbilirubinemia is phototherapy.
3. The premature infant lacks surfactant, which maintains patency of the alveoli, resulting in respiratory distress. Mechanical ventilation and high oxygen concentration can damage alveoli, which results in bronchopulmonary dysplasia.

   Stress or hypoxia during pregnancy can cause the fetus to pass meconium into the amniotic fluid, which the fetus can inhale and aspirate into the alveoli.

POWERPOINT LECTURE SLIDES

(NOTE: The number on each PPT Lecture Slide directly corresponds with the Concepts for Lecture.)

1 High-Risk Newborn
- Cardiovascular conditions
  - Congenital anomalies
  - Hemorrhage
  - Hemolytic disorders

2 Treatment for Hemolytic Disease (Figure 9-39)

3 Respiratory Conditions
- Congenital anomalies
  - Respiratory distress
  - Bronchopulmonary dysplasia
- Meconium aspiration

3a Treatment for Respiratory Conditions (Figure 9-36)

4 Neurologic Conditions
- Congenital anomalies
- Birth trauma
- Acquired deficits
- Chromosomal abnormalities
- Fetal Alcohol Syndrome

4. Spina bifida and hydrocephalus are two neurologic conditions that are treated with surgery.

   Down syndrome is the most common chromosomal abnormality in which the infant has distinct physical features and is at risk for congenital heart defects, diabetes, and hearing loss.

5. Defects of the gastrointestinal system are the most common of all congenital defects. They require surgical correction before aspiration, malnutrition, or obstruction occurs.

6. The main concern with genitourinary system defects is whether or not the infant is able to urinate.

5 Gastrointestinal Conditions
- Congenital anomalies
  - Cleft lip and palate
  - Esophageal atresia and tracheoesophageal fistula
  - Imperforate anus
  - Omphalocele
  - Pyloric stenosis
  - Hernia

5a Gastrointestinal Conditions (Figure 9-40)

6 Genitourinary Conditions
- Congenital anomalies
  - Urethral malposition
  - Phimosis
  - Ambiguous genitalia
  - Extrophy of the bladder

6a Genitourinary Conditions (Figure 9-44)

6b Nursing Care of High-Risk Newborn
- Maintain airway, breathing, circulation
- Maintain body temperature
- Provide nutrition
- Ensure elimination
- Educate parents

SUGGESTIONS FOR CLASSROOM ACTIVITIES

- Arrange for a neonatal intensive care nurse to speak with students about nursing care of high-risk neonates in the neonatal intensive care unit.
- Have students discuss experiences they have had with a high-risk newborn.

SUGGESTIONS FOR CLINICAL ACTIVITIES

- Arrange for students to observe neonates in a neonatal intensive care unit.

CHAPTER 10
HEALTH PROMOTION IN THE POSTPARTUM PERIOD

RESOURCE LIBRARY

⦿ CD-ROM
Postpartum assessment
Massage a uterine fundus postpartum
Sitz bath

COMPANION WEBSITE
National Adoption Clearinghouse

IMAGE LIBRARY

Figure 10-1 Involution of the uterus.
Figure 10-2 Diastasis recti abdominis, a separation of the abdominal musculature, commonly occurs after pregnancy.
Figure 10-3 As the woman takes hold of her new role, she will begin to perform care activities on the newborn.
Figure 10-4 Mother-child bonding is strengthened as infant and parent look into each other's eyes.
Figure 10-5 The father's intense concentration shows engrossment in his new child.
Figure 10-6 The uterine fundus becomes displaced and deviated to the right when the bladder is full.
Figure 10-7 (A) Position of hands to palpate the uterus, assess its firmness, and promote contraction. (B) Nurse palpating uterus.

Figure 10-8 Suggested guidelines for assessing lochia volume.
Figure 10-9 Complete uterine prolapse with inversion of the vagina.
Figure 10-10 Nurse removing clots from uterus.
Figure 10-11 Intact perineum with hemorrhoids.
Figure 10-12 (A) Nurse assessing client's foot for edema. (B) Assessing for thrombosis
Figure 10-13 Postpartum flow sheet of physical and psychological assessment and possible educational needs of the client.
Figure 10-14 A sitz bath promotes healing and provides relief from perineal discomfort during the initial weeks following birth.
Figure 10-15 Postpartal exercises.

LEARNING OUTCOME 1

Describe physical changes in the mother during the postpartum period.

CONCEPTS FOR LECTURE

1. The postpartum or puerperium period begins immediately after birth of the baby and continues for 6 weeks or until the woman's body systems change again and return to a near prepregnant state.

   Involution is the return of the uterus to a nonpregnant state.

   Lochia is the discarding of blood, mucus, and tissue. It is classified by its appearance: lochia rubra, lochia serosa, and lochia alba.

   Exfoliation is healing of the placenta site by the shedding of tissue instead of scar formation, which would prevent uterine attachment of future pregnancies.

2. Within 3 weeks, the tissue of the vagina, cervix, and perineum heals.

   The return of breast tissue to a prepregnant state depends on whether the mother is breastfeeding or not and for the length of time breastfeeding lasts.

POWERPOINT LECTURE SLIDES

(NOTE: The number on each PPT Lecture Slide directly corresponds with the Concepts for Lecture.)

1 Physical Changes during the Postpartum Period
- Reproductive system
  - Uterus
    - Involution
    - Lochia
    - Exfoliation

2 Physical Changes during the Postpartum Period (Figure 10-1)

2a Physical Changes during the Postpartum Period
- Reproductive system
  - Vagina
  - Breasts
  - Ovaries
    - Ovulation and menstruation resume in 2 to 3 months

Ovulation and menstruation usually returns in 2 to 3 months, longer for the breastfeeding woman.

3. Abdominal muscles take several months of exercise to regain muscle tone.

The cartilage of the pelvis regains its firmness, but the diameter of the pelvis remains widened.

4. Stool softeners, high-fiber diet, and adequate fluid are advised to relieve or prevent constipation. With a cesarean section, diet is advanced from liquids when bowel sounds return.

5. After delivery, puerperal diuresis occurs. Swelling of the perineum and surrounding structures and decreased sensation of bladder filling may make urination difficult.

6. Due to dehydration and physical exertion, the temperature may rise to 100.4°F. After delivery, the woman may experience a postpartum chill due to the increased temperature. The temperature should return to normal within 24 hours after delivery.

Blood values may be abnormal for first few days after delivery. Due to activation of blood coagulation factors, the woman is at risk for thrombosis.

7. Hormone changes take place after delivery with a gradual return to normal levels.

3 Physical Changes during the Postpartum Period
- Musculoskeletal system
  - Abdominal muscles
  - Diastasis recti abdominis
  - Pelvis

3a Physical Changes during the Postpartum Period (Figure 10-2)

4 Physical Changes during the Postpartum Period
- Gastrointestinal system
  - Diet
  - Peristalsis
  - Bowel sounds

5 Physical Changes during the Postpartum Period
- Renal system
  - Puerperal diuresis
  - Difficult urination

6 Physical Changes during the Postpartum Period
- Cardiovascular system
  - Temperature
    - Postpartal chill
  - Blood pressure
  - Blood values
    - Thrombosis

7 Physical Changes during the Postpartum Period
- Endocrine system
  - Estrogen and Progesterone
  - Prolactin
  - Oxytocin

SUGGESTIONS FOR CLASSROOM ACTIVITIES

- Discuss physical changes the client undergoes during the postpartum period using case studies to demonstrate body system changes.
- Invite a panel of women who recently delivered babies to discuss postpartum changes they experienced.

SUGGESTIONS FOR CLINICAL ACTIVITIES

- Arrange for students to accompany a public health nurse on postpartum visits. Have them develop a concept map or care plan addressing the physical changes noted on a postpartum client.

LEARNING OUTCOME 2

Discuss psychological changes in the mother during the postpartum period.

CONCEPTS FOR LECTURE

1. Adjustment to the role of mother takes place in the stages of taking-in and taking-hold.

2. A client giving a baby up for adoption may experience feelings of grief and will require emotional care by the nurse.

Postpartum blues is a mild depression beginning a few days after delivery and may last for 2 weeks. It may be associated with hormone changes and psychological adjustment to motherhood.

POWERPOINT LECTURE SLIDES

(NOTE: The number on each PPT Lecture Slide directly corresponds with the Concepts for Lecture.)

1 Psychological Changes during the Postpartum Period
- Taking-In Stage
  - Taking-in information about baby
  - Recalling delivery experience
  - Storing information to memory
  - Dependent on others

3. Bonding is an emotional attachment between the mother and the infant.

    The nurse must identify negative feelings and help the family explore these feelings.

    The baby's father will demonstrate engrossment in interactions with the infant.

1a Psychological Changes during the Postpartum Period
- Taking-Hold Stage
  - Controls care of self and baby
  - Preoccupied with body functions
  - Begins to assume role of mother
  - Social interactions important

1c Psychological Changes during the Postpartum Period (Figure 10-3)

2 Psychological Changes during the Postpartum Period
- Adoption
  - Feelings of grief
- Postpartum Blues
  - Mild depression
  - Begins on 3rd or 4th day postdelivery
  - Lasts up to 2 weeks

3 Psychological Changes during the Postpartum Period
- Attachment
  - Bonding
- Negative feelings
  - Disappointment
- Fathers, siblings, others
  - Engrossment, bonding

SUGGESTIONS FOR CLASSROOM ACTIVITIES

- Compare the taking-in stage with the taking-hold stage of psychological adjustment of the postpartum client.
- Arrange for a social worker to speak to the class about adoptions and counseling the postpartum client who gave a baby up for adoption or who is having problems adjusting to having a newborn.

SUGGESTIONS FOR CLINICAL ACTIVITIES

- Have students identify what stage of psychological adjustment their assigned client is in.
- Have students observe bonding with the client and newborn and for engrossment of the father with the newborn.

LEARNING OUTCOME 3

Discuss important aspects of postpartum assessment and nursing care.

CONCEPTS FOR LECTURE

1. The nurse is responsible to advocate for the rights of the client and family based on their cultural beliefs.

    The LPN/LVN must know the normal findings to report abnormal readings to the charge nurse or primary care provider.

    The mnemonic BUBBLE helps the nurse to remember the important areas to examine during the postpartum assessment.

    The mnemonic REEDA is used to assess incisions, lacerations, episiotomies.

POWERPOINT LECTURE SLIDES

(NOTE: The number on each PPT Lecture Slide directly corresponds with the Concepts for Lecture.)

1 Postpartum Assessment
- Culture
  - Hygiene
  - Food choices
  - Activity
  - Family roles

1a Postpartum Assessment
- Postpartum vital signs
  - Return to normal by 24 hours after delivery
- Pain
  - With afterpains
  - With breastfeeding

1b Postpartum Assessment
- Breasts
  - Palpate for softness or fullness if breastfeeding
- Abdomen
  - Fundus should be firm and midline
  - Measure fundus in fingerbreadths above or below umbilicus

1c Postpartum Assessment (Figure 10-7)

1d Postpartum Assessment (Figure 10-8)

1e Postpartum Assessment (Figure 10-11)

1f Postpartum Assessment
- Perineum
  - Void every 2 to 4 hours after delivery
  - Prevent constipation

1g Postpartum Assessment
- Lower extremities
  - Negative Homan's sign
- Psychological assessment
  - Assess attitude, feelings, bonding

SUGGESTIONS FOR CLASSROOM ACTIVITIES

- Assign students to research a culture and report to the class on the beliefs of the culture in regard to postpartum care.
- Have students view a video on postpartum assessments. Explain BUBBLE and REEDA mnemonics to assess postpartum clients.

SUGGESTIONS FOR CLINICAL ACTIVITIES

- Have students practice postpartum assessment skills on models in the laboratory.
- Assist students to perform postpartum assessments on assigned clients on the postpartum unit.

LEARNING OUTCOME 4

Describe the complications commonly seen during the postpartum period.

CONCEPTS FOR LECTURE

1. The first priority for nursing care in the postpartum period is to assess for complications to prevent serious life-threatening conditions.

   While assessing the client, the nurse has the opportunity to teach normal body changes and signs of complications to report to the physician.

   Using the BUBBLE assessment as a guide for postpartum assessment, the LPN/LVN can identify abnormalities to report to the charge nurse or primary care provider.

   The mnemonic REEDA is used as a guide for assessing incisions and/or lacerations.

POWERPOINT LECTURE SLIDES

(NOTE: The number on each PPT Lecture Slide directly corresponds with the Concepts for Lecture.)

1 Postpartum Complications
- Vital signs
  - Temperature above 100.4°F after 24 hours may be infection
  - Tachycardia may indicate hemorrhage
  - Tachypnea indicates respiratory distress
  - Blood pressure elevation may indicate PIH

1a Postpartum Complications
- Pain
  - Report increases in pain
- Breasts
  - Report redness, heat, pain
- Abdomen
  - Massage boggy fundus
  - Assess cesarean section incision for REEDA

1b Postpartum Complications (Figure 10-6)

1c Postpartum Complications
- Lochia
  - Report large amount and large clots
  - Report foul smelling
- Perineum
  - Observe discoloration, bruising, swelling
  - Assess episiotomy or laceration for REEDA
  - Assess hemorrhoids for bleeding, tenderness

1d Postpartum Complications
- Elimination
  - Report urinary retention, painful urination
  - Assess for constipation
- Lower extremities
  - Note redness, swelling or tenderness
  - Report positive Homan's sign

1e Postpartum Complications (Figure 10-12)

1f Postpartum Complications
- Psychological assessment
  - Assess for fatigue
  - Note attachment problems

SUGGESTIONS FOR CLASSROOM ACTIVITIES

- Review pain medications used to relieve pain after delivery. See Table 10-2 for oral pain medications.
- Explain BUBBLE and REEDA mnemonics to identify complications in the postpartum period.
- Review treatments for complications experienced by the postpartum client.

SUGGESTIONS FOR CLINICAL ACTIVITIES

- Have students demonstrate BUBBLE and REEDA assessments on postpartum clients in the clinical setting.

LEARNING OUTCOME 5

Discuss topics for client teaching about self-care in the postpartum period.

CONCEPTS FOR LECTURE

1. The second priority for nursing care in the postpartum period is to teach the mother how to care for herself and her infant.

   Daily hygiene is important to prevent infections. Showers are preferred over tub baths to prevent cross-contamination.
2. Sitz baths are used to relieve perineal swelling and discomfort.
3. A balanced diet and ambulation promote healing and prevent complications.
4. A support system and healthy patterns of living will help the mother recover without complications

POWERPOINT LECTURE SLIDES

(NOTE: The number on each PPT Lecture Slide directly corresponds with the Concepts for Lecture.)

1 Client Teaching
- Hygiene
  - Daily bath, preferably shower
  - Wash nipples without soap and air dry
  - Rinse perineum after each toileting
  - Pat perineum dry front to back

2 Client Teaching
- Sitz Bath (Figure 10-14)

3 Client Teaching
- Postpartum Nutrition
  - High fiber and fluid diet
  - Decrease daily caloric intake by 300 kcal if not breastfeeding

- If breastfeeding, add 500 kcal, 1000 mL fluids, 65 g protein, 1000 mg calcium per day
- Prenatal vitamins with iron for 3 months

3a Client Teaching
- Exercise (Figure 10-15)

3b Client Teaching
- Postpartum Immunizations
  - RhoGAM
    – Rh negative mother with Rh positive baby
    – Administer within 72 hours after delivery
  - MMR

4 Client Teaching
- Support network and healthy patterns
  - Assist mother at home
  - Encourage good eating, exercise, and rest
  - Respect rest periods
  - Simplify routines, no major changes
  - Discuss concerns or anxieties about parenting

SUGGESTIONS FOR CLASSROOM ACTIVITIES

- Have students develop a discharge instruction sheet to give clients when discharged. Review Box 10-4 with students to discuss self-care after discharge.
- Review the use of immunizations after delivery. See Table 10-3 for information on immunizations.

SUGGESTIONS FOR CLINICAL ACTIVITIES

- Arrange for students to attend a discharge teaching class on the postpartum unit.
- Have students observe a nurse do discharge teaching with the postpartum client.

LEARNING OUTCOME 6

Discuss client teaching about warning signs in infants in the postpartum period.

CONCEPTS FOR LECTURE

1. The mother needs to understand warning signs of complications in infants to report them to the physician.

POWERPOINT LECTURE SLIDES

(NOTE: The number on each PPT Lecture Slide directly corresponds with the Concepts for Lecture.)

1 Warning Signs in Infants
- Axillary temperature above 100.4° F or below 97.8° F
- Projectile or frequent vomiting
- Refusal to eat for 2 feedings or 6 hours
- Listlessness or difficulty waking baby
- Excessive fussiness

1a Warning Signs in Infants
- Increasing jaundice
- Two or more loose black or green watery stools
- Fewer than 6 wet diapers in 24 hours
- Call 911 if baby is blue or not breathing

SUGGESTIONS FOR CLASSROOM ACTIVITIES

- Divide students into groups and assign one group to discuss the warning signs of complications in infants and another group to discuss the warning signs of complications in postpartum clients. Have groups present to each other. Refer to Box 10-5.
- Develop a case study of an infant with warning signs of complications. Have students identify the warning signs and discuss appropriate treatment of the newborn.

SUGGESTIONS FOR CLINICAL ACTIVITIES

- Have students observe the nurse doing discharge teaching on the warning signs of complications in the infant.

CHAPTER 11
LIFE SPAN GROWTH AND DEVELOPMENT

RESOURCE LIBRARY

CD-ROM

Infancy: Major life transition
Handling temper tantrums
Teens: Mental + spiritual health

COMPANION WEBSITE

Internet safety
Apprehending child predators

IMAGE LIBRARY

Figure 11-1 Illustration showing growth and development direction in a small child.

Figure 11-2 Infants learn to sit by about 6 months.

Figure 11-3 Freud saw the vast importance of the unconscious in people's lives.

Figure 11-4 In the first year, reflex actions gradually evolve into deliberate actions.

Figure 11-5 (*Top*) Typical eruption of deciduous ("baby") teeth. (*Bottom*) The school-age child loses teeth at a rate of 4 a year and, by age 12, has 26 of the permanent teeth.

Figure 11-6 Toilet training requires consistency and commitment on the part of the caregiver to schedule regular trips to bathroom.

Figure 11-7 School-age children have fine motor coordination and higher cognitive ability.

Figure 11-8 Teens typically engage in high-risk behaviors and exhibit an attitude of "it can't happen to me."

Figure 11-9 Today's more health-conscious middle and older adults may be more than just observers of their grandchildren's activities.

LEARNING OUTCOME 1

Differentiate growth from development.

CONCEPTS FOR LECTURE

1. Growth is the process of increasing in physical size. Growth and development progress from simple to complex.

2. Development is the process of maturation, which includes the refinement of body systems, thought processes, and judgment.

   Development is cephalocaudal, proceeding from head to toe, and proximodistal, center to periphery and general to specific.

POWERPOINT LECTURE SLIDES

(NOTE: The number on each PPT Lecture Slide directly corresponds with the Concepts for Lecture.)

1 Growth
   • Process of increasing physical size
   • Progresses from simple to complex

2 Development
   • Process of maturation
   • Refinement of body systems, thought processes, judgment
   • Progresses from simple to complex
   • Cephalocaudal
   • Proximodistal

2a Development (Figure 11-1)

SUGGESTIONS FOR CLASSROOM ACTIVITIES

• Compare and contrast growth with development, giving examples of each. See Box 11-1.

SUGGESTIONS FOR CLINICAL ACTIVITIES

• Have students observe children of different age groups and compare how growth patterns differ between differing age groups.

LEARNING OUTCOME 2

List factors that influence growth and development.

CONCEPTS FOR LECTURE

1. Inherited characteristics from ancestors are determined at conception through combinations of genes.

   Due to the mobility of society today, nationality, race, and cultural customs are blending, which has resulted in changes in growth and developmental patterns.

   The order of birth or ordinal position influences development as parents are learning to parent with the oldest child, learning from parents and the older child influence the middle child, and the youngest child may be babied and slower in development.

   An only child may develop faster intellectually or may be spoiled and develop slower.

   Development and maturation occur at different rates between males and females, due to different expectations and cultural influences.

   Family structure influences development of the child through differences in roles of the mother and father, alternative family situations, poverty, lack of nutrition, and limited access to health care.

   A secure and stable environment allows the child to focus energy toward healthy growth and development. An unloved and insecure environment with limited nutrition and health care interferes with growth and development.

POWERPOINT LECTURE SLIDES

(NOTE: The number on each PPT Lecture Slide directly corresponds with the Concepts for Lecture.)

 Factors Influencing Growth and Development
- Heredity
- Nationality, race, culture
- Order of birth
- Gender
- Family structure
- Physical and emotional environment

SUGGESTIONS FOR CLASSROOM ACTIVITIES

- Assign groups of students a different factor of growth and development to research. Have them share their findings with the rest of the class.
- Divide students according to their ordinal position in their families. Have first born students stand together by the door because they are older and more responsible. Have last born students stand in the back of the room, as they are the babies and more likely to get into something. Have middle born students stand anywhere in the middle of the room. Have "only" children stand together. Have the students list what is special about their particular ordinal position and what they like and dislike about their ordinal position. Have them guess the instructor's ordinal position.

SUGGESTIONS FOR CLINICAL ACTIVITIES

- Have students share the factors of growth and development they noted in their own family situations. Have students from different race or culture background discuss differences in their family.

LEARNING OUTCOME 3

Describe Piaget's stages of cognitive development.

CONCEPTS FOR LECTURE

1. Children are born with an innate cognitive ability that must be developed.

    Jean Piaget proposed four levels of cognitive development: sensorimotor, preoperational, concrete operational, and formal operations.

    Sensorimotor, from birth to 2 years, interacts with the environment through reflex responses.

    Preoperational level, ages 2 to 7 years, progresses from using symbolism to symbols.

    Concrete operational, ages 7 to 11 years, is oriented to the present and in concrete terms, such as "black or white" or "right or wrong."

    Formal operations, ages 11 to 16 years, is able to predict the future and to learn abstract comprehension.

POWERPOINT LECTURE SLIDES

(NOTE: The number on each PPT Lecture Slide directly corresponds with the Concepts for Lecture.)

1 Piaget's Stages of Cognitive Development
- Sensorimotor
  - Birth to 2 years
  - Interacts with environment by reflex response
- Preoperational
  - Ages 2 to 7
  - Interacts with environment through use of symbols

1a Piaget's Stages of Cognitive Development
- Concrete operational
  - Ages 7 to 11
  - "Black or white," "right or wrong"
- Formal operations
  - Ages 11 to 16
  - Abstract comprehension

SUGGESTIONS FOR CLASSROOM ACTIVITIES

- Discuss Piaget's levels of cognitive development and give examples of each level to increase students' understanding. See Table 11-1.
- Relate physical growth with cognitive development in different age groups.

SUGGESTIONS FOR CLINICAL ACTIVITIES

- Have students select a client in the clinical setting and identify which stage of cognitive development best describes the client. Discuss how the cognitive development stage affects their disease process, hospitalization, and implications for nursing care.

LEARNING OUTCOME 4

Describe Erikson's levels of psychosocial development.

CONCEPTS FOR LECTURE

1. Erikson described eight stages of psychosocial development: infancy, early childhood, late childhood, school age, adolescence, young adult, middle years, and older adult.

    Infancy level, newborn to 1 year of age, is the development of trust versus mistrust. The ability to trust as an infant influences to the ability to trust as an adult. Inability to trust develops mistrust in relationships.

    Early childhood, ages 1 to 3 years, is the level of autonomy versus shame and doubt. Feelings of trust in successes help the child develop confidence in learning by autonomy. Negative reinforcement develops shame and doubt in abilities.

2. Late childhood, ages 3 to 6 years, is the level of initiative versus guilt. Through positive reinforcement, the child will take initiative to meet needs and not feel a failure.

    School age, ages 6 to 12 years, is the level of industry versus inferiority. The child is learning to apply what he learns, becoming industrious. If the child is unsuccessful or is not praised for what he accomplishes, the child becomes inferior.

POWERPOINT LECTURE SLIDES

(NOTE: The number on each PPT Lecture Slide directly corresponds with the Concepts for Lecture.)

1 Erikson's Levels of Psychosocial Development
- Infancy
  - Newborn to 1 year
  - Trust versus mistrust
- Early Childhood
  - Ages 1 to 3 years
  - Autonomy versus shame and doubt

4 Erikson's Levels of Psychosocial Development
- Late Childhood
  - Ages 3 to 6 years
  - Initiative versus guilt
- School Age
  - Ages 6 to 12 years
  - Industry versus inferiority

6 Erikson's Levels of Psychosocial Development
- Adolescence
  - Ages 12 to 20 years
  - Identity versus role confusion

3. Adolescence, ages 12 to 20 years, is the level of identity versus role confusion, which is becoming independent, separating from parents, and making decisions about self. Inferiority and guilt lead to role confusion and an inability to develop relationships and independence.

   Young adult, ages 20 to 40 years, is the level of intimacy versus isolation. It is a time of developing relationships and making decisions about life's work. Difficulty finding companionship leads to isolation.

4. Middle years, ages 40 to 65 years, is the level of generativity versus self-absorption and stagnation. It is a time of sharing life experiences and becoming a contribution to society. Inability to complete this level leads to not seeing any value or meaning in life.

   Older adult, ages 65 and older, is the level of ego integrity versus despair. It is a time of looking at accomplishments of life and having a "good life." A life of inability to accomplish other levels leads to bitterness and isolation.

- Young Adult
  - Ages 20 to 40 years
  - Intimacy versus isolation
- **8** Erikson's Levels of Psychosocial Development
  - Middle Years
    - Ages 40 to 65 years
    - Generativity versus self-absorption and stagnation
  - Older Adult
    - Ages 65 and older
    - Ego integrity versus despair

SUGGESTIONS FOR CLASSROOM ACTIVITIES

- Discuss Erikson's stages of development and give examples of each stage to increase students' understanding of the stages. See Table 11-2.
- Have students identify the level of psychosocial development they are in. Discuss the implications of their level.

SUGGESTIONS FOR CLINICAL ACTIVITIES

- Have students select a client in the clinical setting and identify the level of psychosocial development in which the client fits. Discuss how psychosocial development affects their disease process, hospitalization, and implications for nursing care.
- Arrange for students to attend a child day care center or an adult day care center to observe the levels of psychosocial development. Have them write a paper on their observations.

LEARNING OUTCOME 5

Describe Freud's stages of psychosexual development.

CONCEPTS FOR LECTURE

1. Freud believed that early childhood experiences led to unconscious motivation for actions later in life and that sexual instincts were important for personality development.

2. The personality has three parts: id, which is the drive to seek pleasure; ego, which is acceptable methods to meet pleasure; and the superego, which is the conscience.

   Freud identified five stages of psychosexual development. See Table 11-3.

   Freud theorized that behavior is motivated and is often unconscious, and defense mechanisms are used to protect the ego from threatening or painful life experiences.

POWERPOINT LECTURE SLIDES

(NOTE: The number on each PPT Lecture Slide directly corresponds with the Concepts for Lecture.)

- **1** Freud's Stages of Psychosexual Development
  - Personality (Figure 11-3)

- **3** Freud's Stages of Psychosexual Development
  - Five stages
  - Behavior is motivated and often unconscious
  - Defense mechanisms protect the ego

SUGGESTIONS FOR CLASSROOM ACTIVITIES

- Discuss Freud's stages of psychosexual development and give examples to improve student's understanding. See Table 11-3.
- Identify and discuss the cultural relevance of Freud's psychosexual development.

SUGGESTIONS FOR CLINICAL ACTIVITIES

- Have students select a client in the clinical setting and identify what level of psychosexual development applies to the client. Discuss how psychosexual development affects their disease process, hospitalization, and implications for nursing care.
- Have students identify the defense mechanisms used by children on the pediatric unit in the clinical setting. Refer to Table 11-4. Have students identify defense mechanisms they may have used.

LEARNING OUTCOME 6

Describe Kohlberg's levels of moral development.

CONCEPTS FOR LECTURE

1. Kohlberg established three levels of moral development, which range from a desire to please others and to avoid punishment, to learning rules and following ethical standards.

POWERPOINT LECTURE SLIDES

(NOTE: The number on each PPT Lecture Slide directly corresponds with the Concepts for Lecture.)

1. Kohlberg's Levels of Moral Development (Table 11-5)

SUGGESTIONS FOR CLASSROOM ACTIVITIES

- Assign groups of students to present Kohlberg's levels of moral development. Have them provide examples to explain the assigned level. See Table 11-5.
- Provide students with ethical issues in health care. Have them identify how moral development affects how ethical decisions are made and what the implications are for nursing care.

SUGGESTIONS FOR CLINICAL ACTIVITIES

- Have students select a child in the pediatric setting and identify what level of moral development fits the child's progress. Discuss how moral development affects their disease process, hospitalization, and implications for nursing care.

LEARNING OUTCOME 7

Describe the usual physical development for each age group.

CONCEPTS FOR LECTURE

1. Infancy is a time of rapid growth and developmental changes. Weight triples and height grows 12 inches in the first year. Body systems mature and teeth erupt at about 6 months of age.
2. Cognitive development in the infant matures from reflexes to purposeful interaction with the environment, noises to words in speech development, and wakefulness increases.
3. In the toddler years, physical growth slows but many developmental changes take place with developing independence and learning to walk, run, and toilet train.
4. The toddler's cognitive development shows growth in language abilities and socialization but experiences separation anxiety when separated from parents and throws temper tantrums to communicate needs.
5. The preschool child steadily grows physically and becomes more independent and self-disciplined.

POWERPOINT LECTURE SLIDES

(NOTE: The number on each PPT Lecture Slide directly corresponds with the Concepts for Lecture.)

1. Stages of Physical Growth and Development
   - Infant (Birth to 1 Year)
     - Doubles birth weight by 5 months
     - Triples birth weight by 12 months
     - Height grows by 12 inches
     - Head growth slows, torso and limbs grow
     - Body systems mature
     - Teeth erupt at about 6 months

2. Stages of Cognitive Development
   - Infant
     - Reflexes to interacting with environment
     - Speech develops from noises to words
     - Sleeps 20 to 22 hours per day
     - Increases wakefulness to 2 to 3 hours at a time

6. Cognitive development in the preschooler shows gender identification, understanding relationships, and continued development of language skills.

7. The school-age growth continues to change to a more adult-like appearance, and most of the permanent teeth have erupted.

8. In cognitive development, the school-age child develops confidence in self, learns to cooperate with others, begins to question family roles and values, and joins clubs and teams.

9. Adolescence is a time for maturing from childhood to adulthood. Females mature faster than males, and hormones guide physical changes.

10. Cognitive development in adolescents progresses from concrete to abstract comprehension. Adolescents may be very self-centered or "immortal," and peers influence behavior.

11. Young adults are at the peak of physical efficiency. As aging continues into middle age, the body gradually decreases in its abilities.

12. Cognitive skills are used to develop a productive life with career, relationships, becoming parents and grandparents, planning for retirement and becoming the sandwich generation.

13. In the older adult there is a slowing or decreasing in the function of all body systems.

14. Cognitive deficits are noted in the older adult, such as loss of memory.

3 Stages of Physical Growth and Development
- Toddler (1–3 years)
  - Walk to run, climb, stand on one foot
  - Ride bicycle
  - Growth slows, pot-bellied abdomen
  - Cuts up to 20 teeth, feeds self

4 Stages of Cognitive Development
- Toddler
  - Vocabulary increases to 1,000 words
  - Parallel play
  - Separation anxiety
  - Temper tantrums

5 Stages of Physical Growth and Development
- Preschool Child (3–6 years)
  - Learns to obey rules
  - Uses imagination
  - Height increases by 2 to 2½ inches
  - Weight increases 4 to 5 pounds a year
  - Gains muscle strength and coordination

6 Stages of Cognitive Development
- Preschool Child
  - Knows name and age
  - Develops understanding of relationships
  - Identifies with gender
  - Vocabulary increases to 2,000 words
  - Follows three simple commands

7 Stages of Physical Growth and Development
- School-Age Child (6–12 years)
  - Height increases 2 inches a year
  - Weight increases 2 pounds a year
  - Body proportions change
  - Loses teeth and gains 26 permanent teeth

8 Stages of Cognitive Development
- School-Age Child
  - Learns to compromise and cooperate with others
  - Learns to reason
  - Learns to understand cause and effect
  - Vocabulary increases to 2,500 words
  - Questions family rules and traditions
  - Joins clubs and teams

9 Stages of Physical Development
- Adolescent (12 to 20 years)
  - Height increases earlier in females
  - Weight increases earlier in females
  - Increase in sex hormones cause physical changes
  - Tanner's stages of sexual maturity

10 Stages of Cognitive Development
- Adolescent
  - Concrete to abstract comprehension
  - Self-centered, strong identity
  - Hormonal changes, sexuality development
  - Peers have positive or negative influence
  - Feelings of immortality

11 Stages of Physical Development
- Adult (18 to 65 years)
  - Young adults are resilient
  - Young adults are at peak efficiency
  - Middle adults gradually decrease abilities
    - Presbyopia and presbycusis develop
    - Menopause, midlife crisis

12 Stages of Cognitive Development
- Adult
  - Cognitive skills for productive life
    - Career, relationships
    - Parents, grandparents
  - Plan for retirement
  - Sandwich generation

13 Stages of Physical Development
- Older Adult (over 65 years)
  - Slowing or decreasing of all body systems

14 Stages of Cognitive Development
- Older Adult
  - Cognition declines
    - Loss of memory
  - Look at meaning of life

SUGGESTIONS FOR CLASSROOM ACTIVITIES

- Have each student develop a poster with pictures comparing stages of physical growth and development.
- Have students discuss how to determine readiness for toilet training and what experiences they have had with toilet training. See hints in Box 11-4.

SUGGESTIONS FOR CLINICAL ACTIVITIES

- Arrange for students to attend a day care center with age groups through school-age children. Have students practice communication skills with the different age groups. See Box 11-5 for guidelines.
- Have students perform physical assessments on children of different age groups on the pediatric unit in the clinical setting, paying particular attention to height, weight, dentition, stages of puberty, and differences in gender. Complete growth charts to compare normal and abnormal deviations.
- Arrange for students to attend a nursing home or adult day care center to practice communication skills and observe physical and cognitive developmental patterns of the older adult.

LEARNING OUTCOME 8

Describe characteristic milestones and deviations from the norm for each age group.

CONCEPTS FOR LECTURE

1. Health assessment and promotion of activities to assist the client meet developmental milestones.

    Deviations from meeting milestones at the appropriate age are warning signs for further assessment and interventions.

POWERPOINT LECTURE SLIDES

(NOTE: The number on each PPT Lecture Slide directly corresponds with the Concepts for Lecture.)

1 Milestones and Deviations
- Infancy
  - Roll over
  - Grasp
  - Sit alone, crawl, stand

1a Milestones and Deviations (Figure 11-4)

1b Milestones and Deviations
- Toddler
  - Runs, jumps
  - Dress and undress self
  - Communication advances
  - Toilet training begins

1c Milestones and Deviations (Figure 11-5)

1d Milestones and Deviations
- Preschooler
  - Toilet trained
  - Ride bicycle
  - Begins to write
  - Tie shoes

1e Milestones and Deviations (Figure 11-6)

1f Milestones and Deviations
- School-Age
  - Reads
  - Plays sports
  - Loses and erupts teeth

1g Milestones and Deviations (Figure 11-7)

1h Milestones and Deviations
- Adolescence
  - Well-developed skills
  - Puberty changes

1i Milestones and Deviations (Figure 11-8)

1j Milestones and Deviations (Table 11-12)

SUGGESTIONS FOR CLASSROOM ACTIVITIES

- Identify appropriate milestones for various age groups. Discuss nursing care that is provided for clients how deviate from normal development. See Tables 11-4, 11-5, 11-6, 11-7, 11-8, 11-9, and 11-10.
- Identify nursing diagnoses and nursing interventions for clients with growth and development deviations.

SUGGESTIONS FOR CLINICAL ACTIVITIES

- Arrange for students to observe physical assessments in the pediatric nurse practitioner or physician's office.
- Arrange for students to attend a physical therapy or rehabilitation unit to observe care for clients with deviations from accomplishing appropriate milestones.

LEARNING OUTCOME 9

Provide some guidelines for age-appropriate teaching to each age group.

CONCEPTS FOR LECTURE

1. Establish a therapeutic relationship with client.
2. Communicate appropriately for age, stage of development, and cognitive level.
3. Be sensitive to developmental issues and allow client to express feelings.
4. Refer to appropriate resources or support groups.

POWERPOINT LECTURE SLIDES

(NOTE: The number on each PPT Lecture Slide directly corresponds with the Concepts for Lecture.)

 Age-Appropriate Teaching Guidelines
- Establish therapeutic relationship
- Communicate appropriately
- Be sensitive to developmental issues
- Refer to appropriate resources
- Refer to support groups

SUGGESTIONS FOR CLASSROOM ACTIVITIES

- Develop scenarios that reflect growth and development of various age groups. Have students role-play the scenarios for how to teach health promotion to these age groups.
- Have students research what resources or support groups are available in the area where they reside.

SUGGESTIONS FOR CLINICAL ACTIVITIES

- Arrange for students to participate in a health fair to educate the public on growth and development and health promotion for all age groups.

CHAPTER 12
ILLNESS PREVENTION, HEALTH PROMOTION, AND NUTRITION IN CHILDREN

RESOURCE LIBRARY

 CD-ROM

Health promotion and health maintenance
Children and overweight

 COMPANION WEBSITE

Learning styles
Nutriition guides

📖 IMAGE LIBRARY

Figure 12-1 The nurse begins assessment of the infant's family when they are seen in the waiting room and called in for care.

Figure 12-2 (A) Adults teach children the proper technique for washing and drying hands. (B) When preschoolers and kindergarten children share snacks or supplies, there is always the potential for transmitting infection. (C) Many respiratory infections are transmitted by droplets from person to person.

Figure 12-3 Immunization schedule.

Figure 12-4 One effective discipline method is to move the child to an isolated area where no interaction with children or adults can occur and no toys are present.

Figure 12-5 Preschoolers develop eye–hand coordination in a variety of settings.

Figure 12-6 Food pyramid.

Figure 12-7 Adjustable mirrors are available to allow the driver to see the infant via the car's rearview mirror.

Figure 12-8 Bottle mouth.

Figure 12-9 It is important to be consistent in use of safety-approved car seats for infants and children.

Figure 12-10 Body proportions at various ages.

Figure 12-11 The home needs to be childproofed for safety.

Figure 12-12 (A) Infants and toddlers can easily lose their balance in a bathtub, and they do not have the muscle strength and coordination to pull themselves back up. (B) Toddlers should not be allowed to play in swimming pools or other deep water without a flotation device.

Figure 12-13 In toddler and preschool years, children often participate in parallel play, enjoying each other's presence while having separate playthings.

Figure 12-14 Bit by bit, toddlers learn the complicated task of eating with utensils.

Figure 12-15 Placing hot pots on back burners with handles turned inward is one way to prevent injury to children.

Figure 12-16 Children on motorized bikes are at risk for injury.

Figure 12-17 Teach children never to touch guns without a parent present.

Figure 12-18 Peers are the most important group among teens.

Figure 12-19 Dietary screening for adolescents.

LEARNING OUTCOME 1

Describe techniques for client/family teaching.

CONCEPTS FOR LECTURE

1. Every interaction between the nurse and client and/or family needs to be one of assessment and promoting health teaching.

    The nurse determines specific areas of instruction needed and determines the effectiveness of prior teaching to develop a teaching plan.

    The nurse plans the type of instruction and where instruction is to take place.

2. Instruction needs to be accurate, complete, up-to-date, individualized, and age-specific.

    At the end of the instruction, the nurse must validate understanding of the information taught.

POWERPOINT LECTURE SLIDES

(NOTE: The number on each PPT Lecture Slide directly corresponds with the Concepts for Lecture.)

1 Techniques of Client/Family Teaching
- Determine specific area needing instruction
- Determine effectiveness of prior teaching
- Planned formal teaching
- Spontaneous informal teaching
- One-to-one dialogue
- Distraction-free environment

2 Techniques of Client/Family Teaching
- Age-specific communication
- Audio-visual aids

- Accurate and complete instruction
- Up-to-date research, techniques, technology
- Individualize printed materials
- Validate understanding

SUGGESTIONS FOR CLASSROOM ACTIVITIES

- Review teaching guidelines with students. See Box 12-1.
- Assign students a specific topic in health care and have students develop a teaching plan for this topic.

SUGGESTIONS FOR CLINICAL ACTIVITIES

- Have students use the teaching plan they developed to instruct clients on health care issues while in the clinical setting.

LEARNING OUTCOME 2

Describe illness prevention activities.

CONCEPTS FOR LECTURE

1. Illness prevention can be divided into three categories: primary, secondary, and tertiary prevention. Primary helps to avoid illness. Secondary allows for early detection and treatment. Tertiary involves treating illnesses to prevent complications.
2. Activities, such as well-child visits or administering immunizations, can be performed to prevention illnesses.
3. The nurse promotes healthy individuals, families, and communities by role-modeling healthy behaviors, providing encouragement, reinforcing the need for change, and recognizing efforts of change.

POWERPOINT LECTURE SLIDES

(NOTE: The number on each PPT Lecture Slide directly corresponds with the Concepts for Lecture.)

1 Illness Prevention Categories
  - Primary prevention
    ○ Prevent health problems from developing
  - Secondary prevention
    ○ Early detection and treatment
  - Tertiary prevention
    ○ Preventing complications

2 Illness Prevention Activities
  - Well-child visits
  - Hygiene
  - Immunizations

3 Illness Prevention Activities (Figure 12-2)

SUGGESTIONS FOR CLASSROOM ACTIVITIES

- Divide students into three groups. Assign the groups to primary, secondary or tertiary prevention. Have each group provide examples of the type of prevention they are assigned.
- Review immunizations, including when, how, and why they are to be administered. See Table 12-1, Figure 12-3 on immunizations.

SUGGESTIONS FOR CLINICAL ACTIVITIES

- Arrange for students to observe well-child visits at a pediatrician's office or at the public health agency. Assist the students with administering immunizations.

LEARNING OUTCOME 3

Describe health promotion activities for children in each age group.

CONCEPTS FOR LECTURE

1. Health promotion activities promote lifestyle changes that result in a healthier state for the individual.

    Injuries are the leading cause of death in children ages 1 to 19. Health promotion includes promoting environmental safety.

    To face challenges in a healthy manner, the client needs a high level of self-esteem.

POWERPOINT LECTURE SLIDES

(NOTE: The number on each PPT Lecture Slide directly corresponds with the Concepts for Lecture.)

1 Health Promotion Activities
  - Environmental safety
    ○ Injuries
  - Psychosocial health
    ○ Promoting self-esteem
    ○ Providing discipline
    ○ Promoting play

The nurse can help parents to explore methods of discipline and effective consequences for bad behavior.

Through play, the child learns skills necessary to function throughout their life span.

1a Providing Discipline (Figure 12-4)

1b Health Promotion Activities
- Infant
  - Falls
  - Choking
  - Car safety
  - Trust
  - Appropriate toys

1c Health Promotion Activities (Figure 12-7)

1d Health Promotion Activities
- Toddler
  - Injuries
  - Toilet training
  - Discipline
  - Play
  - Appropriate toys

1e Health Promotion Activities
- Preschooler
  - Injuries, car seats
  - Strangers
  - Organized learning
  - Discipline
  - Play and appropriate toys

1f Health Promotion Activities
- School-Age
  - Pedestrian and bicycle safety
  - Latch-key children
  - Promote self-esteem
  - Play, school sports
  - Discipline

1g Health Promotion Activities (Figure 12-16)

1h Health Promotion Activities
- Adolescent
  - Risk-taking behaviors
  - Health education
    - Sexual contact, substance abuse
  - Self-esteem
  - Play, peers
  - Discipline

SUGGESTIONS FOR CLASSROOM ACTIVITIES

- Have students discuss methods of discipline and relate how their parents used discipline. Review theories of discipline—see Box 12-3.
- Have students role-play how to communicate with children to increase their self-esteem and not criticize children.
- Have students develop a pamphlet on car safety to teach parents and children about safe use of car seats and seat belts.

SUGGESTIONS FOR CLINICAL ACTIVITIES

- Have students observe children as they play and discuss how types of play change as the child ages.
- Arrange for students to teach a group of children about safe play in the environment.
- Arrange for students to teach parents safety issues for children from infancy through adolescence at a low-income housing project. See Boxes 12-5, 12-6, 12-7, 12-8, 12-9, and 12-10.

LEARNING OUTCOME 4

Discuss important aspects of nutrition for each age group.

CONCEPTS FOR LECTURE

1. 15.3% of American children are considered clinically obese. A type of malnutrition in the United States is obesity.
2. A priority in nursing is to monitor the client's weight, height, nutritional status, nutritional intake, and environmental factors affecting diet.
3. Nurse should teach parents and children adequate nutrition and the risks of inadequate nutrition.
4. Good oral health begins in infancy. Fluoride supplements may be needed if fluoride levels in water are less than 0.6 ppm. Dental visits should begin with toddlers.

POWERPOINT LECTURE SLIDES

(NOTE: The number on each PPT Lecture Slide directly corresponds with the Concepts for Lecture.)

1 Nutrition
- Obesity
  - Malnutrition in U.S.
  - High fat, carbohydrate, sodium diets
  - Low fruit, vegetables, fiber, and water diets

2 Nutrition
- Nurse should monitor:
  - Weight, height
  - Nutritional status
  - Nutritional intake
  - Environmental factors

3 Nutrition
- Nurse should teach:
  - Adequate nutrition
  - Risks of inadequate nutrition

4 Nutrition (Figure 12-6)

4a Nutrition
- Infant
  - Breastfeeding
  - Bottle-feeding
  - Solid foods
  - Food allergies
  - Oral health

4b Nutrition (Figure 12-8)

4c Nutrition
- Toddler
  - One tablespoon of food per age
  - Cow's milk
  - Feeds self
  - Oral health

4d Nutrition
- Preschooler
  - Three meals and two snacks per day
  - Nutritious foods
  - Begin to assist with meals
  - Oral health, dental care

4e Nutrition
- School-Age
  - Eat one meal per day away from home
  - Nutritious snacks and meals
  - Proper etiquette
  - Increased appetite
  - Oral health

4f Nutrition
- Adolescent
  - 2,000 to 3,000 calories per day
  - Increase need for iron, calcium, zinc, vitamins

- Three nutritious meals and snacks
- Prepare own foods
- Oral health, dental care
- Piercings

 Nutrition (Figure 12-19)

SUGGESTIONS FOR CLASSROOM ACTIVITIES

- Compare breastfeeding and bottle-feeding the infant. Discuss dangers of bottle propping and bottle mouth.
- Review the food pyramid for children and discuss ways to encourage children to eat more fruits and vegetables and to drink more milk and less carbonated beverages.
- Discuss the amount of recommended calories infants and children need to maintain optimal nutrition. Plan a daily menu and calculate the calories to obtain the recommended amount of calories.

SUGGESTIONS FOR CLINICAL ACTIVITIES

- Arrange for students to spend a day with a Lactation Consultant to observe breastfeeding and discuss breastfeeding problems.
- Have students teach parents about well-balanced nutrition and dental care when in the clinical setting.

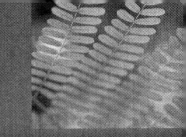

CHAPTER 13
ADAPTING PROCEDURES IN THE CARE OF CHILDREN

RESOURCE LIBRARY

 CD-ROM

Child physical assessment
Blood pressure
Health care teaching aids

Gavage tube
Tracheostomy

📖 IMAGE LIBRARY

Figure 13-1 A family-centered care policy permits parents to be present during a procedure performed on their child.

Figure 13-2 Position for inserting thermometer when tympanic route is used.

Figure 13-3 Measuring oral temperature.

Figure 13-4 (A) Thermometers within pacifiers may be used by some parents. (B) A chemically treated tape can provide temperature readings when pressed firmly against a clean, dry forehead.

Figure 13-5 Measuring the axillary temperature.

Figure 13-6 Taking a rectal temperature reading from an infant.

Figure 13-7 The sites used to assess pulses in children.

Figure 13-8 Assessing the apical heart rate.

Figure 13-9 Place the fingerpads firmly over each point to evaluate the pulsation.

Figure 13-10 Blood pressure cuffs are available in various types and sizes for pediatric clients.

Figure 13-11 With the cuff snugly wrapped around the arm, hold the arm with the cubital fossa at the level of the heart and place the stethoscope against the artery with the dominant hand.

Figure 13-12 Wong-Baker Pain Rating Scale for children 3 to 7 years.

Figure 13-13 Measure an infant's length carefully from the crown of the head to the heel.

Figure 13-14 Standing height measurements are taken routinely at each well-child visit to assess the child's rate of growth.

Figure 13-15 Measure chest circumference with the tape flat and at an even distance under the axillae.

Figure 13-16 To restrain an uncooperative child, place the child supine on the examining table.

Figure 13-17 Child on a papoose restraint board.

Figure 13-18 Making a mummy restraint.

Figure 13-19 Infant with elbow restraints.

Figure 13-20 Vacutainer® is used in collecting blood specimens.

Figure 13-21 Venipuncture procedure.

Figure 13-22 (A) Attaching the urine collection bag. (B) Urine cup.

Figure 13-23 Equipment for a stool specimen. In the case of an infant or toddler, the specimen could be collected from a soiled diaper.

Figure 13-24 A long cotton-tipped applicator can be used as a throat swab or wound swab.

Figure 13-25 Child supplying a sputum specimen.

Figure 13-26 (A) Infant positioned for a lumbar puncture. (B) Child positioned for a lumbar puncture.

Figure 13-27 Measuring for nasogastric tube placement.

Figure 13-28 Nasogastric tube taped securely in place.

Figure 13-29 Gravity assists the flow of a gavage feeding to this hospitalized infant.

Figure 13-30 Enema equipment, suppositories, and laxatives.

Figure 13-31 (A) Insertion of a deflated tube bulb syringe. (B) Removal of a reinflated bulb syringe.

Figure 13-32 Tracheostomy tube suctioning.

Figure 13-33 (A) Simple face mask. (B) Nasal cannula. (C) Oxygen tent.

Figure 13-34 (A) Pulse oximeter on finger. (B) Pulse oximeter on infant's foot.

Figure 13-35 (A) Peak expiratory flow rate (PERF) meter. (B) Child using PEFR meter.

Figure 13-36 (A) Estimating the size of an oropharyngeal airway. (B) Estimating the size of a nasopharyngeal airway.

Figure 13-37 Administering an ophthalmic medication.

Figure 13-38 Administering an otic medication.

Figure 13-39 The suppository is inserted gently just past the internal sphincter (about 1 in. or 2.5 cm in children; about 1/2 in. or 1.25 cm in infants).

Figure 13-40 Intramuscular injection sites.

Figure 13-41 The child is restrained by staff while an injection is being administered.

Figure 13-42 Buretrol device.

Figure 13-43 This intravenous site on a hand has been placed on an armboard, securely wrapped, and covered with part of a plastic cup to prevent the child from disrupting the line.

LEARNING OUTCOME 1

Define key terms.

CONCEPTS FOR LECTURE

1. Parents participate in the health care of the child in family-centered care.
2. Assessment is a collection of data and interpretation of the findings to make a decision regarding nursing care of the client.
3. Obtaining vital signs includes temperature, pulse, respirations, and blood pressure. Point of maximal impulse is the site where the heart rate can be best heard.
4. A Vacutainer is hollow, plastic device used to collect blood specimens from veins.
5. When administering gastric feedings, the residual amount or amount remaining in the stomach from last feeding needs to be measured prior to administering a feeding.

POWERPOINT LECTURE SLIDES

(NOTE: The number on each PPT Lecture Slide directly corresponds with the Concepts for Lecture.)

1 Family-Centered Care
  - Parental participation in care
  - Parents provide security and comfort

1a Family-Centered Care (Figure 13-1)

2 Assessment
  - Collection of data
  - Interpretation of findings
  - Decisions regarding care

3 Vital Signs
  - Temperature, pulse, respirations
  - Blood pressure
  - Point of maximal impulse

4 Vacutainer (Figure 13-20)

5 Residual volume
  - Amount of feeding remaining in stomach
  - Check prior to administering tube feeding

SUGGESTIONS FOR CLASSROOM ACTIVITIES

- Develop a word search puzzle. List definitions under word search puzzle and have students figure out the word that matches the definition and find the words in the puzzle.

SUGGESTIONS FOR CLINICAL ACTIVITIES

- None

LEARNING OUTCOME 2

Describe why procedures need to be adapted in the care of children.

CONCEPTS FOR LECTURE

1. Most procedures are the same for children as for adults but modifications or adaptations must be adapted to the size, age, and developmental level of the child.

   To increase cooperation, small children are given limited information about the procedure directly before performing the procedure, whereas parents are informed about procedures ahead of time.
2. Older children and adolescents will cooperate better if they are informed about a procedure ahead of time and given an explanation of the purpose of the procedure.

POWERPOINT LECTURE SLIDES

(NOTE: The number on each PPT Lecture Slide directly corresponds with the Concepts for Lecture.)

1 Procedures Adapted in Care of Children
  - Infants and Young Children
    ○ Parents need to be informed
    ○ Simple explanations defining rationale
    ○ Outline steps of procedure
    ○ Describe how parent can assist
    ○ Allow child to touch or play with equipment

3 Procedures Adapted in Care of Children
  - Older children
    ○ Simple explanation of procedure
    ○ Explain immediately before procedure
    ○ Allow opportunity to ask questions
    ○ Allow to discuss fears
    ○ Sign consent form with parents

LEARNING OUTCOME 3

Identify specific adaptations for selected procedures in the care of children.

CONCEPTS FOR LECTURE

1. Children will often feel safer if the nurse makes a self-introduction to the parent first, and then introduce themselves to the child.

2. Organize assessment to perform least comfortable or most invasive procedures last. Appropriate teaching and emotional support helps to alleviate fear of procedures. While child is quiet, obtain pulse and respirations before beginning body systems assessment.

3. Pain is subjective, but children are not able to verbalize pain. Physiological responses and other indicators such as restlessness, facial grimacing, and crying are used to assess pain in children.

4. Growth measurements are plotted on standardized growth charts. Protect child's privacy and modesty when obtaining measurements.

5. Restraints should be used to ensure safety of the child during procedures. Use restraints as the last resort after other methods of protecting child have failed. Use the least restrictive type of restraint for shortest period of time possible.

6. Specimen collection may be a challenge to complete. Age-specific instruction is essential. Assistance from parents or coworkers may be obtained.

7. The nurse may need to be present at meals to encourage intake. Offering choices reinforces independence and protects dignity. Forcing child to eat may result in aspiration from crying or struggling.

8. Age-specific instructions are essential when administering a suppository or enema. A second nurse may be needed to restrain the child to ensure child's safety during the procedure.

9. Maintaining a patent airway is the nurse's highest priority in client care. High levels of oxygen over prolonged time can cause retinal damage and lung disorders. Aspiration is avoided by proper positioning and feeding methods.

10. The pharmacokinetics of drug administration differ from adults due to immature body systems; therefore, adverse effects and allergic reactions may be more severe.

11. All medication dosages and calculations must be checked for accuracy. Use appropriate size syringes and needles.

POWERPOINT LECTURE SLIDES

(NOTE: The number on each PPT Lecture Slide directly corresponds with the Concepts for Lecture.)

1 Common Procedure Steps
- Check physician's order
- Gather equipment
- Introduce self to child and family
- Identify client by identification band

1a Common Procedure Steps
- Explain procedure
- Obtain consent, if necessary
- Provide privacy
- Wash hands
- Don gloves according to standard precautions

2 Obtaining Vital Signs
- Temperature
  - Axillary, rectal, oral
  - Use electronic or tympanic thermometer, or chemical tapes
  - Normal temperature ranges are same as for adult

2a Obtaining Vital Signs
- Pulse
  - Accurate pulses may be difficult to obtain
    - Radial, carotid, popliteal, pedal pulses
  - Take apical pulse for one minute
  - Adult range reached by age 16 years

2b Apical pulse (Figure 13-2)

2c Obtaining Vital Signs
- Respirations
  - Observe abdomen for diaphragmatic respirations
  - Report respirations greater than 60
  - Adult ranges reached by 16 years

2d Obtaining Vital Signs
- Blood pressure
  - Cuff should cover 2/3 upper arm, thigh, calf
  - Too large cuff gives false low
  - Too small cuff gives false high
  - Adult ranges reached by age 16 years

2e Blood pressure (Figure 13-11)

The nurse must be vigilant in assessing intravenous rates, condition of intravenous sites, and systemic effects of intravenous infusion.

3 Pain
- Physiological responses to pain
  - Tachycardia, tachypnea, pupil dilation, pallor
- Indicators of pain
  - Restlessness, short attention span, sleep disturbance
  - Facial grimacing, crying, posturing, anorexia

3a Pain (Figure 13-12)

4 Growth Measurements
- Height
- Weight
- Body Mass Index
  - Ages 2 through adolescence

4a Growth Measurements (Figure 13-14)

4b Growth Measurements
- Head circumference
  - Under 36 months or neurological defect
  - Largest diameter of infant's head
  - Equal to or 2 cm > chest until 2 years
- Chest circumference
- Abdominal girth

5 Restraining Child
- Consider age, size, condition of child
- Obtain physician's order
- Use least restrictive type for shortest time period
- Avoid requiring parents to restrain
- Monitor skin integrity
- Assess neurologic intactness

5a Restraining Child (Figure 13-16)

6 Specimen Collection
- Age-specific instruction
- Assistance from parents or co-workers
- Cleanse puncture sites with alcohol or povidine-iodine
- Apply bandage after completing puncture procedure
- Use 3 cleansing swabs prior to urinary collection
- Talk quietly and gently to child during procedures

7 Nutrition
- Encourage and assist with intake
- Cut food in bite-sized pieces
- Risk of aspiration if force feedings
- Offer choices and favorite foods
- Limit distractions
- Use praise for eating

Nutrition
- Tube feedings
  - Check placement prior to feeding
  - Check residual volume prior to feeding
  - Position in Fowler's or high Fowler's position
  - Administer liquids at room temperature
  - If residual volume is ≥ feeding per hour, stop feeding
  - If volume remains high, notify primary care provider.

 Tube feedings (Figure 13-27)

8 Elimination
- Promote diet adequate in fiber and fluids
- Age-specific instructions
- Assistance may be needed to restrain child
- Avoid raising enema container higher than 12 to 18 inches
- Choose smallest size catheter for indwelling catheter

9 Respiratory
- Maintain patent airway
- Bulb suction infant's mouth, then nose
- Preoxygenate prior to suctioning
- Apply suction 5–10 seconds
- Use pulse oximeter to monitor oxygen
- Use apnea monitor to measure breathing patterns

 Oxygen Administration (Figure 13-33)

10 Medication Administration
- Monitor adverse effects and allergic reactions
- Measure and calculate drugs accurately
- Mix oral medications with food
- Do not leave medications at bedside

 Medication Administration
- Administer liquid medications with syringe or dropper
- Administer IM medication into vastus lateralis in infant through 3 years
- Use appropriate size needle and syringe

 Medication Administration (Figure 13-39)

 Medication Administration (Figure 13-40)

11 Intravenous Infusion
- Ensure proper dilution of medication
- Assess rate of infusion
- Assess condition of intravenous site
- Monitor for systemic effects
- Lock infusion pumps

 Intravenous Infusion (Figure 13-43)

SUGGESTIONS FOR CLASSROOM ACTIVITIES	SUGGESTIONS FOR CLINICAL ACTIVITIES
• Compare vital signs ranges for age groups. See Table 13-2. • Have students practice drug calculations and temperature conversions. See Boxes 13-2, 13-3.	• Have students perform procedures on a pediatric unit, including vital signs, pain assessment, growth measurements, specimen collection, feeding, suctioning, and intravenous infusions. • Assign students to administer medications to children. Have students calculate drug dosages and intravenous rate infusions.

LEARNING OUTCOME 4

Discuss the role of the LPN/LVN in adapting procedures in the care of children.

CONCEPTS FOR LECTURE

1. Scope of practice varies between states and facilities, LPN/LVNs must follow the State Board of Nursing Rules and facility policies of where they practice. Common sense, coupled with nursing judgment, should guide decisions when adjustment to procedures is needed.
2. The nurse's primary responsibility during procedures is the child's safety. Safety includes performing procedures correctly, restraining the child when necessary, and observing child's well-being following the procedure.
3. Correct documentation includes date and time procedure was performed, objective information about the procedure, results of the procedure, condition of the child following the procedure, and any further nursing measures related to the procedure.
4. Provide support to parents and child through providing information, allowing verbalization of feelings, maintaining consistency of care, giving choices when possible, and providing a calm environment.

POWERPOINT LECTURE SLIDES

(NOTE: The number on each PPT Lecture Slide directly corresponds with the Concepts for Lecture.)

 Role of LPN/LVN in Adapting Procedures
 • Scope of practice varies between states and facilities
 • Safety is primary responsibility
 • Correct documentation
 • Provide support to parents and child
 • Display caring behaviors
 • Teach factual information

SUGGESTIONS FOR CLASSROOM ACTIVITIES	SUGGESTIONS FOR CLINICAL ACTIVITIES
• Have students view the Web site for the State Board of Nursing to read the Scope of Practice for LPN/LVNs. • Have students research where to find factual information for parents. Look at facility resources, professional pamphlets, and legitimate Web sites.	• Have students find a specific policy and procedure in the policy and procedure manual of the health care facility where they have clinical practice. • Have students practice documentation of procedures. Assist them with the actual documentation of procedures on client charts. • In postconference, discuss safety issues they noted throughout the day in the clinical setting.

CHAPTER 14
CARE OF THE HOSPITALIZED OR CHRONICALLY ILL CHILD

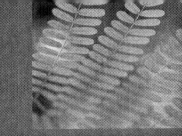

RESOURCE LIBRARY

 CD-ROM

Client pain assessment

Tracheostomy

📖 IMAGE LIBRARY

Figure 14-1 Portion of a pediatric admission form showing developmental level and habits of children.

Figure 14-2 Children and their families need to be actively involved in decisions about care when appropriate.

Figure 14-3 A child specialist works with children being treated for cancer.

Figure 14-4 Role-playing is one type of therapeutic play.

Figure 14-5 This child has brought a favorite toy from home to make the hospital environment feel more secure and familiar.

Figure 14-6 This child is old enough to understand the need to take glucose tablets or another form of rapidly absorbed sugar when her blood glucose level is low.

Figure 14-7 The nurse can use a simple gender-specific drawing of a child's body to encourage children to draw what they think about their medical problems.

Figure 14-8 A hard bubble-top crib protects a climbing child from injury.

Figure 14-9 (A) Infants and toddlers are transferred in high-topped cribs. (B) This child, who is getting tube feedings or other infusions during the day, can be easily and safely transported in a wheelchair equipped with a safety harness.

Figure 14-10 When painful procedures are planned, use EMLA cream to anesthetize the skin where the painful stick will be made.

Figure 14-11 The older child is able to regulate a PCA pump.

Figure 14-12 The incentive spirometer is an excellent method of promoting lung expansion in school-age and older children.

Figure 14-13 Play areas can give the child a welcome diversion from the hospital room.

Figure 14-14 It important that the hospitalized child does not fall behind in schoolwork.

Figure 14-15 The presence of the parent is an important part of pain management.

Figure 14-16 (A) It is often desirable from a family and cost perspective to provide health care in the home, and advances in technology have made this possible. (B) Daily caregiving demands of the child who is medically fragile continue 24 hours a day, 7 days a week.

Figure 14-17 This child requires use of a nebulizer during school hours.

Figure 14-18 (A) Rehabilitation units provide an opportunity for the child to relearn such tasks as walking and climbing stairs. They provide an important transition from hospital to home and community. (B) The nurse can help the child and family accept and adjust to new circumstances.

Figure 14-19 Shriner's Hospital in Spokane, Washington, has a special room and teachers for children undergoing lengthy hospital stays, enabling them to remain current with their schoolwork.

LEARNING OUTCOME 1

Define key terms.

CONCEPTS FOR LECTURE

1. Illness is a state of disease or sickness that may be physical or psychological.
2. Illness is characterized as acute (rapid onset, severe symptoms, short course), chronic (long-lasting, slowly progressing), or terminal (final, fatal).

POWERPOINT LECTURE SLIDES

(NOTE: The number on each PPT Lecture Slide directly corresponds with the Concepts for Lecture.)

1 Illness
- State of disease or sickness
- Physical or psychological

2 Illness Characteristics
- Acute
  - Having rapid onset, severe symptoms, short course

3. Therapeutic play is play that allows the individual to deal with fears associated with the health care experience.
4. A child life specialist is a trained professional who plans therapeutic activities for the hospitalized child.
5. Separation anxiety is apprehension due to parents or personal items not being present in the child's environment. The three stages of separation anxiety are: protest, despair, and detachment.
6. Client-controlled analgesia (PCA) is a device, attached to an intravenous line, which allows the client to release pain medication as needed.
7. Conscious sedation is the administration of intravenous medication to produce an impaired level of consciousness to safely perform therapeutic or diagnostic procedures outside the operating room.
8. Deep sedation is a controlled state of depressed consciousness or unconsciousness in which the child is unable to maintain protective reflexes. It is used during surgical procedures and is administered and maintained by an anesthesiologist and nurse anesthetist.
9. A chronically ill child may have a hereditary condition, which is a genetic inheritance from a parent or both parents, or may have a congenital condition, which is a condition present from birth that results in a chronic disorder.
10. An individualized education plan is an interdisciplinary plan that pinpoints the special needs of a client with a chronic condition and establishes a plan for meeting the client's needs.

- Chronic
  - Long-lasting, slowly progressing
- Terminal
  - Final, fatal

3 Therapeutic play
- Allows the individual to deal with fears
- Fears associated with health care experiences

4 Child Life Specialist
- Trained professional
- Plans therapeutic activities for hospitalized child

4a Child Life Specialist (Figure 14-3)

5 Separation Anxiety
- Apprehension due to parents not present
- Three stages:
  - Protest
  - Despair
  - Detachment

6 Client-Controlled Analgesia Pump
- Attached to intravenous line
- Allows release of pain medication as needed
- For short-term treatment after surgery
- Programmed to deliver medication at intervals
- Has "lock-out interval" to prevent overdose

6a Client-Controlled Analgesia Pump (Figure 14-10)

7 Conscious sedation
- Administration of intravenous medication
- Produces impaired level of consciousness
- Used outside operating room
- To perform therapeutic or diagnostic procedures
- Administered by skilled registered nurse

8 Deep Sedation
- Controlled state of depressed consciousness
- Controlled state of unconsciousness
- Unable to maintain protective reflexes
- Used for surgical procedures
- Administered and maintained by anesthesiologist/nurse anesthetist

9 Chronically Ill Child
- Hereditary Condition
  - Genetic inheritance
  - From one or both parents
- Congenital condition
  - Condition present at birth
  - Results in chronic disorder

10 Individualized Education Plan
- Interdisciplinary plan for meeting needs
- Special education needs
- Specialized services
- Specialized medical needs
- Transport needs

LEARNING OUTCOME 2

Describe how to prepare children for hospitalization.

CONCEPTS FOR LECTURE

1. The age of the child, reason for hospitalization, length of hospitalization and past experiences determine the method and amount of preparation needed for preparing the child for hospitalization.

   The needs of the individual child and family must be assessed to develop an interdisciplinary plan of care.

   The child's limited understanding of what is happening to the child produces anxiety over hospitalization, diagnostic, and therapeutic procedures.

   It is important for the nurse to help relieve stress by providing age-specific preparation for hospitalization and every procedure the child will experience.

POWERPOINT LECTURE SLIDES

(NOTE: The number on each PPT Lecture Slide directly corresponds with the Concepts for Lecture.)

1 Preparing Child for Hospitalization
- Infant
  - Parents and sibling need instruction
  - Reassurance is provided
  - Comfort infant after procedure
  - Family or hospital personnel in attendance

1a Preparing the Child for Hospitalization
- Infant
  - Separation anxiety
    - Stages of separation
  - Parental involvement to promote security
  - Honest communication to develop trust
  - Requires supervision unless sleeping

1b Preparing the Child for Hospitalization
- Toddler
  - Identifies body parts for pain
  - Uses magical thinking
  - Give brief instruction prior to procedure
  - Tell child if procedure is painful
  - Separation anxiety present
  - Requires supervision unless sleeping

1c Preparing Child for Hospitalization
- Preschooler
  - Follow rituals and routine practices
  - Need reassurance illness is not their fault
  - Frightened by new people and experiences
  - Encourage parents to participate in care
  - Parents reinforce instructions provided by nurse
  - Have familiar objects for security

1d Preparing Child for Hospitalization (Figure 14-5)

1e Preparing Child for Hospitalization
- School-Age
  - Can participate in care and treatment
  - Understand written and verbal instructions

○ Need parent support
○ Brings favorite item from home for comfort
○ Participate in variety of activities
○ Can be left alone for brief periods

1f Preparing Child for Hospitalization (Figure 14-7)

1g Preparing Child for Hospitalization
- Adolescent
  ○ Active participant in care
  ○ Reassure modesty and provide privacy
  ○ Understands instructions
  ○ Encourage questions
  ○ Encourage visits from friends

1h Admission Process
- Use variety of resources to prepare child
  ○ Books
  ○ Drawings
- Orient to hospital environment and routines
- Complete and document assessment
- Determine problems and develop care plan

1i Admission Process (Figure 14-1)

1j Preparation for Procedures
- Provide instruction
- Obtain informed consent
- Administer medications
- Assess health status and document care
- Use therapeutic play
- Transfer safely in hospital

1k Preparation for Procedures (Figure 14-9)

Suggestions for Classroom Activities

- Show a video in class on preparing a child for hospitalization.
- Explain to students the importance of maintaining confidentiality with any client they observe in the health care setting. Discuss any situations in which confidentiality cannot be guaranteed.
- Present case studies on hospitalized children to the class and have them critically think about the appropriate interventions for the children, considering safety issues, medication administration, therapeutic play, teaching needs, and anxieties and fears.

Suggestions for Clinical Activities

- Assign children of various ages with different disease processes to the students in the acute care setting each week. Have them develop a care plan or concept map each week on one of the children.
- Have students discuss how they used therapeutic play to interact with children being hospitalized.

LEARNING OUTCOME 3

Describe how to prepare parents for their child's hospitalization.

CONCEPTS FOR LECTURE

1. The nurse must determine the amount and quality of preparation the child and family have received when the child is hospitalized.

   The nurse needs to establish a positive relationship with the child and family, answer questions, and reduce fear and anxiety.

POWERPOINT LECTURE SLIDES

(NOTE: The number on each PPT Lecture Slide directly corresponds with the Concepts for Lecture.)

1. Parental Preparation for Child's Hospitalization
   - Establish a positive relationship
   - Answer questions
   - Provide emotional support
   - Orient to hospital environment

SUGGESTIONS FOR CLASSROOM ACTIVITIES

- Discuss ways to prepare parents for a child's hospitalization.
- Have students develop a teaching sheet for parents to answer questions to prepare for a child's hospitalization.

SUGGESTIONS FOR CLINICAL ACTIVITIES

- Have students use their teaching sheet when interacting with parents of children being hospitalized.
- Have students research books and resources about child's surgery for parents. Have them develop a list of this information and deliver it to admissions offices or primary care provider's offices for use in teaching parents how to prepare their children for hospitalization.

LEARNING OUTCOME 4

Describe the preoperative and postoperative care of children.

CONCEPTS FOR LECTURE

1. The LPN/LVN provides input into the individualized care plan for the preoperative and postoperative care of the child.

   The physical and psychological preparation of the child before and after surgery is similar to the care of the adult.

   The LPN/LVN assists the registered nurse in the implementation and evaluation of preoperative and postoperative nursing care of the child.

POWERPOINT LECTURE SLIDES

(NOTE: The number on each PPT Lecture Slide directly corresponds with the Concepts for Lecture.)

1. Preoperative Care of Children
   - Prepare psychologically to relieve fear
   - Introduce to key personnel
   - Show surgical attire
   - Allow therapeutic play with dolls and equipment
   - Sign informed consent

1a. Preoperative Care of Children (Figure 14-4)

1b. Preoperative Care of Children
   - Maintain nothing by mouth
   - Empty bladder
   - Initiate intravenous infusion
   - Administer preoperative medications
   - Use local or topical anesthetics
   - Instruct in client-controlled analgesia device

1c. Preoperative Care of Children (Figure 14-11)

1d. Postoperative Care of Children
   - Recovery room
     - Maintain airway
     - Assess level of consciousness
     - Record vital signs
     - Assess dressings and drainage tubes
     - Monitor intravenous fluids, pain

1e Postoperative Care of Children
- Client room
  - ◦ Routine postoperative care
  - ◦ Teach postoperative exercises
  - ◦ Teach use of incentive spirometer

1f Care of Child Undergoing Conscious Sedation
- Maintain patent airway
- Maintain protective reflexes
- Maintain response to physical and verbal stimuli
- One-to-one observation until stable vital signs
- Parents instructed in discharge instructions

SUGGESTIONS FOR CLASSROOM ACTIVITIES

- Show a video in class on the preoperative and postoperative care of children.
- Review information needed to complete a preoperative informed consent. Refer to Table 14-3.
- Review the medications used for conscious sedation, especially adverse effects and nursing considerations for administration. Refer to Table 14-4.
- Review postoperative nursing care of a child. Refer to Box 14-2.

SUGGESTIONS FOR CLINICAL ACTIVITIES

- Arrange for students to observe children's procedures performed in an ambulatory surgery center or outpatient care center. Have them observe conscious sedation being administered. Discuss the nursing care provided before and after the procedure.
- Arrange for a student to follow a child into surgery and to the recovery room after surgery. Have the student write a paper on their observations, including the duties of the surgical nurse, circulating nurse, and recovery room nurse.

LEARNING OUTCOME 5

Describe how to prepare parents and children for discharge.

CONCEPTS FOR LECTURE

1. The LPN/LVN assists the registered nurse to prepare the parents and children for discharge.

POWERPOINT LECTURE SLIDES

(NOTE: The number on each PPT Lecture Slide directly corresponds with the Concepts for Lecture.)

 1 Preparation for Discharge
- Assist with discharge teaching
- Answer questions
- Demonstrate proper techniques of care
- Make follow-up and referral telephone calls
- Complete documentation

SUGGESTIONS FOR CLASSROOM ACTIVITIES

- Arrange for students to attend an interdisciplinary discharge planning meeting.

SUGGESTIONS FOR CLINICAL ACTIVITIES

- Have students provide an in-service for the nursing staff and families on preparing for discharge.
- Assist a nurse with discharge teaching and documentation of the teaching.

LEARNING OUTCOME 6

Describe important aspects of care for the chronically ill child and the family.

CONCEPTS FOR LECTURE

1. Chronically ill children may have a disorder caused by a hereditary condition or a congenital condition.

   Some chronically ill children are able to use adaptive equipment that allows them to lead a relatively normal life.

   Parents need direction and support from nurses to learn how to care for the chronically ill child at home.

POWERPOINT LECTURE SLIDES

(NOTE: The number on each PPT Lecture Slide directly corresponds with the Concepts for Lecture.)

[1] Chronically Ill Child
- Hereditary condition
- Congenital condition
- Use of adaptive equipment
- Give parents direction and support

SUGGESTIONS FOR CLASSROOM ACTIVITIES

- Have students identify chronic illnesses caused by hereditary conditions versus chronic illnesses caused by congenital conditions. Discuss the differences in care administered in these conditions.
- Have students research types of adaptive equipment used for chronically ill children.

SUGGESTIONS FOR CLINICAL ACTIVITIES

- Arrange for students to visit a health care supply company to see types of adaptive equipment used by chronically ill clients. Arrange for a demonstration of how to use the equipment.

LEARNING OUTCOME 7

Describe the role of the LPN/LVN in caring for children with acute or chronic disorders.

CONCEPTS FOR LECTURE

1. The role of the LPN/LVN is to assist in the care of the child with an acute or chronic disorder in a physician's office or clinic, a school system, and an acute care setting.

   The nurse can use therapeutic play to help children deal with the fears associated with the health care experience and to encourage health promotion activities.

   The nurse provides verbal and written explanations about plans for discharge.

POWERPOINT LECTURE SLIDES

(NOTE: The number on each PPT Lecture Slide directly corresponds with the Concepts for Lecture.)

[1] Role of the LPN/LVN in the Office or Clinic
- Assist in care of the child
- Collects data about child and family
- Assists with diagnostic procedures
- Provides instruction for home care
- Provides instruction for hospitalization

[1a] Role of the LNPN/LVN in the School
- Assist with health screenings
- Administers prescribed medications
- Cares for ill child until parents arrive
- Provides health teaching in classroom

[1b] Role of LPN/LVN in the Hospital
- Provides care by assisting with ADLs
- Administers medications
- Collects data for admission
- Helps child through therapeutic play
- Reinforces rehabilitation therapies
- Encourages health promotion activities

[1c] Role of LPN/LVN in the Hospital (Figure 14-1)

[1d] Role of LPN/LVN in the Hospital
- Provide age-appropriate instructions to child
- Provides written and verbal instructions for discharge
- Involve family in care of child
- Creative to prevent isolation of deaf child
- Have adequate resources to meet needs of children

LEARNING OUTCOME 8

Discuss how to care for children in the home or in long-term care settings.

CONCEPTS FOR LECTURE

1. The chronically ill or disabled child may require care at home, at school, in a rehabilitation center, or in a long-term care facility. Nurses in these areas must be prepared to meet the child's physical and developmental needs.

   Teaching must be provided to the child, parents, and members of the community who will be responsible for aspects of care.

   Caregivers need support to prevent fatigue and burnout.

POWERPOINT LECTURE SLIDES

(NOTE: The number on each PPT Lecture Slide directly corresponds with the Concepts for Lecture.)

1 Care for Chronically Ill Children
- Care at home
  ◦ Special equipment
  ◦ House accommodations
  ◦ 24-hour care or supervision
  ◦ Caregiver support
  ◦ Therapeutic communication
  ◦ Resources available

1a Care for Chronically Ill Children (Figure 14-16)

1b Care for Chronically Ill Children
- Care at school
  ◦ Teach school personnel to care for child
  ◦ Transport responsibility
  ◦ Infection control
  ◦ Individualized education plan
  ◦ Altered classrooms
  ◦ Health-related data collection

1c Care for Chronically Ill Children (Figure 14-17)

1d Care for Chronically Ill Children
- Rehabilitation
  ◦ Plan and implement physical care
  ◦ Meet growth and development needs

1e Care for Chronically Ill Children (Figure 14-18)

1f Care for Chronically Ill Children
- Long-term care
  ◦ Extensive physical and mental disabilities
  ◦ Emotional and financial drain on family
  ◦ Age-specific activities
  ◦ Education specific to disabled child
  ◦ Consistent approach to care
  ◦ Supervision of unlicensed personnel

1g Care of the Caregiver
- Address caregiver role strain
- Explore feelings of family members
- Develop plan to prevent burnout
- Obtain respite support system
- Referrals to resources as needed

SUGGESTIONS FOR CLASSROOM ACTIVITIES

- Have a rehabilitation nurse give a talk about the responsibilities of caring for a chronically ill child.
- Arrange for a chronically ill child and caregiver to visit the classroom to talk about experiences in caring for the child.
- Have students explore what resources are available for children and families in the community where they live.

SUGGESTIONS FOR CLINICAL ACTIVITIES

- Arrange for students to observe an alternative classroom in a school to see how chronically ill children are mainstreamed into the school setting. Have them discuss how the children are cared for and discuss their feelings about the experience.
- Arrange for students to visit a rehabilitation center or a rehabilitation unit in a health care setting to observe therapy sessions. Have them share their observations with the clinical groups.

CHAPTER 15
CARE OF THE CHILD WITH FLUID, ELECTROLYTE, AND ACID-BASE DISORDERS

RESOURCE LIBRARY

CD-ROM

Fluid
Hyperkalemia
Evaluate deep tendon reflex

COMPANION WEBSITE

Asphyxiation as a game

IMAGE LIBRARY

Figure 15-1 Percentage of water by body weight changes dramatically from 75% in infants to about 50% to 55% in adults.

Figure 15-2 When fluid is inside the body's arteries, veins, and capillaries (*vasculature*), it is plasma.

Figure 15-3 (A) Osmosis. (B) Diffusion. (C) Filtration is the process by which water and solutes move across capillary membranes driven by fluid pressure. (D) Active transport.

Figure 15-4 The intake–output chart is an important tool for monitoring fluid status.

Figure 15-5 A urine collection device can be placed in the toilet for children who are out of diapers.

Figure 15-6 The body's response to fluid loss involves several body systems.

Figure 15-7 Multisystem effects of fluid volume deficit (FVD).

Figure 15-8 Pediatric access sites are more difficult to use because of the small size of the veins.

Figure 15-9 If isotonic fluid containing sodium is given too rapidly or in too large an amount, an extracellular fluid volume excess will develop.

Figure 15-10 Multisystem effects of hypokalemia.

Figure 15-11 The child with hypocalcemia may exhibit increased deep tendon reflexes.

Figure 15-12 The normal ratio of bicarbonate to carbonic acid is 20:1.

Figure 15-13 Buffer response to acid-base.

Figure 15-14 Positioning to facilitate chest expansion.

Figure 15-15 Teaching parents to use safety latches on cabinets to keep aspirin away from small children can prevent one cause of metabolic acidosis.

LEARNING OUTCOME 1

Discuss fluid and electrolyte balance in children.

CONCEPTS FOR LECTURE

1. Children have a high percentage of water; therefore, fluid and electrolyte imbalances are much more dangerous in pediatric clients than in adults.
2. Homeostasis is achieved by balance of fluid and electrolytes, as well as fluid intake, hormonal regulation, and fluid output.
3. Body fluids are in two distinct compartments: intracellular and extracellular. The extracellular compartment includes plasma and interstitial fluid.
4. Body fluids contain solutes. A solute is a substance dissolved in a fluid or a solvent. A solution is formed when one or more solutes are dissolved in a solvent.
5. Fluids and electrolytes move across cell membranes by one of four methods: osmosis, diffusion, filtration, and active transport.

POWERPOINT LECTURE SLIDES

(NOTE: The number on each PPT Lecture Slide directly corresponds with the Concepts for Lecture.)

1 Fluid and Electrolyte Balance
- Percent of water varies with age
  - Newborn—75% body weight is water
  - Infant—60% body weight is water
  - Child—50% body weight is water
  - Adult—50-55% body weight is water

2 Principles Related to Fluid and Electrolytes
- Homeostasis
  - Balance of fluid and electrolytes
  - Balance of acids and bases
  - Fluid intake regulated by thirst
  - Hormones
  - Fluid output to rid excess fluid

6. Electrolytes are solutes within the body fluid. Cations are positively charged electrolytes, such as potassium (K^+), sodium (Na^+), and calcium (Ca^+). Anions are negatively charged electrolytes, such as chloride (Cl^-), bicarbonate (HCO_3^-), and sulfate (SO_4^-).

3 Body Fluids
- Intracellular
- Extracellular
  - Plasma
- Interstitial
- Solution
  - Solute dissolved in solvent

4 Body Fluids (Figure 15-2)

5 Movement of Body Fluids (Figure 15-3)

6 Electrolytes
- Solutes within body fluid
- Cations
  - Positive charged electrolytes
- Anions
  - Negative charged electrolytes

SUGGESTIONS FOR CLASSROOM ACTIVITIES

- Review key terms with students. Develop a quiz with key terms in left column and definitions in right column. Have students match terms with definitions.

SUGGESTIONS FOR CLINICAL ACTIVITIES

- None
- Have students list their assigned client's electrolytes and point out whether the results are "high" or "low." Have students explain why the client may have these results in relation to their diagnosis.

LEARNING OUTCOME 2

Discuss acid-base balance in children.

CONCEPTS FOR LECTURE

1. Homeostasis applies to the balance of hydrogen ion concentration within the body.

   Acidosis develops when there is an increase of hydrogen ion concentration.

   Alkalosis develops when there is a decrease of hydrogen ion concentration.
2. Three body mechanisms that compensate for abnormal pH levels leading to acidosis or alkalosis are the buffer system, the respiratory system, and the renal system.
3. Arterial blood gas (ABG) analysis determines functioning of the respiratory system to detect acid-base imbalances. The ABG analyzes pH, $PaCO_2$, and HCO_3 values.
4. The nurse must be able to analyze ABG results accurately by reviewing pH, CO_2, and HCO_3 values.

POWERPOINT LECTURE SLIDES

(NOTE: The number on each PPT Lecture Slide directly corresponds with the Concepts for Lecture.)

1 Acid-Base Balance
- Homeostasis
  - Balance of hydrogen ion concentration
- Acidosis
  - Increase in hydrogen ion concentration < 7.36
- Alkalosis
  - Decrease in hydrogen ion concentration > 7.44

4 Compensation for Abnormal pH
- Buffer System
  - Chemical reactions
- Respiratory system
  - Retain or "blow off" CO_2 in respirations
- Renal system
  - Increase or decrease urine output adjusts hydrogen

4a Compensation for Abnormal pH (Figure 15-13)

5 Arterial Blood Gas Analysis
- Determines functioning of respiratory system
- Detects acid-base imbalances
- Analyzes pH, $PaCO_2$, HCO_3

SUGGESTIONS FOR CLASSROOM ACTIVITIES

- Divide the students into three groups. Assign each group a different buffer system. Have them illustrate the compensation mechanisms that work to return the pH to a normal balance.
- Review how to determine an arterial blood gas analysis in Box 15-5. Have students practice examples of arterial blood gas analysis.

SUGGESTIONS FOR CLINICAL ACTIVITIES

- Have students find arterial blood gas analysis results in client's chart. Have them analyze the results and discuss appropriate treatment.

LEARNING OUTCOME 3

Identify alterations in fluid and electrolyte and acid-base balance in children.

CONCEPTS FOR LECTURE

1. During illnesses, body fluids and electrolytes may become imbalanced through losses or gains of fluid.

   Dehydration can be classified by three types: isotonic, hypotonic, and hypertonic.

2. When the balance of hydrogen ion concentration within the body becomes disturbed, acidosis or alkalosis conditions develop.

POWERPOINT LECTURE SLIDES

(NOTE: The number on each PPT Lecture Slide directly corresponds with the Concepts for Lecture.)

1 Alterations in Fluid and Electrolyte Balance
- Fluid volume deficit (dehydration)
  - Deficient fluid volume
  - Sodium imbalance
  - Three types
    - Isotonic, hypotonic, hypertonic

2 Alterations in Fluid and Electrolyte Balance
- Fluid volume excess (hypervolemia)
  - Overload of fluid
  - Low protein intake
  - High sodium intake

2a Alterations in Fluid and Electrolyte Balance
- Sodium imbalance
  - Hyponatremia
    - Excessive water intake
    - Excessive sodium loss

2b Alterations in Fluid and Electrolyte Balance
- Sodium imbalance
  - Hypernatremia
    - Excessive water loss
    - Excessive sodium intake

2c Alterations in Fluid and Electrolyte Balance
- Potassium imbalance
  - Hypokalemia
    - Increased excretion
    - Decreased intake

2d Alterations in Fluid and Electrolyte Balance
- Potassium imbalance
  - Hyperkalemia
    - Excessive intravenous intake
    - Renal dysfunction and failure
    - Burns, sickle cell anemia, acidosis
    - Blood transfusions, prematurity
    - Severe hypovolemia, lead poisoning

2e Alterations in Fluid and Electrolyte Balance
- Calcium imbalance
  - Hypocalcemia
    - Poor dietary intake

– Lack of vitamin D intake
– Lack of exposure to sunlight
– Surgical removal of parathyroid
– Acute pancreatitis, steatorrhea

 Alterations in Fluid and Electrolyte Balance
- Calcium imbalance
  - Hypercalcemia
    - Hyperparathyroidism
    - Prolonged immobilization
    - Leukemia, bone tumors
    - Excessive calcium intake

 Alterations in Acid-Base Balance
- Respiratory acidosis
  - Hypoventilation, altered perfusion
  - Inadequate respiratory diffusion
  - Airway obstruction, respiratory diseases
  - Central nervous system injuries
  - Anesthesia, narcotics, sedatives

 Alterations in Acid-Base Balance
- Respiratory alkalosis
  - Hyperventilation
  - Anxiety, fear, panic
  - Pain
  - Salicylate poisoning, altitude sickness
  - Meningitis, septicemia, mechanical overventilation

 Alterations in Acid-Base Balance
- Metabolic acidosis (ketoacidosis)
  - Process of metabolism, starvation
  - Loss of bicarbonate through urine
  - Loss of bicarbonate through gastrointestinal fluids
  - Excess ketone bodies, diabetes, renal failure

 Alterations in Acid-Base Balance
- Metabolic alkalosis
  - Vomiting, hypokalemia
  - Nasogastric suction
  - Cystic fibrosis
  - Inappropriate use of diuretics
  - Overdose of antacids, blood transfusions

 Alterations in Acid-Base Balance (Figure 15-15)

SUGGESTIONS FOR CLASSROOM ACTIVITIES

- Develop flash cards of electrolytes and acid-base disorders. Place the name on one side and the cause on the other side.
- Compare types of dehydration and treatment for each type. Refer to Table 15-2.
- Have students bring examples of foods to class and have them identify the electrolytes present in the foods. Show students how to read labels to identify the nutrient content of the food.

SUGGESTIONS FOR CLINICAL ACTIVITIES

- Have students do a 24-hour diet recall on a child. Have them identify the nutrients ingested and the amount of fluid intake. Compare this data with the recommended intake for the child.
- Have students identify clients at risk for fluid and electrolyte imbalance or acid-base balance. Have them provide the rationale for the imbalance

---

LEARNING OUTCOME 4

Describe appropriate assessment and interventions related to fluid and electrolyte and acid-base imbalances.

CONCEPTS FOR LECTURE

1. Careful measuring of intake and output, accurate measurement of the child's weight, and monitoring lab values are essential in identifying fluid and electrolyte imbalances.

   The treatment of dehydration requires rehydration. This may be accomplished with oral or intravenous fluids based on the degree of dehydration.

2. Fluid restriction is a necessary treatment for fluid volume excess. The nurse must take care to explain the fluid restriction in terms the child can understand and to involve parents and child in the plan.

3. Expected outcomes for a child with fluid and electrolyte imbalances are the return of adequate hydration, weight gain or loss, and intact skin.

4. Children experiencing an acid-base imbalance are at risk for ventilation and oxygenation difficulties, neurologic difficulties, and cardiac difficulties.

POWERPOINT LECTURE SLIDES

(NOTE: The number on each PPT Lecture Slide directly corresponds with the Concepts for Lecture.)

1 Fluid Volume Deficit
- Assessment
  - Weight loss
  - Rapid, thready pulse and decreased blood pressure
  - Decreased urinary output, lack of tears
  - Dry mucous membranes, poor skin turgor
  - Impending signs of shock

1a Fluid Volume Deficit
- Diagnosis
  - Increased urine specific gravity
  - Increased blood urea nitrogen and creatinine
  - Elevated hemoglobin and hematocrit
  - Elevated glucose and protein

1b Fluid Volume Deficit
- Treatment
  - Fluid replacement
    - Oral rehydration fluid
    - Intravenous fluid replacement

1c Fluid Volume Deficit (Figure 15-7)

2 Fluid Volume Excess
- Assessment
  - Acute weight gain, edema
  - Pulse fast and bounding
  - Increased blood pressure and respiratory rate
  - Dyspnea, crackles
  - Increased urine output

2a Fluid Volume Excess
- Diagnosis
  - Decreased hematocrit
  - Decreased urine specific gravity
  - Decreased blood urea nitrogen
  - Fluid in lungs on x-ray

2b Fluid Volume Excess
- Treatment
  - Sodium and fluid restriction
  - Diuretic administration
  - Hemodialysis
  - Daily weight
  - Elevate head of bed, oxygen if dyspneic

2c Fluid Volume Excess (Figure 15-9)

3 Sodium Deficit
- Assessment
  - Headaches
  - Lethargy, confusion

- Muscle weakness
- Decreased deep tendon reflexes
- Seizures, coma

 Sodium Deficit
- Diagnosis
  - Decreased sodium levels
  - Decreased urine specific gravity
  - Serum osmolality > 280 mOsm/kg

 Sodium Deficit
- Treatment
  - Fluid restriction
  - Oral sodium supplements
  - Isotonic intravenous solutions
  - Hypertonic intravenous solution
  - Diet high in sodium, diuretics

 Sodium Excess
- Assessment
  - Thirst
  - Restlessness, confusion, stupor
  - Seizures, coma
  - Dry mucous membranes, low grade fever
  - Oliguria, flushed skin

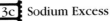 Sodium Excess
- Diagnosis
  - Increased sodium levels
  - Increased or decreased urine specific gravity

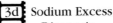 Sodium Excess
- Treatment
  - Oral and intravenous rehydration
  - Low sodium diet
  - Diuretics
  - Oral hygiene and moisturizer
  - Seizure precautions

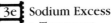 Potassium Deficit
- Assessment
  - Weakness, fatigue
  - Intestinal distention
  - Polyuria
  - Cardiac Irregularities

 Potassium Deficit (Figure 15-10)

 Potassium Deficit
- Diagnosis
  - Decreased potassium levels
  - Symptoms exhibited

 Potassium Deficit
- Treatment
  - Oral or intravenous potassium replacement
  - Increase potassium in diet
  - Avoid life-threatening complications
  - Monitor pulse and respiratory rate and rhythm
  - EKG monitoring, strict intake and output

3j Potassium Excess
- Assessment
  - Anxiety
  - Hypotension, dysrrhythmias
  - Diarrhea
  - Weakness
  - Cardiac arrhythmias leading to cardiac arrest

3k Potassium Excess
- Diagnosis
  - Increased potassium levels
  - Symptoms exhibited

3l Potassium Excess
- Treatment
  - Restrict potassium intake
  - Administer Kayexalate, peritoneal dialysis
  - Intravenous calcium gluconate
  - Insulin, sodium bicarbonate
  - Monitor pulse and respiratory rate and rhythm

3m Calcium Deficit
- Assessment
  - Numbness and tingling in fingers and around mouth
  - Muscle cramps
  - Pathological fractures
  - Increased deep tendon reflexes
  - Congestive heart failure in newborns

3n Calcium Deficit (Figure 15-11)

3o Calcium Deficit
- Diagnosis
  - Decreased calcium levels

3p Calcium Deficit
- Treatment
  - Oral or intravenous calcium
  - Vitamin D supplementation
  - Diet high in calcium
  - Cardiac monitoring
  - Seizure precautions

3q Calcium Excess
- Assessment
  - Decreased muscle tone
  - Nausea, vomiting
  - Decreased level of consciousness
  - Renal calculi
  - Cardiac arrhythmias, cardiac arrest

3r Calcium Excess
- Diagnosis
  - Increased calcium levels

3s Calcium Excess
- Treatment
  - Hydration

  ○ Administer diuretics and glucocorticoids
  ○ Dialysis
  ○ Strain urine for calculi
  ○ Prevent falls due to weakness

4 Respiratory Acidosis
- Assessment
  ○ Disorientation, lethargy, headaches
  ○ Unconsciousness
  ○ Tachycardia, hypotension, ventricular fibrillation
  ○ Muscle weakness or convulsions
  ○ Rapid and shallow respirations

4a Respiratory Acidosis
- Diagnosis
  ○ Deceased serum pH
  ○ Increased PCO_2
  ○ Normal bicarbonate
  ○ Increased bicarbonate with compensation
  ○ Decreased urine pH with compensation

4b Respiratory Acidosis
- Treatment
  ○ Administration of bronchodilators, antibiotics
  ○ Administration of oxygen
  ○ Chest physiotherapy, mechanical ventilation
  ○ Removal of airway obstruction
  ○ Elevate head of bed, avoid sedation

4c Respiratory Acidosis (Figure 15-14)

4d Respiratory Alkalosis
- Assessment
  ○ Tingling of fingers and toes
  ○ Rapid, deep respiratory rate
  ○ Lightheadedness, confused, anxious, unable to concentrate
  ○ Tachycardia, dysrrhythmias
  ○ Tetany, numbness, hyperreflexia

4e Respiratory Alkalosis
- Diagnosis
  ○ Increased serum pH
  ○ Decreased PCO_2
  ○ Normal bicarbonate
  ○ Decreased bicarbonate with compensation

4f Respiratory Alkalosis
- Treatment
  ○ Administer oxygen
  ○ Administer sedatives, antianxiety agents
  ○ Breathe into paper bag or cupped hands
  ○ Mechanical ventilation
  ○ Anxiety-reducing techniques, pain relief

4g Metabolic Acidosis
- Assessment
  ○ Hyperventilation, Kussmaul respirations

    ◦ Hypotension, ventricular fibrillation
    ◦ Dull headache, muscle weakness
    ◦ Nausea and vomiting
    ◦ Abdominal pain, malaise to unconsciousness

4h Metabolic Acidosis
- Diagnosis
    ◦ Decreased pH and bicarbonate
    ◦ Normal PCO_2
    ◦ Decreased urine pH if compensated

4i Metabolic Acidosis
- Treatment
    ◦ Administer insulin, IV sodium bicarbonate
    ◦ Dialysis
    ◦ Administer antidiarrheal drugs
    ◦ Proper positioning, oral hygiene
    ◦ Protect skin, conserve energy

4j Metabolic Acidosis

4k Metabolic Alkalosis
- Assessment
    ◦ Abdominal distention, constipation, polyuria
    ◦ Cardiac arrhythmias
    ◦ Decreased rate and depth of respirations
    ◦ Tetany, seizures
    ◦ Weakness, confusion, lethargy, coma

4l Metabolic Alkalosis
- Diagnosis
    ◦ Increased serum pH
    ◦ Increased HCO_3
    ◦ Normal PCO_2
    ◦ Increased PCO_2 when compensated

4m Metabolic Alkalosis
- Treatment
    ◦ Administer normal saline intravenous infusion
    ◦ Administer acetazolamide
    ◦ Assist with effective respirations
    ◦ Monitor neurologic status
    ◦ Strict monitoring of intake and output

Suggestions for Classroom Activities

- Review assessment procedures for infants and children to determine fluid and electrolyte status. Refer to Table 15-1.
- Review laboratory study results for infants and children, including complete blood count, electrolytes, and arterial blood gases. Refer to Table 15-3.
- Develop case studies with a fluid and electrolyte imbalance and an acid-base imbalance. Have students discuss appropriate treatment and nursing interventions for the fluid and electrolyte imbalance and acid-base imbalance.

Suggestions for Clinical Activities

- Utilize actual client data from assigned client charts to discuss electrolyte imbalances and discuss interventions in postconference.
- Have students develop a teaching plan for the child with an electrolyte disorder or an acid-base disorder.

CHAPTER 16
CARE OF THE CHILD WITH NEUROLOGIC AND SENSORY DISORDERS

RESOURCE LIBRARY

CD-ROM

Down syndrome
Conjunctivitis
Otitis media

COMPANION WEBSITE

ALS
Palliative care

IMAGE LIBRARY

Figure 16-1 Structures of the neuron.

Figure 16-2 The developing brain.

Figure 16-3 Transverse section of the brain and spinal cord.

Figure 16-4 (A) The four major regions of the brain: cerebrum, cerebellum, diencephalon, and brainstem. (B) Lobes of the cerebrum and functional areas of the cerebral cortex.

Figure 16-5 (A) Anterior dermatomes of the body. (B) Posterior dermatomes of the body.

Figure 16-6 Autonomic nervous system and the organs it affects.

Figure 16-7 Gate control theory of pain perception.

Figure 16-8 (A) Meningocele. (B) Myelomeningocele. (C) The infant with a myelomeningocele is placed prone or in a side-lying position, and the exposed sac is protected carefully and kept moist.

Figure 16-9 (A) Infant with hydrocephalus. (B) A ventriculoperitoneal shunt, which allows fluid to leave the cranial cavid and so reduced intracranial pressure, is usually placed at 3 to 4 months of age.

Figure 16-10 A child who has a seizure when standing should be gently assisted to the floor and placed in a side-lying position.

Figure 16-11 A child with cerebral palsy has abnormal muscle tone and lack of physical coordination.

Figure 16-12 Central nervous system infections.

Figure 16-13 (A) The child with bacterial meningitis assumes an opisthotonic position (lying with the neck and head hyperextended) to relieve discomfort. (B) Kernig's and Brudzinski's signs are common findings in meningitis. (C) To test for Brudzinski's sign, flex the child's head while the child is supine.

Figure 16-14 Intracranial hematomas.

Figure 16-15 (A) Decorticate posturing, characterized by rigid flexion, is associated with lesions above the brainstem in the corticospinal tracts. (B) Decerebrate posturing, distinguished by rigid extension, is associated with lesions of the brainstem.

Figure 16-16 Flowchart of near-drowning in fresh- or saltwater.

Figure 16-17 Sites of brain tumors in children.

Figure 16-18 This child with Down syndrome has typical characteristics, including Mongolian slant, short wide neck, and a protruding tongue.

Figure 16-19 (A) Internal structure of the eye. (B) External structure of the eye.

Figure 16-20 Acute conjunctivitis.

Figure 16-21 Periorbital cellulitis is an infection of the eyelid and surrounding tissues, not of the eye itself.

Figure 16-22 Small pieces of debris or foreign objects can be visualized more readily by rolling the eyelid up over a cotton swab.

Figure 16-23 (A) Hyperopia. (B) Myopia. (C) Astigmatism.

Figure 16-24 Snellen letter chart.

Figure 16-25 (A) The Snellen E chart is often used for young school-age children. (B) The Snellen picture chart is used for very young children who can talk.

Figure 16-26 Strabismus.

Figure 16-27 An eye patch is used with nystagmus ("lazy eye") to strengthen the weaker eye.

Figure 16-28 Congenital cataract.

Figure 16-29 Congenital glaucoma can be seen in this child's right eye as a cloudy film.

Figure 16-30 (A) Ear anatomy. (B) Difference in the Eustachian tube between an infant and an adult.

Figure 16-31 The correct placement of the external ears is found by drawing an imaginary line through the medial and lateral canthi of the eye toward the ear.

Figure 16-32 Listening to loud music with headphones or at rock concerts is a frequent cause of hearing loss among teenagers and young adults.

Figure 16-33 (A) Structure and positioning of cochlear implant. (B) Child with cochlear implant.

Figure 16-34 (A) This young child is pulling at an ear and acting fussy, two important signs of otitis media. (B) Acute otitis media is characterized by pain and a red, bulging nonmobile tympanic membrane.

Figure 16-35 (A) This tympanogram demonstrates normal hearing as evidenced by the curve showing the tympanic membrane's movement when a sound wave is emitted into the ear canal. Mobility is between 0.2 and 1.0 mL, the normal range. (B) In contrast, note the flat pattern in the second tympanogram, which shows restricted mobility of the tympanic membrane in response to sound.

LEARNING OUTCOME 1

Discuss the anatomy and physiology of the pediatric neurological system.

CONCEPTS FOR LECTURE

1. The nurse needs to understand the anatomy and physiology of the child's nervous system to have an understanding of the disorders of the neurological system.
2. The nurse needs to recognize early and late signs of increased intracranial pressure to initiate appropriate interventions.
3. The nurse needs to understand the anatomy and physiology of the sensory system to have an understanding of the disorders of the sensory system.

   The eye is composed of internal and external structures that relay light impulses to the occipital area of the brain.

   The ear is composed of three sections: the external ear, middle ear, and the inner ear.

POWERPOINT LECTURE SLIDES

(NOTE: The number on each PPT Lecture Slide directly corresponds with the Concepts for Lecture.)

1 Anatomy and Physiology of the Neurological System
- Central Nervous System
  - Neurons
    - Nerve cells
    - Axon, dendrite
    - Cell body
    - Myelin sheath

1a Anatomy and Physiology of the Neurological System (Figure 16-2)

1b Anatomy and Physiology of the Neurological System
- Central Nervous System
  - Brain
    - Cerebrum
    - Diencephalons
    - Brain stem
    - Cerebellum

1c Anatomy and Physiology of the Neurological System
- Central Nervous System
  - Cranium
  - Spinal cord
  - Cerebral spinal fluid

1d Anatomy and Physiology of the Neurological System (Figure 16-3)

2 Anatomy and Physiology of the Neurological System
- Increased Intracranial Pressure
  - Early signs
    - Headache, vomiting
    - Level of consciousness changes
    - Asymmetrical pupils
    - Seizures

2a Anatomy and Physiology of the Neurological System
- Increased Intracranial Pressure
  - Infants
    - High-pitched cry

– Bulging fontanels
– Dilated scalp veins
– Irritability

 Anatomy and Physiology of the Neurological System
- Increased Intracranial Pressure
  - Late signs
    – Changes in level of consciousness
    – Respiratory distress, bradycardia
    – Increased systolic blood pressure
    – Fixed and dilated pupils, death

2c Anatomy and Physiology of the Neurological System
- Peripheral Nervous System
  - Spinal nerves—31 pairs
  - Cranial nerves—12 pairs
  - Somatic reflexes
  - Autonomic reflexes

2d Anatomy and Physiology of the Neurological System
- Peripheral Nervous System
  - Autonomic nervous system
    – Sympathetic nervous system
    – Parasympathetic nervous system

2e Autonomic Nervous System (Figure 16-6)

3 Anatomy and Physiology of the Eye (Figure 16-19)

3a Anatomy and Physiology of the Eye
- Six muscles for movement
- Vision
  - Light comes in to cornea
  - Passes through lens
  - Is focused by ciliary muscle onto retina
  - Rods and cones relay light to optic nerve

3b Anatomy and Physiology of the Ear
- External ear
- Middle ear
  - Eustachian tube—shorter, wider, more horizontal
- Inner ear

3c Anatomy and Physiology of the Ear (Figure 16-30)

Suggestions for Classroom Activities

- Hand out a diagram of the brain and spinal cord. Have students label the anatomy on the diagram. Review the physiology of each part of the brain and spinal cord.
- Compare the body responses to stimulation of sympathetic nervous system with stimulation of the parasympathetic nervous system.
- Discuss incidences when to observe for increased intracranial pressure.

Suggestions for Clinical Activities

- Using a skeleton model in the clinical laboratory, demonstrate the areas innervated by the spinal nerves and the levels of cranial nerves and the areas innervated by each. Use a dermatone chart for reference. See Figure 16-5.
- Using ear and eye models in the clinical laboratory, view the anatomy of the eye and ear parts and discuss areas where various disorders affect.

LEARNING OUTCOME 2

Describe neurological disorders to include seizures, cerebral palsy, meningitis, spina bifida, hydrocephalus, and Guillain-Barré syndrome.

CONCEPTS FOR LECTURE

1. Congenital neurologic disorders are disorders of the nervous system that are present at birth.
2. Nervous system disorders may be caused by a pathologic condition or may be a genetic factor.
3. Nervous system infections may be caused by a bacteria or virus. Bacterial infections are more serious, causing neurological damage and death.

POWERPOINT LECTURE SLIDES

(NOTE: The number on each PPT Lecture Slide directly corresponds with the Concepts for Lecture.)

1 Congenital Neurologic Disorders
- Spina Bifida
  - Incomplete closure of vertebrae and neural tube
  - Genetic predisposition with folic acid deficiency
  - Probability of clubfoot, hip defects, hydrocephalus

1a Congenital Neurologic Disorders
- Hydrocephalus
  - Increased production cerebral spinal fluid
  - Decreased absorption of cerebral spinal fluid
  - Blockage of flow of cerebral spinal fluid
  - Chari II malformation
  - Dandy-Walker syndrome

1b Congenital Neurologic Disorders
- Amyotrophic Lateral Sclerosis
  - Progressive, degenerative neurologic disease
  - Familial link to chromosome 21 defects

2 Nervous System Disorders
- Seizures
  - Sudden discharge of electrical activity in brain
  - Epilepsy
    - Chronic, repeated seizure activity
  - Status epilepticus
    - Continuous seizure > 30 minutes

2a Nervous System Disorders
- Cerebral Palsy
  - Affects motor function and posture
  - Causes of disorder
    - Lesions or anomalies of brain
    - Hypoxic damage
    - Birth trauma

2b Nervous System Disorders
- Fibromyalgia
  - Musculoskeletal pain and fatigue
  - Irritable bowel syndrome, skin sensitivities
  - Chronic headaches, impaired coordination
  - Temporomandibular joint dysfunction
  - PMS in adolescence

3 Nervous System Infections
- Meningitis and Encephalitis
  - Inflammation of meninges and brain
  - Bacterial or viral
  - May result in significant neurological deficits

3a Nervous System Infections (Figure 16-12)

3b Nervous System Infections
- Reye's Syndrome
  - Acute encephalitis
  - Complication of viral infection
  - Associated with salicylate use during viral infection

3c Nervous System Infections
- Guillain-Barré Syndrome
  - Acute viral infection
  - Ascending, then descending paralysis
  - Resolves in 2 to 4 weeks

SUGGESTIONS FOR CLASSROOM ACTIVITIES

- Develop a word search puzzle. Describe the condition and have the student find the disorder that matches the condition in the word search.
- Arrange for a parent of a child with cerebral palsy to speak to the students about the daily routine with the child.

SUGGESTIONS FOR CLINICAL ACTIVITIES

Have students visit a drugstore to read labels of over-the-counter products to identify products containing salicylate. Have them develop a teaching sheet for parents regarding Reye's syndrome, including the products containing salicylate.

LEARNING OUTCOME 3

Explain appropriate nursing interventions for children with neurological disorders.

CONCEPTS FOR LECTURE

1. Neurologic assessments include the Glasgow Coma Scale, which is used to evaluate a child's level of consciousness and verbal and motor response to stimuli.

   Pain in the child can be difficult to assess. Management of pain in children includes both the use of pharmacologic and nonpharmacologic methods of pain relief.
2. Spina bifida defects can occur anywhere along the spinal column and can cause a variety of pathologies such as hydrocephalus and seizures.
3. During a seizure, the first priority is to establish a safe environment for the child.
4. Amyotrophic lateral sclerosis may result in death in 2 to 5 years from respiratory failure.
5. Cerebral palsy damage can occur during the prenatal, perinatal, and postnatal periods and up to 2–3 years of age. It is more common in very-low-birth weight and small-for-gestational age infants.
6. Fibromyalgia is a disorder characterized by widespread musculoskeletal pain and fatigue.
7. The majority of meningitis cases in children occur before 5 years of age. Encephalitis is usually caused by a virus but may occur after vaccination with the measles, mumps, and rubella vaccine.
8. Parents should be taught to avoid using salicylates for viral infections due to the possibility of developing Reye's syndrome.
9. Guillain-Barré syndrome is most commonly seen in children between 4–9 years of age.

POWERPOINT LECTURE SLIDES

(NOTE: The number on each PPT Lecture Slide directly corresponds with the Concepts for Lecture.)

1 Neurologic Assessment
- History, physical examination
- Glasgow Coma Scale
- Pain assessment

1a Neurologic Assessment (Table 16-1)

2 Spina Bifida
- Manifestations
  - Meningocele
  - Myelomeningocele
  - Flaccid paralysis
  - Bowel and bladder incontinence
  - Sensory deficits

2a Spina Bifida (Figure 16-8)

2b Spina Bifida
- Treatment and Nursing Interventions
  - Surgical correction
  - Shunt if hydrocephalus
  - Observe for signs of infection
  - Monitor bowel and bladder function
  - Observe movement of extremities

2c Spina Bifida
- Preoperative interventions
  - Moist saline dressings to sac
  - Prone or side position
  - Keep warm

- Emotional care, tactile stimulation
- Feeding

 Spina Bifida
- Postoperative interventions
  - Observe for infection, neurological changes
  - Position prone, side lying, hold upright
  - Passive range of motion exercises
  - Monitor for bowel and bladder retention
  - Clean intermittent catheterization

 Hydrocephalus
- Manifestations
  - Head circumference greater than normal
  - Top of head out of proportion
  - Bulging anterior fontanel, "setting sun" sign
  - Irritable or lethargic
  - Nausea and vomiting

 Hydrocephalus (Figure 16-9)

 Hydrocephalus
- Treatment and Nursing Interventions
  - Surgical placement of ventriculoperitoneal shunt
  - Measure head circumference regularly
  - Monitor for increased intracranial pressure
  - Prevent skin breakdown, proper positioning
  - Give small, frequent feedings

3 Seizures
- Manifestations
  - Involuntary muscle activity
  - Change in level of consciousness
  - Altered behavior and sensory manifestation
  - Febrile seizure
    - Rapid temperature elevation > 102° F

 Seizures
- Focal seizure
  - Blank stare, facial movement, hear abnormal sounds
- Generalized seizure
  - Tonic-clonic movement
  - Loss of consciousness
  - Aura before, postictal period following seizure

 Seizures
- Treatment and Nursing Interventions
  - Administer anticonvulsants
  - Lower fever
  - Maintain seizure precautions
    - Pad side rails, suction equipment
  - Position on side, assess airway, LOC

3c Seizures (Figure 16-10)

4 Amyotrophic Lateral Sclerosis
- Manifestations
  - Muscle weakness and wasting

- Respiratory failure
- Death

 Amyotrophic Lateral Sclerosis
- Treatment and Nursing Interventions
  - Give respiratory and nutritional support
  - Teach hygiene, medication administration
  - Provide end-of-life care
  - Show support for client and family
  - Give referrals to community resources

 Cerebral Palsy
- Manifestations
  - Abnormal muscle tone
  - Lack of coordination
  - Delayed growth and development milestones
  - Hearing loss, visual defects, speech delay
  - Seizures, mental retardation

 Cerebral Palsy
- Treatment and Nursing Interventions
  - Teach devices to assist motor function
  - Use physical, occupational , speech therapy
  - Surgical procedures to improve motor function
  - Administer anticonvulsant, antispasmodic medications
  - Refer to appropriate resources

 Fibromyalgia
- Manifestations
  - Pain
  - Fatigue

 Fibromyalgia
- Treatment and Nursing Interventions
  - Exercise, water therapy
  - Minimize pain
  - Conserve energy

 Meningitis and Encephalitis
- Manifestations
  - Fever, change in appetite, vomiting, diarrhea
  - Lethargic or irritable
  - Headache, photophobia, nuchal rigidity
  - Positive Kernig and/or Brudzinski signs
  - Hemorrhagic rash

 Meningitis and Encephalitis (Figure 16-13)

 Meningitis and Encephalitis
- Treatment
  - Administer oral or intravenous fluids
  - Administer broad-spectrum antibiotics
  - Administer nonsteroidal anti-inflammatory drugs
  - Arrange long-term rehabilitation
  - Refer to appropriate resources

Meningitis and Encephalitis
- Nursing Interventions
  - Monitor vital signs and LOC
  - Measure head circumference daily
  - Monitor for seizures, respiratory distress
  - Monitor for sensory or movement deficiencies
  - Private, darkened room, respiratory precautions

 Reye's Syndrome
- Manifestations
  - Encephalitis symptoms
  - 1 to 3 weeks after viral infection

 Reye's Syndrome
- Treatment and Nursing Interventions
  - Same as encephalitis treatment
  - Teach to avoid products containing salicylates

 Guillain-Barré Syndrome
- Manifestations
  - Pain and weakness lower extremities
  - Paralysis progressing upward
  - Respiratory difficulty
  - Difficulty talking, chewing, swallowing
  - Dysfunction of autonomic nervous system

 Guillain-Barré Syndrome
- Diagnosis
  - Lumbar puncture
  - CSF evaluation
  - Electroconduction tests
  - Presenting symptoms

9b Guillain-Barré Syndrome
- Treatment and Nursing Interventions
  - Maintain respiratory function
  - Prevent malnutrition
  - Prevent complications associated with immobility
  - Provide emotional support
  - Teach family home care

Suggestions for Classroom Activities

- Develop a case study of a child with spina bifida who has hydrocephalus and a seizure disorder. Have students identify clinical manifestations and nursing interventions.
- Review medications used for cerebral palsy clients to decrease spasticity of muscles. Provide information on using a pump to deliver medication rather than administering oral medications. Discuss the advantages of this type of drug administration.
- Compare meningitis and encephalitis infections and prioritize nursing interventions. Refer to Table 16-3.

Suggestions for Clinical Activities

- Have students demonstrate Kernig and Brudzinski signs as a part of neurological assessment.
- Assign students to provide care for children with seizure disorders. Have them observe electroencephalogram studies. Review what preparation is needed to complete these studies. Review nursing interventions to perform if the child has a seizure.
- Have students assess pain in assigned children in the clinical setting. Use the PQRST mnemonic as a guide to charting pain assessment. Refer to Box 16-3.

Describe disorders of the eye and ear in children.

CONCEPTS FOR LECTURE

1. Eye infections are caused by bacteria, viruses, allergies, or trauma. They may be highly contagious. Prompt treatment prevents damage to the eye.

   Structures of the eye are not well protected. Penetrating or nonpenetrating eye injuries may occur.

   Visual impairment can cause learning difficulties or decreased vision.

   Hearing impairment may be congenital or acquired resulting in slight hearing loss to total deafness.

   Ear infections have increased incidence with upper respiratory infections, cleft palate, immunodeficiencies, bottle feeding, pacifier use, and exposure to cigarette smoking.

POWERPOINT LECTURE SLIDES

(NOTE: The number on each PPT Lecture Slide directly corresponds with the Concepts for Lecture.)

1 Eye Conditions
- Acute conjunctivitis
  - Acute inflammation of the conjunctiva
  - Caused by allergies, bacteria, viruses
  - Bacterial and viral are contagious

1a Acute Conjunctivitis (Figure 16-20)

1b Eye Conditions
- Stye
  - Infection of sebaceous gland of eye lid
  - Caused by *Staphylococcus*

1c Eye Conditions
- Periorbital Cellulitis
  - Inflammation of subcutaneous tissue of eyelid
  - Caused by preexisting infection, insect bite, trauma

1d Eye Injuries
- Penetrating Injuries
  - Object projected into eye
- Nonpenetrating Injuries
  - Corneal abrasion, chemical burn
  - Foreign object hits not penetrates eye
  - Hypema—hemorrhage into eye

1e Visual Impairments
- Hyperopia
  - Farsightedness
- Myopia
  - Nearsightedness
- Astigmatism
  - Uneven focusing results in blurred images

1f Visual Impairments (Figure 16-23)

1g Visual Impairments
- Strabismus
  - Uncoordinated eye muscles "cross-eyed"
  - Failure to maintain proper eye alignment
  - Esotropia
  - Exotropia
  - Hypertropia

1h Visual Impairments
- Amblyopia
  - Reduction of vision in one eye
  - "Lazy-eye"
- Dyslexia
  - See mirror images of letters, numbers
  - See mirror images of symbols

1i Visual Impairments
- Cataracts
  - Opacities of the lens

- Glaucoma
  - ○ Increased intraocular pressure
  - ○ Inadequate drainage of aqueous humor

1j Hearing Impairment
- Slight hearing loss to total deafness
- Congenital or acquired
- Sound waves not transmitted to brain correctly
- Foreign object in ear

1k Ear Infection
- Otitis Media
  - ○ Inflammation of the middle ear
  - ○ Accompanied by fluid in middle ear

SUGGESTIONS FOR CLASSROOM ACTIVITIES

- Develop a jeopardy game with eye and ear terminology on one side of card and definition on other side. Tape the cards with terminology side up to a whiteboard with the category written across the top of the white-board and money amounts written down the side. Have a student chose a card by picking a category and money amount. The student with the highest score wins.

SUGGESTIONS FOR CLINICAL ACTIVITIES

- Arrange for students to observe at an eye clinic or ophthalmologist office. Have students write a paper on the conditions they observed.
- Arrange for students to observe at an EENT office. Have students write a paper on their observations.

LEARNING OUTCOME 5

Explain appropriate nursing interventions for children with disorders of the eye and ear.

CONCEPTS FOR LECTURE

1. When assessing the eye, use terminology the child will understand and ask parents if the child has any difficulty seeing.
   To prevent transferring eye infections to others, frequent handwashing needs to be practiced.
2. Penetrating and nonpenetrating injuries need prompt treatment.
3. The Snellen letter chart, picture chart, and E chart are available to screen for visual acuity.
4. Dyslexia is a common learning disability. This condition makes speaking, writing, memorizing, working math problems, reading, and spelling difficult due to seeing mirror images of letters, numbers, and symbols.
5. Cataracts may be acquired through infections, trauma, or congenital as an inherited autosomal dominant trait.
6. Glaucoma has the potential to cause retinal damage, compression of the optic disc tissue, resulting in decreased visual fields or blindness.
7. When assessing a child's hearing, the difference in the anatomical shape of the eustachian tube of young children is important to understand. The shape increases risk of otitis media infections.

POWERPOINT LECTURE SLIDES

(NOTE: The number on each PPT Lecture Slide directly corresponds with the Concepts for Lecture.)

1 Eye Assessment
- History of eye problems
- Physical assessment
  - ○ Inspect conjunctivae, sclera, iris, pupils
  - ○ PERRLA
  - ○ Visual acuity

1a Acute Conjuctivitis
- Manifestations
  - ○ Eye irritation, redness, inflammation
  - ○ Photophobia, drainage
  - ○ Pruritis

1b Acute Conjunctivitis
- Diagnosis
  - ○ Cultures of drainage
- Treatment
  - ○ Administer ophthalmic antibiotics or antivirals
  - ○ Apply cool compresses
  - ○ Administer antihistamines

1c Acute Conjunctivitis
- Nursing Interventions
  - ○ Teach frequent handwashing
  - ○ Teach ophthalmic medication administration
  - ○ Change clean linens frequently

CONCEPTS FOR LECTURE *continued*

8. Because care of the child with otitis media is in the home, parents need to be taught proper medication administration and prevention methods.

   Delayed speech and language development may be the result of poor hearing acuity. Early detection of hearing loss identifies children in need of early interventions.

POWERPOINT LECTURE SLIDES *continued*

○ Teach to avoid rubbing eyes
○ No school or day care while infected

1d Stye
- Manifestations
  ○ Pain, redness, edema of eyelid
  ○ Enlarged preauricular lymph nodes

1e Stye
- Treatment
  ○ Administer ophthalmic antibiotic ointment
  ○ Apply warm, moist compresses

1f Periorbital Cellulitis
- Manifestations
  ○ Fever, malaise
  ○ Decreased visual acuity

1g Periorbital Cellulitis
- Diagnosis
  ○ Elevated white blood cell count
- Treatment
  ○ Administer intravenous antibiotics

1h Periorbital Cellulitis (Figure 16-21)

2 Penetrating and Nonpenetrating Injuries
- Manifestations
  ○ Intense eye pain
  ○ Excessive tearing
  ○ Light sensitivity
  ○ Changes in vision

2a Penetrating Injuries
- Treatment
  ○ Sedate child until removal of object
  ○ Administer ophthalmic ointment
  ○ Patch affected eye
  ○ Administer tetanus booster

2b Nonpenetrating Injuries
- Treatment
  ○ Remove foreign object
  ○ Use cotton-tipped applicator to remove
  ○ Administer ophthalmic antibiotic ointment
  ○ Perform water or saline irrigation for chemical

2c Nonpenetrating Injuries (Figure 16-22)

3 Hyphema
- Treatment
  ○ Apply patch to both eyes
  ○ Place on bedrest

3a Hyperopia, Myopia, Astigmatism
- Diagnosis
  ○ Snellen Letter Chart
  ○ Snellen E or Picture Chart
- Treatment
  ○ Corrective lenses

3b Strabismus
- Manifestations
  - Difficulty seeing objects clearly, clumsy
  - Close one eye to see better
- Diagnosis
  - Cover test

3c Strabismus
- Treatment
  - Use corrective lenses
  - Use eye patching
  - Perform orthoptics or eye exercises
  - Administer miotic medications
  - Perform surgery

3d Amblyopia
- Diagnosis
  - Detected in routine visual screen
- Treatment
  - Give referral to ophthalmologist or optometrist
  - Use corrective lenses, eye patch
  - Perform orthoptics

3e Amblyopia (Figure 16-27)

4 Dyslexia
- Manifestations
  - Learning difficulties
- Treatment
  - Specialized learning assistance

5 Cataracts
- Manifestations
  - Distorted or absent red reflex
  - Unable to focus on close objects
  - Demonstrate nystagmus
  - Report blurred vision

5a Cataracts
- Treatment
  - Remove surgically
  - Use corrective lenses
  - Have artificial lens implants

5b Cataracts (Figure 16-28)

6 Glaucoma
- Manifestations
  - Increased tearing, eyelid spasms
  - Buphthalmos, photophobia
  - Bump into objects
  - Difficult peripheral vision
  - Halos around objects

6a Glaucoma
- Diagnosis
  - Tonometer
- Treatment
  - Perform surgery (goniotomy)

7 Ear Assessment
- History of ear problems, hearing loss

- Physical Assessment
  - Inspect ear placement
  - Inspect external ear
  - Palpate for pain and tenderness
  - Assess for hearing acuity

7a Hearing Impairment
- Manifestations
  - No startle reflex in infant
  - Does not imitate sounds
  - Does not respond to name called
  - Uses nonverbal language instead of verbal
  - Asks for repeat of instructions

7b Hearing Impairment
- Diagnosis
  - Hearing acuity screening
    - Pure Tone Audiometry
    - Tympanometry

7c Hearing Impairment
- Treatment
  - Use speech therapy, sign language, lip reading
  - Use a hearing aid
  - Perform cochlear implant

7d Hearing Impairment (Figure 16-33)

7e Foreign Object in Ear
- Diagnosis
  - Otoscopic examination
- Treatment
  - Irrigate ear
  - Use sterile forceps to remove object
  - Administer otic medications

8 Otitis Media
- Manifestations
  - Upper respiratory infection symptoms
  - Fever, ear pain (otalgia), pulling at ear
  - Irritability, vomiting, diarrhea

8a Otitis Media
- Diagnosis
  - Symptoms exhibited
  - Opthalmic examination
    - Red and bulging tympanic membrane
    - Light reflex diminished or absent

8b Otitis Media (Figure 16-34)

8c Otitis Media
- Treatment
  - Administer antibiotics, decongestants, analgesic, antipyretics
  - Perform surgery—myringotomy
- Interventions
  - Teach proper administration of medications
  - Teach prevention methods

LEARNING OUTCOME 6

Discuss clinical manifestations, diagnostic procedures, medical management, and nursing interventions related to neurological trauma.

CONCEPTS FOR LECTURE

1. Neurological trauma is defined as any injury to the head or spinal cord due to force, anoxia, or penetration. Closed head injuries are the result of head trauma from external force or internal force.
2. Hematoma is blood trapped within the brain tissue or bruising from injury to the spinal cord.
3. Concussions are caused by a temporary impairment, such as a blunt injury or shaking that stretches, compresses, or tears nerve fibers near the brain.
4. Drowning is loss of life within 24 hours following submersion in a liquid. Near-drowning is suffocation from submersion in liquid of a person who survives for the first 24 hours following the incident.
5. Brain tumors are the most common solid tumor in children and the second most common malignancy after leukemia. Nursing care requires a multidisciplinary approach.
6. Mental retardation is a disability characterized by specific limitations in conceptual, social, and practical adaptive skills. It may be associated with disorders, infections, hypoxia, neurological trauma, or ingestion of poisons.
7. Down syndrome is the most common chromosomal abnormality, causing mental retardation and developmental delays.

POWERPOINT LECTURE SLIDES

(NOTE: The number on each PPT Lecture Slide directly corresponds with the Concepts for Lecture.)

1 Neurological Trauma
- Injury to head or spinal cord
- Caused by force, anoxia, penetration
- Closed head injury
  - Shaken baby syndrome

2 Hematoma
- Manifestations
  - Loss of consciousness
  - Amnesia, headache, nausea, vomiting
  - Fixed and dilated pupils
  - Decorticate or decerebrate posturing
  - Alteration in reflexes, seizures

2a Hematoma (Figure 16-15)

2b Hematoma
- Diagnosis
  - History and physical
  - Neurological assessment
  - X-rays
  - CT scan
  - MRI

2c Hematoma
- Treatment
  - Provide oxygen, intubation
  - Administer diuretics, sedatives
  - Provide decreased stimuli

2d Hematoma
- Nursing Interventions
  - Manage open airway
  - Assess for increased intracranial pressure
  - Maintain skin integrity
  - Teach caregivers safety issues
  - Allow parents to vent feelings

3 Concussion
- Manifestations
  - Altered mental status, loss of consciousness
  - Nausea, vomiting

- ○ Headache, dizziness
- ○ Amnesia

 Concussion
- • Diagnosis
  - ○ Skull x-ray
  - ○ Calculate Glasgow Coma Scale
- • Treatment
  - ○ Observe for decreased LOC, disorientation
  - ○ Awaken every 1 to 2 hours to check LOC

 Drowning or Near-Drowning
- • Manifestations
  - ○ Restlessness, loss of consciousness, vomiting
  - ○ Cyanosis, tachypnea, tachycardia
  - ○ Hypotension, hypothermia, death
  - ○ Risk for pneumonia
  - ○ Electrolyte imbalance if in salt water

 Drowning or Near-Drowning
- • Diagnosis
  - ○ Blood gases, serum chemistries
  - ○ Blood cultures
  - ○ Head or lung x-rays

 Drowning or Near-Drowning
- • Treatment
  - ○ Administer CPR
  - ○ Correct hypothermia, electrolyte imbalance
  - ○ Prevent hyper- or hypovolemic shock
  - ○ Monitor for neurological dysfunction, respiratory status
  - ○ Administer vasopressor, antibiotic medications

 Drowning or Near-Drowning
- • Nursing Interventions
  - ○ Improve neurologic function
  - ○ Provide oxygenation
  - ○ Decrease risk of infection
  - ○ Encourage to verbalize fear of water
  - ○ Teach water safety to parents/child

 Brain Tumors (Figure 16-17)

Brain Tumors
- • Manifestations
  - ○ Slight behavior change
  - ○ Poor school performance
  - ○ Change in coordination
  - ○ Diabetes insipidus
  - ○ Growth abnormalities

Brain Tumors
- • Diagnosis
  - ○ CT scan
  - ○ MRI
  - ○ PET scan, SPECT scan
  - ○ Lumbar puncture
  - ○ Bone marrow aspiration, bone scan

5c Brain Tumors
- Treatment
  - Perform surgery
  - Administer radiation
  - Administer chemotherapy

5d Brain Tumors
- Nursing Interventions
  - Coordinate multidisciplinary care
  - Teach parents home care
  - Provide support to child and family

6 Mental Retardation
- Manifestations
  - Infant
    - Unresponsive to contact, irritable
    - No eye contact during feeding
  - Child
    - Developmental delays
    - Learning difficulties

6a Mental Retardation
- Diagnosis
  - Chromosomal analyses
  - Blood enzyme levels, toxicology screens
  - Cranial imaging
  - Standardized tests

6b Mental Retardation
- Treatment
  - Coordinate multidisciplinary plan of care
  - Adapt education programs
  - Increase visual and physical stimulation
  - Provide job training if appropriate
  - Provide financial assistance and alternative living

6c Mental Retardation
- Nursing Interventions
  - Assist family with grief and coping
  - Provide appropriate referrals
  - Teach safety to prevent physical harm
  - Encourage child to care for own needs
  - Discuss sexuality issues, living options

7 Down Syndrome
- Manifestations
  - Short head, flat forehead, short limbs
  - Short wide neck, protruding tongue
  - Epicanthal folds, simian crease, Brushfield spots
  - Sluggish reflexes as infant
  - Mental retardation

7a Down Syndrome (Figure 16-18)

7b Down Syndrome
- Diagnosis
  - Chromosomal analysis
  - X-ray or ultrasound for cardiac defects
  - Clinical findings

Down Syndrome
- Treatment
  - Provide surgery to correct deformities
  - Assist parents in coping
  - Arrange referrals to community resources

 Down Syndrome
- Nursing Interventions
  - Provide emotional support
  - Model loving and positive response
  - Assist with "mainstreaming" into schools
  - Provide information
  - Coordinate referrals

SUGGESTIONS FOR CLASSROOM ACTIVITIES

- Arrange for a trauma nurse to speak to the students about experiences with providing nursing care for neurologic trauma clients.
- Have students search the Internet for cases of shaken baby syndrome. Discuss the treatment and outcomes in class.

SUGGESTIONS FOR CLINICAL ACTIVITIES

- Assign students to provide care for a child with a brain injury or a spinal injury. Have them identify the level of injury or disorder, the clinical manifestations exhibited, and nursing interventions.
- Arrange for students to observe in a school that "mainstreams" children with conditions such as Down syndrome and mental retardation. Have them write a paper on their observations and the role of a nurse in the school.

CHAPTER 17
CARE OF THE CHILD WITH MUSCULOSKELETAL DISORDERS

RESOURCE LIBRARY

CD-ROM
Skeleton

COMPANION WEBSITE
Strength training

IMAGE LIBRARY

Figure 17-1 These images show the remarkable development of bone as children grow.

Figure 17-2 The three sections of the long bone are the epiphysis, metaphysis, and diaphysis.

Figure 17-3 Posture.

Figure 17-4 (A) Genu valgum, or knock-knees. (B) Genu varum, or bowlegs.

Figure 17-5 Steps for Pavlik harness application.

Figure 17-6 Clubfoot, with the midfoot directed downward, the hindfoot turned inward, and the forefoot curled toward the heel and upward.

Figure 17-7 Gower's maneuver in child with muscular dystrophy.

Figure 17-8 Toronto brace used for Legg–Calvé–Perthes disease.

Figure 17-9 Scoliosis, showing deviation of the spine to the left.

Figure 17-10 In severe scoliosis, the child may wear a halo brace, shown here, to hold the body in position after surgery.

Figure 17-11 Osgood–Schlatter disease often occurs in school-age children involved in running sports such as soccer.

Figure 17-12 Fracture of the bone is defined as any disruption in the bone itself.

Figure 17-13 Salter–Harris classification system for fractures involving the epiphyses (growth plates).

Figure 17-14 Types of traction used for children.

Figure 17-15 Cast care.

Figure 17-16 Crutches should fit comfortably under the axillae so they do not rub against the skin.

Figure 17-17 The skin of the extremities should be warm.

Figure 17-18 Osteomyelitis.

Figure 17-19 With an above-the-knee amputation, a figure-eight bandage is wrapped around the waist, then brought down over the stump and back up around the hip.

Figure 17-20 A role model can provide support and encouragement to a child learning to adapt to life with a prosthetic limb.

LEARNING OUTCOME 1

Discuss the anatomy and physiology of the pediatric musculoskeletal system.

CONCEPTS FOR LECTURE

1. The muscular system is essentially complete at birth. Growth in length and circumference continues as the child grows.
2. Injuries to a child's bones may be due to the fact that the growth plate is still open and the child's long bones are less dense than the adult's.
3. Postural changes occur as the child grows and the musculoskeletal system matures.

POWERPOINT LECTURE SLIDES

(NOTE: The number on each PPT Lecture Slide directly corresponds with the Concepts for Lecture.)

 Anatomy and Physiology of the Musculoskeletal System
- Muscles
  - 3 types of body muscles
  - Skeletal muscles are striated
    - Assists in movement, maintains posture
- Tendons
  - Attach bones to muscles

2 Anatomy and Physiology of the Musculoskeletal System
- Skeleton
  - Ossification almost complete at birth
  - 3 sections of bone
  - Epiphyseal plate (growth plates)
  - Hematopoiesis

2a Anatomy and Physiology of the Musculoskeletal System (Figure 17-2)

3 Anatomy and Physiology of the Musculoskeletal System
- Postural changes with growth
  - Cervical and lumbar areas become concave
  - Bowed legs (genu varum) in infant
  - Knock knees (genu valgum) in preschool child
  - Resolve with growth

3a Anatomy and Physiology of the Musculoskeletal System (Figure 17-4)

Suggestions for Classroom Activities

- Develop flash cards to review the bones and muscles of the body.
- Review changes in the musculoskeletal system that occur as the child's musculoskeletal system grows and developments.

Suggestions for Clinical Activities

- Using a model of the bones in the clinical laboratory, review the sections of the bones and demonstrate where growth plates are and hematopoiesis takes place.

Learning Outcome 2

Describe musculoskeletal disorders to include developmental hip dysplasia, scoliosis, muscular dystrophy, osteomyelitis, osteosarcoma, and musculoskeletal injuries.

Concepts for Lecture

1. Skeletal defects can be minor and easy to correct or major malformations requiring long-term therapy.
2. Musculoskeletal disorders are due partly to changes in bone structure during periods of rapid growth and partly to injuries.
3. Musculoskeletal trauma, such as fractures, is a common occurrence in childhood due to play, sporting activities, and taking risks.
4. Musculoskeletal infections may be the result of injury or having surgery.
5. Periods of rapid growth are the most common time for musculoskeletal tumors to develop.

PowerPoint Lecture Slides

(NOTE: The number on each PPT Lecture Slide directly corresponds with the Concepts for Lecture.)

1 Congenital Hip Disorders
- Developmental Dysplasia of the Hip
  - Developmental hip abnormality
  - Involves femoral head, acetabulum, or both.

1a Congenital Hip Disorders
- Talipes (Clubfoot)
  - Congenital twisting of the foot
  - Unilateral or bilateral
  - Usually inward twisting

2 Musculoskeletal Disorders
- Muscular Dystrophy
  - Inherited sex-linked recessive disease
  - Carried by mother and passed to sons
  - Muscle degeneration and wasting
  - Most common is Duchenne muscular dystrophy

2a Musculoskeletal Disorders
- Legg-Calvé-Perthes Disease
  ○ Femoral head dies
  ○ Lack of blood supply to femoral head
  ○ Necrotic bone reabsorbed
  ○ Vascularized granulation tissue forms
  ○ Ossification occurs forming new femoral head

2b Musculoskeletal Disorders
- Scoliosis
  ○ Lateral S- or C-shaped curve of spine
  ○ Rotation of spine and ribs
  ○ Right-sided thoracic curve
  ○ Left-sided lumbar curve
  ○ More common in girls

3 Musculoskeletal Trauma
- Osgood-Schlatter Disease
  ○ Overgrowth of tibial epiphysis
  ○ Due to recurring inflammatory episodes
  ○ Bony prominence at knee

3a Musculoskeletal Trauma
- Fracture
  ○ Altered continuity of bone

4 Musculoskeletal Infection
- Osteomyelitis
  ○ Infection of bone
  ○ May spread to surrounding tissue
  ○ Caused by bacteria, virus, fungi
  ○ Follows injury or surgery

5 Musculoskeletal Tumors
- Osteosarcoma
  ○ Bone tumor
  ○ Most common in adolescent boys
  ○ Found in distal femur, proximal tibia
  ○ Found in proximal humerus

5a Musculoskeletal Tumors
- Ewing's Sarcoma
  ○ Malignant tumor of bone
  ○ Affects mostly Caucasians and Hispanics
  ○ Affects children 10 to 20 years

SUGGESTIONS FOR CLASSROOM ACTIVITIES

- Develop a matching quiz with the musculoskeletal disorder terminology on the left and a definition on the right. Have students match the correct terminology with the correct definition.
- Arrange for a client who has had an amputation to speak to the students about the care of the stump and their feelings regarding loss of a limb.

SUGGESTIONS FOR CLINICAL ACTIVITIES

- Arrange for students to assist with a scoliosis screening at a school.

LEARNING OUTCOME 3

Discuss clinical manifestations, diagnostic procedures, and medical management related to musculoskeletal disorders.

CONCEPTS FOR LECTURE

1. Obtaining the birth history is an essential part of the assessment as trauma or hypoxia during the birthing process may develop musculoskeletal difficulties.
2. Musculoskeletal defects require correction for normal support and movement to occur.
3. There is no cure for muscular dystrophy. Respiratory infections need to be treated promptly, and death occurs from respiratory paralysis during adolescence.
4. Assistive devices may be used for musculoskeletal disorders and injuries. Proper placement and prevention of complications need to be taught.
5. Infections of the bone require long-term antibiotic treatment. Intravenous antibiotics may be administered at home with assistance from a home health nurse.
6. Musculoskeletal tumors may result in loss of a body part. Feelings and concerns need to be addressed.

POWERPOINT LECTURE SLIDES

(NOTE: The number on each PPT Lecture Slide directly corresponds with the Concepts for Lecture.)

1 Assessment of the Musculoskeletal System
- Review history of birth, injuries, deformities
- Determine activity level, developmental delays
- Inspect posture and gait
- Note symmetry of structure, curves of spine
- Assess for full range-of-motion of joints
- Assess muscle strength

2 Developmental Dysplasia of Hip
- Manifestations
  - Partial or complete dislocation of hip joint
  - Shortening of femur
  - Uneven thigh and gluteal folds
  - Limited abduction on the affected side

2a Developmental Dysplasia of the Hip
- Diagnosis
  - Physical examination of hip
  - Allis sign
  - Ortolani-Barlow maneuver

2b Developmental Dysplasia of Hip
- Treatment
  - Small abnormality—apply three diapers
  - Apply Pavlik harness for 3–4 months
  - Place in skin traction for older children
  - Perform surgery followed by hip spica cast

2c Developmental Dysplasia of Hip (Figure 17-5)

2d Talipes (Clubfoot)
- Manifestations
  - Equines or midfoot directed downward
  - Varus or hindfoot turns inward
  - Forefoot curls toward heel and upward
  - Smaller foot, shortened Achilles tendon
  - Atrophies muscles of lower leg

2e Talipes
- Diagnosis
  - Observation of symptoms
  - X-ray
- Treatment
  - Apply cast to correct foot position
  - Change cast every 1–2 weeks for 3 months
  - Perform surgical correction if casting fails

3 Muscular Dystrophy
- Manifestations
  - Delayed walking, tires easily
  - Muscles degenerate over time

- Positive Gower's sign
- Develops scoliosis, respiratory difficulty
- Develops malnutrition, respiratory infection, respiratory paralysis

3a Muscular Dystrophy (Figure 17-7)

3b Muscular Dystrophy
- Diagnosis
  - Observation of clinical manifestations
  - Elevated serum creatine kinase
  - Muscle biopsy with low dystrophin
  - Electromyography

3c Muscular Dystrophy
- Treatment
  - Surgically correct scoliosis
  - Treat respiratory infections promptly
  - Physical therapy
  - Use of braces and wheelchairs

4 Legg-Calvé-Perthes Disease
- Manifestations
  - Mild hip and anterior thigh pain
  - Limp, worse with activity
  - Muscle wasting
  - Decreased mobility

4a Legg-Calvé-Perthes Disease
- Diagnosis
  - X-rays, bone scans, MRIs
- Treatment
  - Relieve pain
  - Apply Toronto brace or Scottish-Rite brace

4b Legg-Calvé-Perthes Disease (Figure 17-8)

4c Scoliosis
- Manifestations
  - Shoulders and hips different heights
  - Rotation of vertebrae and ribs
  - One-sided rib hump, prominent scapula
  - Asymmetrical posterior chest

4d Scoliosis (Figure 17-9)

4e Scoliosis
- Diagnosis
  - *Moire photography*
  - Spinal x-ray

4f Scoliosis
- Treatment
  - Mild scoliosis
    - Exercise, chiropractic adjustments
  - Moderate scoliosis
    - Boston or Milwaukee brace

○ Severe scoliosis
- Surgery with rods, wires, halo brace

 Osgood-Schlatter Disease
- Treatment
  ○ Resting joint until healing occurs
  ○ Apply cast to knee
  ○ Exercise to strengthen muscles
  ○ Perform knee surgery if indicated

 Fractures
- Manifestations
  ○ Pain, abnormal positioning, edema
  ○ Discoloration, abnormal movement
  ○ Broken skin, bleeding
- Diagnosis
  ○ X-rays of injured area

 Fractures (Figure 17-13)

 Fractures
- Treatment
  ○ Realign by closed reduction
  ○ Realign by open reduction
  ○ Apply traction
  ○ Immobilize with external fixators or immobilizers
  ○ Apply plastic or plaster cast

 Osteomyelitis
- Manifestations
  ○ Constant pain in affected area
  ○ Edema
  ○ Decreased mobility of joint
  ○ Refuse to use limb, limp extremity
  ○ Redness at site of injury, fever

 Osteomyelitis
- Diagnosis
  ○ History of trauma
  ○ Increased white blood cell count
  ○ Increased erythrocyte sedimentation rate
  ○ X-rays, bone scans
  ○ Needle aspiration of fluid for culture

 Osteomyelitis
- Treatment
  ○ Hospitalization
  ○ Administer intravenous medication

 Osteosarcoma
- Manifestations
  ○ Pain, swelling, fever
  ○ Mobility or gait problems
- Diagnosis
  ○ Elevated WBC and erythrocyte sedimentation rate
  ○ X-ray, CT, MRI scan, tissue biopsy

Osteosarcoma
- Treatment
  - Perform surgery to remove tumor
  - Perform amputation
  - Administer radiation, chemotherapy
  - Evaluate coping mechanisms

 Ewing's Sarcoma
- Manifestations
  - Pain, swelling, fever
  - Mobility or gait problems
  - Fractures of affected bone
- Diagnosis
  - Biopsy of tumor

Ewing's Sarcoma
- Treatment
  - Administer chemotherapy
  - Administer high-dose radiation
  - Perform surgery to remove bone
  - Referrals for follow-up care

SUGGESTIONS FOR CLASSROOM ACTIVITIES

- Develop a case study of a child with an immobilizing musculoskeletal disorder. Have students identify the clinical manifestations, evaluate diagnostic procedure results, discuss effects of immobilization and appropriate medical treatment.
- Apply moist and dry heat and cold compresses to the arm for 5 minutes. Have students compare the local and systemic responses of each compress. Discuss when warm dressings or cold dressings should be applied. Discuss safety issues of using heat and cold.

SUGGESTIONS FOR CLINICAL ACTIVITIES

- Arrange for students to observe in a pediatric orthopedic office. Have them discuss their experience in postconference.
- Have students practice walking with crutches or a cane, moving about with a makeshift cast or brace, and being confined to a wheelchair to demonstrate the difficulty the client has with these devices.

LEARNING OUTCOME 4

Explain appropriate nursing interventions for children with musculoskeletal disorders.

CONCEPTS FOR LECTURE

1. A priority nursing role when caring for children with musculoskeletal disorders is to promote independence.

   The nurse should teach the child and the parents to prevent complications with a cast by teaching them to keep the cast dry and clean, avoid using powders or lotions, avoid sticking objects into the cast, and cover the edges of the cast to protect the skin from injury.

   An essential assessment for the nurse to make when caring for a child with a cast is observing for compartment syndrome, which occurs when increased pressure in a limited space compromises circulation and nerve innervation.

   When providing instruction to a child who is learning to walk with crutches, the nurse should ensure that the crutches are not pressing on the axilla and that the child is able to maintain a straight spine when walking.

POWERPOINT LECTURE SLIDES

(NOTE: The number on each PPT Lecture Slide directly corresponds with the Concepts for Lecture.)

 Developmental Dysplasia of Hip
- Nursing Interventions
  - Maintain traction
  - Provide cast care
  - Assess lung sounds, neurovascular symptoms, skin
  - Reposition with cast every 2 hours
  - Encourage diet high in fiber, adequate fluids

 Talipes
- Nursing Interventions
  - Assist with cast application
  - Teach parents cast care
  - Administer pain medications
  - Observe for drainage and bleeding

Besides physical care, children in traction need attention to their emotional needs.

The nurse should observe the child with a musculoskeletal disorder for body image disturbance by recognizing certain signs.

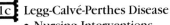

1b Muscular Dystrophy
- Nursing Interventions
  - Administer oxygen, respiratory therapy
  - Administration of medications, tube feedings
  - Monitor for signs of infection
  - Prevent skin breakdown
  - Low-calorie, high protein, high fiber diet

1c Legg-Calvé-Perthes Disease
- Nursing Interventions
  - Teach parents how to apply brace
  - Monitor for skin breakdown
  - Provide skin care
  - Teach to ambulate with brace
  - Support family and child

1d Fractures
- Nursing Interventions
  - Assess neurovascular status using the 5Ps
  - Prevent skin breakdown
  - Maintain proper alignment
  - Traction weights hang freely
  - Administer pin care

1e Fractures (Figure 17-14)

1f Fractures
- Nursing Interventions
  - Assess for compartment syndrome
  - Administer pain medication
  - Teach cast care, orthopedic appliances
  - Teach proper crutch walking
  - Teach to recognize complications, signs of abuse

1g Fractures (Figure 17-15)

1h Osteomyelitis
- Nursing Interventions
  - Administer antibiotics
  - Arrange for home health nurse
    - Administer antibiotics
    - Care of intravenous site

1i Osteosarcoma and Ewing's Sarcoma
- Nursing Interventions
  - Administer preoperative and postoperative care
  - Assess psychological status
  - Teach care of stump
  - Arrange rehabilitation for prosthesis
  - Referrals for financial assistance for appliances

1j Osteosarcoma and Ewing's Sarcoma (Figure 17-19)

Suggestions for Classroom Activities

- Show a video on child abuse. Discuss the appropriate assessment, nursing interventions, and documentation if suspecting child abuse.
- Divide the students into groups. Assign each group to develop a different teaching sheet for parents on care of the child with a cast, brace, or stump. Refer to Box 17-3 and Box 17-8.

Suggestions for Clinical Activities

- Assign students to care for a child with a musculoskeletal disorder. Have them demonstrate a neurovascular assessment. Have them develop a care plan or concept map for the assigned child.
- Arrange for students to observe at a child abuse center. Refer to Box 17-7 for information on assessing for child abuse. Have the student write a paper on the observation.

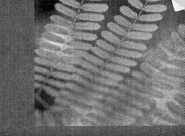

CHAPTER 18
CARE OF THE CHILD WITH RESPIRATORY DISORDERS

RESOURCE LIBRARY

CD-ROM
Lung sounds
Foreign body airway obstruction
Cystic fibrosis
Pulse oximeter
Pneumonia

COMPANION WEBSITE
Asthma

IMAGE LIBRARY

Figure 18-1 The child's airway is clearly smaller and less developed that an adult's.

Figure 18-2 The diameter of an infant's airway is approximately 4 mm; the adult's airway is 20 mm.

Figure 18-3 In children, the trachea is shorter and the angle of the right bronchus at *bifurcation* (place where it splits in two) is more acute than in the adult.

Figure 18-4 Infected tonsils can swell and obstruct the airway.

Figure 18-5 Clearing a foreign object.

Figure 18-6 CPR.

Figure 18-7 Multisystem effects of cystic fibrosis.

Figure 18-8 Sweat test.

Figure 18-9 Positions for postural drainage of different parts of the lung.

Figure 18-10 The cupped-hand position is used to clap against the chest well over the segment to be drained.

Figure 18-11 In croup, the epiglottis swells and occludes the airway (*see inset*).

Figure 18-12 Pneumonia in the lower lung lobes.

Figure 18-13 Positive tuberculin skin test (Mantoux test), showing previous exposure to TB.

Figure 18-14 Respiratory distress syndrome (RDS).

Figure 18-15 Some common triggers of asthma are shown above.

Figure 18-16 When an asthma attack occurs, the bronchi constrict and spasm (*see inset*), and mucus obstructs the airway.

Figure 18-17 (A) Pneumothorax. (B) Mediastinal shift caused by pneumothorax compresses the intact lung, further reducing the oxygen that can be provided to the body.

Figure 18-18 Pleurevac®.

Figure 18-19 Providing support to both the child and the parents is an important part of nursing care during acute episodes of asthma or other respiratory obstruction.

LEARNING OUTCOME 1

Discuss the anatomy and physiology of the pediatric respiratory system.

CONCEPTS FOR LECTURE

1. The respiratory system is divided into the upper respiratory system and the lower respiratory system.

    Mucous membranes produce 125 mL of mucus daily. Nasal sinuses and conchae in the sinuses increase the surface for warming and humidifying the air and trapping foreign objects.

    Eustachian tubes opening into pharynx may promote ear infections.

    Tonsils begin to atrophy in mid-adolescence resulting in lower incidence of tonsillectomy and adenoidectomy after 15 years of age.

    The trachea is smaller in diameter and shorter than the adult's trachea, making it easier to obstruct.

POWERPOINT LECTURE SLIDES

(NOTE: The number on each PPT Lecture Slide directly corresponds with the Concepts for Lecture.)

1 Anatomy of the Upper Respiratory System
- Nose
- Nasal sinuses
  - Conchae
- Pharynx
- Larynx

1a Anatomy of the Lower Respiratory System
- Trachea
- Bronchial tree

2. The mechanisms of respiration are a complex process of changing pressures that takes place 20 to 40 times a minute.

- Lungs
  - Three lobes on right
  - Two lobes on left
- Alveoli

1b Anatomy of the Upper Respiratory System
- Figure 18-1

1c Anatomy and Physiology of the Respiratory System
- Mucous membranes produce 125 mL mucus daily
- Cilia moves mucus toward pharynx

1d Anatomy and Physiology of the Respiratory System
- Sinuses
  - Conchae and nasal sinuses
    - Warm and humidify air
    - Trap foreign particles
  - Four pairs nasal sinuses
    - Frontal, sphenoidal, ethmoidal, maxillary

1e Anatomy and Physiology of the Respiratory System
- Pharynx
  - Eustachian tube open into pharynx
  - Lymphatic tissue or tonsils in walls of pharynx
  - Epiglottis covers larynx during swallowing
- Larynx
  - Contains vocal cords

1f Anatomy and Physiology of the Respiratory System
- Trachea
  - Small diameter, shorter than adult
  - Branches into bronchi and bronchioles
- Bronchioles end in alveoli
  - Gas exchange through capillaries

1g Anatomy and Physiology of the Respiratory System
- Figure 18-3

2 Mechanism of Respiration
- Chemoreceptors sense carbon dioxide elevation
- Chemoreceptors send message to brain
- Brain stimulates diaphragm to contract
- Brain stimulates intercostal muscles to contract
- Increase in chest cavity creates vacuum
- Air is sucked into body

2a Mechanism of Respiration
- Oxygen in alveoli moves into blood
- Carbon dioxide moves into alveoli
- Diaphragm and intercostal muscles relax
- Air is pushed out of lungs
- Takes place 20–40 times a minute

LEARNING OUTCOME 2

Describe respiratory disorders to include upper respiratory infections, tracheoesophageal fistula, cystic fibrosis, asthma, and lower respiratory infections.

CONCEPTS FOR LECTURE

1. Disorders of the respiratory system include congenital malformation, infections, and diseases resulting from chromosomal abnormalities or unknown causes.

   Respiratory infections stimulate the immune system to develop antibodies that will protect the child later in life.

   Cystic fibrosis, an autosomal recessive trait, affects a child's respiratory and gastrointestinal systems. The life expectancy is 30 years.

   With respiratory disorders, the nurse focuses on promoting respiratory function and preparing the family for home care.

   Sudden infant death (SIDS) is more common in Native American or African American descent, low birth weight, and multiple births.

   The stimulus that triggers the inflammatory process in asthma is specific to each individual.

POWERPOINT LECTURE SLIDES

(NOTE: The number on each PPT Lecture Slide directly corresponds with the Concepts for Lecture.)

1 Upper Respiratory Disorders
- Epistaxis
  - Nose bleed
  - Caused by trauma, allergies, forceful blowing, infection

1a Upper Respiratory Infections
- Nasopharyngitis
  - Called rhinitis, coryza, "common cold"
  - Inflammation of nasal mucosa
  - Caused by viral or bacterial infection

1b Upper Respiratory Infection
- Tonsillitis
  - Inflammation of palatine tonsils
  - Caused by viral or bacterial infection

1c Upper Respiratory Infection
- Epiglottitis
  - Inflammation of the epiglottitis
  - Caused by bacterial infection of pharynx and larynx
  - Complete respiratory obstruction can occur

1d Foreign Body Obstructed Airway
- Small object put in mouth and swallowed
- Chokes on food
- Small airway obstructs easily

1e Congenital Respiratory Disorders
- Cystic Fibrosis
  - Inherited recessive disorder of exocrine glands
  - Defective chloride ion and water transport
  - Secretion of thick, tenacious mucus
  - Obstruction of organs with mucus ducts
  - Loss of electrolytes

1f Cystic Fibrosis
- Figure 18-7

1g Lower Respiratory Infections
- Bronchiolitis
  - Infection and inflammation of bronchioles

- Buildup of mucus and swollen mucus membranes
- Wheezing from partial obstruction
- Causative organism is respiratory synctial virus
- Occurs from October to March

1h Lower Respiratory Infections
- Croup
  - Inflammation and swelling larynx, trachea, bronchi
  - Caused by virus or bacteria
  - Laryngotracheobronchitis most common form
  - Swelling of epiglottitis occludes larynx
  - Tracheal edema against cricoid causes obstruction

1i Croup
- Figure 18-11

1j Lower Respiratory Infections
- Pneumonia
  - Inflammation or infection of bronchioles and alveoli
  - Viral in infants and young children
  - Bacterial in premature infants and older children
  - Swelling of mucous membranes
  - Thick mucus, dead cells accumulate in alveoli

1k Lower Respiratory Infections
- Tuberculosis
  - Infection of the respiratory system
  - Caused by bacillus *Mycobacterium tuberculosis*
  - Enters body by droplet from infected person
  - Cause granulomas and scar tissue in lungs
  - May lead to lung damage and CNS involvement

1l Respiratory Disorders
- Neonatal Respiratory Distress Syndrome
  - Inadequate production of surfactant
    - Phospholipids and apoproteins
    - Reduce surface tension in alveoli
  - Common in premature infants

1m Neonatal Respiratory Distress Syndrome
- Figure 18-14

1n Respiratory Disorders
- Bronchopulmonary Dysplasia
  - Chronic lung disease
  - Caused by mechanical ventilation, oxygen toxicity
  - Lung damaged by high ventilator pressures
  - Results in pulmonary inflammation, cellular damage

1o Respiratory Disorders
- Sudden Infant Death Syndrome
  - Sudden unexplained death of infant
  - Most often between 2 and 4 months

⊙ More common in males
⊙ Leading cause of death 1 month to 1 year

1p Respiratory Disorders
- Asthma
  ⊙ Chronic inflammatory disorder of tracheobronchial tree
  ⊙ Caused by allergens, medication, fumes, exercise, stress

1q Asthma
- Figure 18-15

1r Respiratory Disorders
- Pneumothorax
  ⊙ Air in chest cavity
  ⊙ Results from chest trauma or rupture of alveoli
  ⊙ Causes mediastinal shift and shock
  ⊙ Hemothorax if blood in chest cavity

1s Pneumothorax

SUGGESTIONS FOR CLASSROOM ACTIVITIES

- Administer a matching quiz with the respiratory disorder on the left and the definition or cause on the right.
- Have students insert a straw into a deflated balloon. Have them plug their nose and breathe through the straw for 30 seconds to demonstrate the difficulty of breathing through a narrow airway.

SUGGESTIONS FOR CLINICAL ACTIVITIES

- Have students develop a teaching sheet for parents about the structure and function of the respiratory system and how it may relate to a respiratory disease process.

LEARNING OUTCOME 3

Discuss clinical manifestations, diagnostic procedures, medical management, and nursing interventions related to respiratory trauma.

CONCEPTS FOR LECTURE

1. Observation of respiratory patterns and skin color are critical assessments, as the child may not be able to tell the nurse subjective information.

   Viral infections should be treated with supportive care. Antibiotics should only be used for bacterial infections.

   Frequent swallowing after a tonsillectomy is the first sign of bleeding.

   With foreign object obstructed airway, the size of the child determines the position and procedure used for the Heimlich maneuver.

2. Neonatal respiratory distress syndrome is common in premature infants due to inadequate surfactant production which allows alveoli to collapse with each breath.

   Many respiratory disorders begin in early childhood become chronic lifelong disorders.

3. Management of asthma is focused on identifying and avoiding triggers, family education, medication administration, and follow-up care.

POWERPOINT LECTURE SLIDES

(NOTE: The number on each PPT Lecture Slide directly corresponds with the Concepts for Lecture.)

1 Assessment of the Respiratory System
- Breathing patterns
  ⊙ Eupnea
  ⊙ Hypoventilation
  ⊙ Hyperventilation
  ⊙ Dyspnea, apnea
  ⊙ Cheyne-Stokes respirations

1a Assessment of the Respiratory System
- Circumoral cyanosis
- Productive or nonproductive cough
- Lung sounds
  ⊙ Crackles
  ⊙ Rhonchi
  ⊙ Stridor

1b Epistaxis
- Diagnosis
  ⊙ Blood draining from nose or down throat

Health promotion activities (including immunizations, removing pollutants from the environment, infection control measures, and back to sleep for infants) can help to prevent or control pediatric respiratory disorders.

- Treatment
  - Apply direct firm pressure to nares
  - Hold head slightly forward
  - Apply cold cloth to forehead, back of neck

1c Nasopharyngitis
- Manifestations
  - Redness and swelling of mucosa
  - Clear nasal discharge
  - Enlarged tonsils, vesicles, mouth breathing
  - Fever, general discomfort, pain
  - Yellow or green discharge if bacterial

1d Nasopharyngitis
- Diagnosis
  - Symptoms
  - Nasal swab, throat culture
- Treatment
  - Use humidified air, saline nose drops
  - Administer decongestants, antihistamines, antibiotics

1e Tonsillitis
- Manifestations
  - Enlarged tonsils, pain, difficulty swallowing
  - Swollen mucous membranes, otitis media
- Diagnosis
  - Culture tonsils
  - Assess ear for redness and fluid

1f Tonsillitis
- Figure 18-4

1g Tonsillitis
- Treatment
  - Administer acetaminophen, cold nonacidic fluids
  - Use humidifier
  - Gargle with saline solution
  - Antibiotics if bacterial
  - Tonsillectomy for recurrent infections

1h Epiglottitis
- Manifestations
  - High fever, sore throat
  - Muffled or hoarse voice (dysphonia)
  - Difficulty swallowing (dysphonia), inspiratory stridor
  - Drooling, orthopnea
  - Tripod position

1i Epiglottitis
- Diagnosis
  - Symptoms
  - Culture
  - Lateral x-ray neck

1j Epiglottitis
- Treatment
  - No visualization—causes laryngospasm and obstruction
  - Insertion of endotracheal tube or tracheostomy

  ○ Administer intravenous antibiotics
  ○ Administer acetaminophen or ibuprofen
  ○ Admit to intensive care unit

[1k] Foreign Body Obstructed Airway
- Manifestations
  ○ Facial expression
  ○ Ability to talk or not
  ○ Ability to breathe
  ○ Object in back of throat

[1l] Foreign Body Obstructed Airway
- Treatment
  ○ Perform Heimlich maneuver
  ○ Finger sweep if object is visible
  ○ Perform CPR if indicated

[1m] Foreign Body Obstructed Airway
- Figure 18-5

[1n] Cystic Fibrosis
- Manifestations
  ○ Meconium ileus, failure to thrive
  ○ Chronic recurrent respiratory infections
  ○ Constipation, frothy stool, trouble gaining weight
  ○ Chronic productive cough with thick mucus
  ○ Clubbing of fingers

[1o] Cystic Fibrosis
- Diagnosis
  ○ Positive sweat test

[1p] Cystic Fibrosis
- Figure 18-8

[1q] Cystic Fibrosis
- Treatment
  ○ Perform postural drainage
  ○ Treat respiratory infections or allergies aggressively
  ○ Administer pancreatic enzymes, vitamins A, D, E, K
  ○ Encourage diet high in carbohydrates and protein
  ○ Encourage extra fluids and salt

[1r] Bronchiolitis
- Manifestations
  ○ Wheezing and crackles on auscultation
  ○ Breath sounds diminish, retractions
  ○ Nasal stuffiness, fever, cough
  ○ Rapid, labored breathing, nasal flaring
  ○ Refusal to eat, dehydration

[1s] Bronchiolitis
- Diagnosis
  ○ History
  ○ Naspharyngeal secretion cultures
  ○ Chest x-ray

1t Bronchiolitis
- Treatment
  - Begin intravenous fluids
  - Administer humidified oxygen, medications
  - Administer breathing treatments
  - Hospitalize for treatment

1u Croup
- Manifestations
  - Inspiratory stridor
  - Barking "seal-like" cough, hoarseness
  - Onset may be sudden or gradual
  - May or may not have fever
  - Drooling due to pain and swelling

1v Croup
- Diagnosis
  - Clinical findings
  - Chest x-ray
  - Pulse oximetry

1w Croup
- Treatment
  - Administer cool mist by mask or tent
  - Administer antibiotics if bacterial
  - Endotracheal intubation to keep airway open
  - Administer medications to reduce swelling

1x Pneumonia
- Manifestations
  - Fever, malaise, cough
  - Wheezing, diminished or absent breath sounds
  - Tachypnea, labored breathing, dyspnea
- Diagnosis
  - Sputum cultures, chest x-ray

1y Pneumonia
- Treatment
  - Administer antibiotics, fluids, cough suppressants, antipyretics
- Hospitalization
  - Administer oxygen, chest physiotherapy, intravenous fluids

1z Tuberculosis
- Diagnosis
  - Physical findings, sputum culture
  - Positive PPD (Mantoux test), x-rays
- Treatment
  - Administer isoniazid, rifampin, pyrazinamide

2 Neonatal Respiratory Distress Syndrome
- Manifestations
  - Respirations > 60
  - Retractions, nasal flaring, audible grunting
  - Decreased lung sounds

2a Neonatal Respiratory Distress Syndrome
- Diagnosis
  - Clinical symptoms

- Treatment
  - Administer oxygen, assisted mechanical ventilation
  - Administer surfactant
  - Treat atelectasis

 Bronchopulmonary Dysplasia
- Manifestations
  - Wheezing, crackles, retractions, flaring, grunting
  - Failure to thrive
- Diagnosis
  - Chest x-ray

 Bronchopulmonary Dysplasia
- Treatment
  - Progressing weaning from mechanical ventilation
  - Administer oxygen, anti-inflammatory medications
  - May need tracheostomy
  - Support nutrition and caloric intake
  - Complications—asthma, pulmonary infections

 Sudden Infant Death Syndrome
- Manifestations
  - No respirations, no audible cry
  - Blood-tinged frothy fluids mouth and nose
  - Urine and stool in diaper
  - Found clutching blanket
  - Skin white ashen color

 Sudden Infant Death Syndrome
- Diagnosis
  - Clinical findings
  - Autopsy
- Treatment
  - CPR, call Emergency Medical Services
  - Prevention with back to sleep

 Asthma
- Manifestations
  - Fast, labored breathing, productive cough
  - Wheezing on expiration, chest tightness
  - Nasal flaring, intercostal retractions, head bobbing
  - Anxious, suffocating-feeling
  - Status asthmaticus

Asthma
- Figure 18-16

Asthma
- Diagnosis
  - Medical history, physical assessment
  - Pulmonary function tests
  - Peak expiratory flow rates
  - Skin tests for allergens

3c Asthma
- Treatment
  - Avoid triggers
  - Administer medications
  - Teach family care and avoid smoking
  - Obtain follow-up care

3d Pneumothorax
- Manifestations
  - Absent lung sounds
  - Unable to breathe
  - Decrease in oxygen saturation
- Diagnosis
  - Clinical findings, chest x-ray

 3e Pneumothorax
- Treatment
  - Insert chest tube
  - Attach to underwater seal and suction

3f Pneumothorax
- Figure 18-18

SUGGESTIONS FOR CLASSROOM ACTIVITIES

- Have students blow up a new balloon to demonstrate the difficulty of breathing against resistance.
- Have students discuss complementary or alternative ways they have used to treat respiratory disorders. Discuss the medications they have used to treat respiratory disorders.
- Develop case studies of children with various respiratory disorders. Assign groups of students to complete the case study questions for a case study, and then present the case study to the rest of the class.

SUGGESTIONS FOR CLINICAL ACTIVITIES

- Arrange for students to administer PPD tests to clients in the clinical setting or at a clinic. Have them evaluate the results in 72 hours.
- Arrange for students to observe pulmonary function studies in the respiratory department of the acute hospital setting.
- Have students practice respiratory assessments on each other. Review Box 18-5 for assessment of the client with asthma.

LEARNING OUTCOME 4

Explain appropriate nursing interventions for children with respiratory disorders.

CONCEPTS FOR LECTURE

1. Priorities of nursing care for children with respiratory disorders are maintain patent airway, prevent infection, promote healing, and prevent further respiratory damage.

   Pediatric children can be taught to manage their chronic respiratory disorder.

   After discharge teaching is completed, children and families will verbalize understanding of the respiratory disorder, medical treatment and equipment, and medication administration.

POWERPOINT LECTURE SLIDES

(NOTE: The number on each PPT Lecture Slide directly corresponds with the Concepts for Lecture.)

 1 Tonsillitis
- Nursing Interventions
  - Do preoperative teaching
  - Administer postoperative care
    - Administer cold fluids, analgesics
    - Monitor for excessive swallowing
    - Monitor for bleeding

 1a Tonsillitis
- Nursing Interventions
  - Do discharge teaching
  - Encourage soft foods, adequate fluid intake
  - Monitor for bleeding, no straws
  - Teach strong foul odor, no gargling

1b Epiglottitis
- Nursing Interventions
  - Manage airway
  - Administer medications, sedate if needed
  - Maintain hydration with cool mist and fluids
  - Provide emotional support, quiet environment
  - Instruct parents in medications and side effects

1c Cystic Fibrosis
- Nursing Interventions
  - Maintain open airway, administer respiratory therapy
  - Administer antibiotics, pancreatic enzymes, vitamins
  - Encourage normal growth and development
  - Teach parents home care, appropriate referrals

1d Cystic Fibrosis
- Figure 18-9

1e Bronchiolitis
- Nursing Interventions
  - Wear gown and gloves, masks
  - Admit to private room
  - Administer oxygen, monitor oxygen saturation
  - Administer intravenous fluids, medications
  - Reposition every 1/2 hour, monitor respiratory effort

1f Croup
- Nursing Interventions
  - Administer cool mist and oxygen
  - Administer antibiotics, fluids
  - Keep environment quiet, keep from crying
  - Avoid probing throat
  - Discharge teaching for parents

1g Pneumonia
- Nursing Interventions
  - Maintain airway
  - Provide symptom relief for fever, pain
  - Provide support for parents
  - Provide appropriate teaching

1h Tuberculosis
- Nursing Interventions
  - Educate family to adhere to medical regimen
  - Teach to prevent of spread of infection
  - Administer medications
  - Screen all who come in contact

1i Neonatal Respiratory Distress Syndrome
- Nursing Interventions
  - Maintain body temperature
  - Administer oxygen
  - Monitor fluid levels
  - Support parents, teach CPR
  - Teach parents oxygen administration, apnea monitor

[1j] Bronchopulmonary Dysplasia
- Nursing Interventions
  - Teach parents to administer oxygen, medications, nutrition
  - Teach parents to manage required equipment
  - Provide referrals for respiratory supplies, financial support
  - Coordinate follow-up care

[1k] Sudden Infant Death Syndrome
- Nursing Interventions
  - Support family members, provide referrals
  - Educate public about bedding
  - Educate about back to sleep
  - Allow family to hold infant
  - Give parents handprints, footprints, lock of hair

[1l] Asthma
- Nursing Interventions
  - Teach to avoid triggers
  - Teach to administer medication by meter-dose-inhaler
  - Teach to administer medication by continuous nebulizer
  - Teach peak expiratory flow rate monitoring

[1m] Pneumothorax
- Nursing Interventions
  - Set up underwater seal system and tape connections
  - Secure chest tubes to bed and drainage system
  - Remove chest tubes when indicated
  - Maintain patent airway, prevent further damage
  - Administer medications, oxygen, fluids

[1n] Pneumothorax
- Figure 18-18

SUGGESTIONS FOR CLASSROOM ACTIVITIES

- Have students blow on a pinwheel or blow bubbles to demonstrate ways to get children to exercise their lungs.
- Have students write examination questions on nursing interventions with respiratory disorders. Have them share the questions with each other.

SUGGESTIONS FOR CLINICAL ACTIVITIES

- Assign students to provide nursing care to children with respiratory disorders. Have them develop a nursing care plan or concept map with their interventions.
- Check off students suctioning clients, administering oxygen, recording oxygen saturation, teaching incentive spirometry, teaching cough and deep breathing exercises, administering chest physiotherapy, and demonstrating use of metered-dose inhalers.

CHAPTER 19
CARE OF THE CHILD WITH CARDIOVASCULAR DISORDERS

RESOURCE LIBRARY

 CD-ROM

Heart
Congenital heart defects
Heart sounds

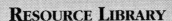 **COMPANION WEBSITE**

Calculating BMI
Hypertension

 IMAGE LIBRARY

Figure 19-1 (A) Fetal circulation. (B) Newborn circulation.

Figure 19-2 The child's circulatory system.

Figure 19-3 Points for auscultating the heart.

Figure 19-4 Atrial septal defect.

Figure 19-5 Patent ductus arteriosus.

Figure 19-6 (A) Septal occluder is used to close an atrial septal defect and less commonly to close a ventricular septal defect. (B) Coil used to close a patent ductus arteriosus.

Figure 19-7 Types of pulse patterns.

Figure 19-8 Ventricular septal defect.

Figure 19-9 Tetralogy of Fallot involves four distinct problems: pulmonary stenosis, ventricular septal defect, right ventricular hypertrophy, and an overriding aorta.

Figure 19-10 (A) A child with cyanotic heart defect squats (assumes a knee-chest position) to relieve cyanotic spells. (B) Clubbing of the fingers is one manifestation of a cyanotic defect in an older child.

Figure 19-11 Coarctation of the aorta. In most instances, the narrowing occurs in the aortic arch.

Figure 19-12 Transposition of the great arteries.

Figure 19-13 Cardiogenic shock.

Figure 19-14 This child has returned for one of her frequent follow-up visits to assess her cardiac status after treatment for Kawasaki syndrome.

Figure 19-15 (A) This child is continuously monitored for congestive heart failure. (B) This child with atrial septal defect repair is placed in a position that assists breathing.

LEARNING OUTCOME 1

Discuss the anatomy and physiology of the pediatric cardiovascular system.

CONCEPTS FOR LECTURE

1. Fetal blood is oxygenated by the placenta. Blood flow to the lungs is decreased by the foramen ovale and the ductus arteriosus.

   The foramen ovale closes shortly after birth causing the right side of the heart to pump blood to the lungs for oxygenation.

   The ductus arteriosus closes shortly after birth to allow oxygenated blood to be pumped out to the body.

2. An infant's heart muscle fibers are not developed fully, and the ventricles are not as compliant to stroke volume; therefore, the infant is very sensitive to volume and pressure overloads.

   Cardiac output is affected by the amount of preload, afterload, and the contractility of the ventricles.

POWERPOINT LECTURE SLIDES

(NOTE: The number on each PPT Lecture Slide directly corresponds with the Concepts for Lecture.)

1 Anatomy and Physiology of the Pediatric Cardiovascular System
- Fetus
  - Blood oxygenated in the placenta
  - Decreased blood flow to lungs
  - Foramen ovale connects atria
  - Ductus arteriosus connects pulmonary artery to aortic arch

1a Anatomy and Physiology of the Pediatric Cardiovascular System
- Figure 19-1

2 Anatomy and Physiology of the Pediatric Cardiovascular System
- Infant
  - Foramen ovale and ductus arteriosus close
  - Left side pressure higher than right side

○ Heart muscle fibers immature
○ Ventricles less compliant to stroke volume
○ Preload, afterload, contractility affect cardiac output

SUGGESTIONS FOR CLASSROOM ACTIVITIES	**SUGGESTIONS FOR CLINICAL ACTIVITIES**
• Have students compare fetal and infant circulation by labeling the parts of the cardiovascular system on diagrams of fetal and infant circulation. • Play a tape or DVD with heart sounds. Have students listen to the sounds through their stethoscopes to identify the different sounds when they perform assessments on clients.	• Have students demonstrate blood flow through the body using a model of the circulatory system.

LEARNING OUTCOME 2

Describe cardiovascular disorders to include both congenital and acquired disorders.

CONCEPTS FOR LECTURE

1. Cardiovascular disorders are serious health threats resulting from congenital heart anomalies or defects or acquired heart diseases.
   Congenital heart defects may arise when the fetus is exposed to infections, such as rubella, alcohol, or drugs in utero.
2. Congenital heart defects can be classified into four groups according to the way the defect affects circulation: defects with increased pulmonary blood flow, defects with decreased pulmonary blood flow, defects that obstruct systemic blood flow, and mixed defects.
3. Congestive heart failure is characterized in children according to the type of heart defect.
   Volume and pressure overloads cause congestive heart failure in infants.
4. Elevated blood pressure in children is often secondary to kidney disease, coarctation of the aorta, hyperthyroidism, increased intracranial pressure, and side effects of certain medications.
5. Kawasaki disease and acute rheumatic fever are inflammatory disorders that can result in damage to the heart.

POWERPOINT LECTURE SLIDES

(NOTE: The number on each PPT Lecture Slide directly corresponds with the Concepts for Lecture.)

1 Cardiovascular Disorders
 • Congenital heart anomalies or defects
  ○ Fetus exposed to infections, genetic inheritance
  ○ Maternal age or disorders
 • Acquired heart diseases
  ○ Diseases or genetic disorders
  ○ Cardiovascular deficits

2 Congenital Heart Anomalies
 • Defects with increased pulmonary blood flow
  ○ Atrial septal defect (ASD)
   – Opening in septum between atria
   – Between left and right atria
   – Foramen ovale
   – Results in right ventricular hypertrophy

2a Atrial Septal Defect
 • Figure 19-4

2b Congenital Heart Anomalies
 • Defects with increased pulmonary blood flow
  ○ Patent Ductus Arteriosus (PDA)
   – Ductus arteriosus fails to close
   – Blood flows from aorta to pulmonary artery
   – Increased blood flow to lungs
   – Causes right ventricular hypertrophy

2c Patent Ductus Arteriosus
 • Figure 19-5

2d Congenital Heart Anomalies
 • Defects with increased pulmonary blood flow
  ○ Ventricular Septal Defect
   – Opening in septum between ventricles
   – Blood flows left to right

2e Ventricular Septal Defect
- Figure 19-8

2f Congenital Heart Anomalies
- Defects with Decreased Pulmonary Blood Flow
  - Tetralogy of Fallot
    - Pulmonary stenosis, narrowing of pulmonary valve
    - Ventricular septal defect
    - Right ventricular hypertrophy
    - Overriding aorta

2g Tetralogy of Fallot
- Figure 19-9

2h Congenital Heart Anomalies
- Defects that Obstruct Systemic Blood Flow
  - Coarctation of the Aorta
    - Narrowing of the aorta
    - Most common site is arch of aorta
    - Leads to congestive heart failure

2i Coarctation of the Aorta
- Figure 19-11

2j Congenital Heart Defects
- Mixed Defects
  - Transposition of the Great Arteries
    - Reversed positions of aorta and pulmonary artery
    - Unoxygenated blood moves in and out of heart
    - Oxygenated blood moves through heart and lungs

2k Transposition of the Great Arteries
- Figure 19-12

3 Acquired Heart Diseases
- Congestive Heart Failure
  - Circulatory deficits
  - Decreased cardiac output
  - Cardiogenic shock
  - Results from congenital or acquired heart defects

3a Congestive Heart Failure
- Figure 19-13

4 Acquired Heart Diseases
- Systemic Hypertension
  - Elevated blood pressure
  - Genetic or family history
  - Secondary to kidney disease, coarctation of aorta
  - Secondary to hyperthyroidism, increased ICP, medications

4a Acquired Heart Diseases
- Hyperlipidemia
  - Increased total cholesterol
  - Low-density lipoproteins, triglycerides
  - Decreased high-density lipoproteins

5 Acquired Heart Diseases
- Kawasaki Disease
  - Acute systemic inflammatory illness
  - Mucocutaneous lymph node syndrome
  - More common in Asian and male children

5a Acquired Heart Diseases
- Acute Rheumatic Fever
  - Inflammatory disorder
  - Follows a group A beta-hemolytic *Streptococcus* infection
  - Autoimmune response damages heart, joints, CNS, skin
  - May recur with further heart damage

SUGGESTIONS FOR CLASSROOM ACTIVITIES

- Administer a matching quiz with the cardiac disorder on the left and the definition or cause on the right.

SUGGESTIONS FOR CLINICAL ACTIVITIES

- Have students develop a teaching sheet for parents about the structure and function of the cardiac system and how it may relate to a cardiac anomaly or disease process.

LEARNING OUTCOME 3

Discuss clinical manifestations, diagnostic procedures, medical management related to cardiovascular disorders.

CONCEPTS FOR LECTURE

1. Children with congenital and acquired heart defects exhibit signs and symptoms of congestive heart failure. It is important for the nurse to monitor vital signs correctly, document accurately, and monitor for changes in status.
2. Congenital anomalies are identified at birth or within the first few weeks of life.
   Anomalies may be repaired immediately or when the child is stronger and able to withstand the surgical procedure.
3. Congestive heart failure affects the cardiac, pulmonary, and metabolic systems and may lead to cardiogenic shock.
4. Systemic hypertension is diagnosed following three separate measurements of elevated blood pressure.
5. Children rarely exhibit symptoms of hyperlipidemia. Diagnosis is based on blood screening for total cholesterol.
6. Kawasaki disease is the most common of acquired heart diseases.
7. Rheumatic fever is more common in children between 6 and 15 years following a strep throat infection.

POWERPOINT LECTURE SLIDES

(NOTE: The number on each PPT Lecture Slide directly corresponds with the Concepts for Lecture.)

1 Assessment of the Cardiovascular System
- History
  - Family history cardiac disease
  - Weakness and fatigue upon physical exertion
  - Cyanosis, edema, dizziness, poor weight gain

1a Assessment of the Cardiovascular System
- Physical
  - Observe child's posture
  - Observe for respiratory difficulty, dehydration
  - Inspect nail beds, sclera, skin tone
  - Monitor vital signs, palpate pulses
  - Auscultate heart and breath sounds

2 Atrial Septal Defect
- Manifestations
  - Asymptomatic in young child/baby
  - Fatigue, delayed growth, congestive heart failure
  - Soft, systolic murmur

2a Atrial Septal Defect
- Diagnosis
  - Echocardiogram
  - Chest x-ray
- Treatment
  - Perform surgical closure or patch
  - Perform cardiac catheterization with septal occluder

2b Atrial Septal Defect
- Figure 19-6

2c Patent Ductus Arteriosus
- Manifestations
  - Full, bounding pulse, dyspnea, tachypnea
  - Delayed growth patterns
  - Continuous systolic murmur
  - Pulmonic thrill at LSB, 2nd to 4th ICS

2d Patent Ductus Arteriosus
- Diagnosis
  - Chest x-ray, ECG, echocardiogram
- Treatment
  - Administer indomethacin or nonsteroidal anti-inflammatory
  - Surgical ligation
  - Surgical closure with transcatheter, obstructive device

2e Ventricular Septal Defect
- Manifestations
  - May be asymptomatic
  - Dyspnea, tachypnea
  - Delayed growth patterns, reduced fluid intake
  - Congestive heart failure, pulmonary disease
  - Systolic murmur

2f Ventricular Septal Defect
- Diagnosis
  - Chest x-ray, ECG, echocardiogram
- Treatment
  - May close spontaneously
  - Perform Rashkind procedure, permanent closure
  - Administer antibiotics

2g Tetralogy of Fallot
- Manifestations
  - Cyanosis, hypoxia
  - Delayed growth, polycythemia, metabolic acidosis
  - Exercise intolerance, clubbing of fingers
  - Systolic murmur

2h Tetralogy of Fallot
- Diagnosis
  - Chest x-ray, ECG, echocardiogram
  - Cardiac catheterization
- Treatment
  - Perform surgical correction of all defects

2i Coarctation of the Aorta
- Manifestations
  - May be asymptomatic, growth patterns unaffected
  - Blood pressure higher in arms than legs
  - Weak pulses in legs
  - Bounding pulses in arms, neck, head
  - Weakness and pain in legs with exercise

2j Coarctation of the Aorta
- Diagnosis
  - Chest x-ray, SCG, MRI
- Treatment
  - Perform balloon dilation, anastomosis
  - Perform surgical resection
  - Teach parents signs and symptoms, may recur

2k Transposition of the Great Arteries
- Manifestations
  - Cyanosis—no improvement with oxygen administration
  - Hypoxia, acidosis, tachypnea, delayed growth
  - Congestive heart failure, fatigue

2l Transposition of the Great Arteries
- Diagnosis
  - Chest-x-ray, echocardiogram
- Treatment
  - Administer Prostaglandin E1 intravenously
  - Perform surgical intervention—arterial switch
  - Balloon atrial septostomy

3 Congestive Heart Failure
- Manifestations
  - Cardiac symptoms
    - Tachycardia, poor capillary refill, peripheral edema
    - Fatigue, restlessness, cardiomegaly

3a Congestive Heart Failure
- Manifestations
  - Pulmonary symptoms
    - Dyspnea, tachypnea, cyanosis, feeding difficulties
    - Crackles, wheezing on auscultation
  - Metabolic symptoms
    - Slow weight gain, perspiration

3b Congestive Heart Failure
- Diagnosis
  - Heart x-ray, symptoms
- Treatment
  - Administer diuretics, potassium supplements, inotropic medications
  - Perform heart transplantation

4 Systemic Hypertension
- Manifestations
  - Headaches, dizziness, visual disturbances
- Diagnosis
  - 3 measurements of elevated blood pressure
  - BUN, creatinine, blood glucose, electrolytes, urinalysis
  - Complete blood count, lipid panel, echocardiogram

4a Systemic Hypertension
- Treatment
  - Encourage weight reduction, regular exercise
  - Encourage diet high in fiber

- ○ Encourage diet low in sodium, fat, calories
- ○ Administer antihypertensive medications
- ○ Teach hazards of smoking, alcohol

5 Hyperlipidemia
- • Manifestations
  - ○ Rare
- • Diagnosis
  - ○ Blood screen for cholesterol, lipoproteins, triglycerides

5a Hyperlipidemia
- • Treatment
  - ○ Encourage low fat, low cholesterol diet
  - ○ Encourage regular exercise program
  - ○ Administer cholesterol lowering medications

6 Kawasaki Disease
- • Manifestations
  - ○ Acute phase
    - – Fever, conjunctival hyperemia, red throat
    - – Swollen hands and feet, rash
    - – Enlarged cervical lymph nodes

6a Kawasaki Disease
- • Manifestations
  - ○ Acute to subacute phase
    - – Skin on lips, hands, feet slough off
    - – Joint pain, thrombosis of heart
    - – Large aneurysms of coronary arteries
    - – Myocardial infarction

6b Kawasaki Disease
- • Manifestations
  - ○ Convalescent phase
    - – Decreased inflammation
    - – Permanent heart damage

6c Kawasaki Disease
- • Figure 19-14

6d Kawasaki Disease
- • Diagnosis
  - ○ Erythrocyte sedimentation rate, platelet count
  - ○ C-reactive protein, white blood cell count
  - ○ Anemia, thrombocytosis, hypoalbuminemia
  - ○ Echocardiogram

6e Kawasaki Disease
- • Treatment
  - ○ Admit to hospital
  - ○ Administer intravenous immunoglobulin, oral aspirin

7 Acute Rheumatic Fever
- • Manifestations
  - ○ Enlarged, painful, inflamed joints (polyarthritis)
  - ○ Fever, tachycardia, red rash (erythema marginatum)
  - ○ Abnormal heart sounds, irregular heart rhythm
  - ○ *Sydenham chorea*

7a Acute rheumatic Fever
- Diagnosis
  - Clinical manifestations, antistreptolysin O titer
- Treatment
  - Administer antibiotics, anti-inflammatories, steroids

SUGGESTIONS FOR CLASSROOM ACTIVITIES

- Have students discuss medications, dosages, and adverse effects of medications used to treat cardiac disorders. Also discuss complementary or alternative medications that may be used to treat cardiac disorders.
- Develop case studies of children with various cardiac disorders. Assign groups of students to complete the case study questions and then present the case study to the rest of the class.

SUGGESTIONS FOR CLINICAL ACTIVITIES

- Arrange for students to observe cardiac surgery in the operating room. Have them share their observations in postconference.
- Have students practice cardiac assessments on each other in the clinical laboratory.

LEARNING OUTCOME 4

Explain appropriate nursing interventions for children with cardiovascular disorders.

CONCEPTS FOR LECTURE

1. Obtaining an accurate blood pressure measure in children with cardiovascular disorders is important. The appropriate size cuff is important.

   Nursing care for children with cardiac disorders should include assessing oxygen status, promoting oxygenation, and energy conservation. Assessment should include fluid and electrolyte balance.

2. Because rheumatic fever most often occurs following a strep infection, the nurse must educate parents on the symptoms and impress on them the need to report these symptoms.

   Polyarthritis of ARF responds better to the anti-inflammatory effects of aspirin than to acetaminophen or ibuprofen. Therefore, parents should administer aspirin only under the supervision of the physician and be instructed to report symptoms of Reye's syndrome.

POWERPOINT LECTURE SLIDES

(NOTE: The number on each PPT Lecture Slide directly corresponds with the Concepts for Lecture.)

1 Congenital and Acquired Heart Disorders
- Nursing Interventions
  - Assess for congestive heart failure, murmurs
  - Promote oxygenation, position to facilitate breathing
  - Administer medications, well-balanced diet
  - Facilitate growth and development, conserve energy
  - Provide teaching for home care and support

1a Congenital and Acquired Heart Disorders
- Figure 19-15

1b Systemic Hypertension
- Nursing Interventions
  - Obtain accurate blood pressure
  - Teach family to take blood pressure
  - Teach family appropriate diet
  - Use herbs and vitamin supplements cautiously

1c Hyperlipidemia
- Nursing Interventions
  - Referral to nutritionist for appropriate diet
  - Assist child and family to make lifestyle changes
  - Encourage aerobic activity, 3 to 4 times/week

1d Kawasaki Disease
- Nursing Interventions
  - Take temperature every four hours
  - Administer large doses of aspirin
  - Assess for bleeding
  - Monitor conjunctiva, oral mucosa, skin
  - Assess for dehydration, malnutrition

PowerPoint Lecture Slides *continued*

 Kawasaki Disease
- Nursing Interventions
  - Auscultate heart every four hours
  - Provide oral and bath care gently
  - Administer intravenous fluids, soft foods
  - Maintain bed rest with repositioning and exercises
  - Teach parents home care

 Acute Rheumatic Fever
- Nursing Interventions
  - Assessment of symptoms
  - Acute phase
    - Assess temperature, heart every 4 hours
    - Administer intravenous fluids, prevent overload
    - Administer antibiotics, aspirin
    - Provide quiet activities, prevent fatigue

2a Acute Rheumatic Fever
- Nursing Interventions
  - Recovery phase
    - Teach parents home care
    - Provide limited activities
    - Administer long-term antibiotic therapy
    - Administer prophylactic antibiotics for invasive procedures

---

Suggestions for Classroom Activities

- Have students develop a teaching sheet for parents of children with Kawasaki disease or acute rheumatic fever. Have them hand out the sheet in the clinical setting. Refer to Box 19-3.
- Have students write examinations questions on nursing interventions with cardiac disorders. Have them share the questions with each other.

Suggestions for Clinical Activities

- Assign students to provide nursing care for children with congenital or acquired cardiac defects or deficits in the acute care setting. Have them develop a care plan or concept map on the care they administered.
- Arrange for students to perform blood pressure checks in schools. Have them compare the blood pressures they obtained with normal blood pressure ranges. Have them teach proper diet and exercise to the children.

CHAPTER 20
CARE OF THE CHILD WITH HEMATOLOGIC OR LYMPHATIC DISORDERS

RESOURCE LIBRARY

💿 CD-ROM
Lymphatic system
Sickle cell anemia

📖 IMAGE LIBRARY

Figure 20-1 Types of blood cells: leukocytes (white blood cells).

Figure 20-2 Lymph system in the child.

Figure 20-3 (A) The lymph nodes in the neck are often palpated to determine the presence of infection. (B) Care provider assessing the lymph nodes in a young client.

Figure 20-4 Nonpalpable purpura with bleeding into the tissue below the skin.

COMPANION WEBSITE
Leukemia
Hair loss

Figure 20-5 Multisystem effects of anemia.

Figure 20-6 Pathophysiology of sickle cell anemia.

Figure 20-7 Hodgkin's disease.

Figure 20-8 Acute lymphoblastic leukemia is the most common type of leukemia in children and the most common cancer affecting children younger than 5 years.

Figure 20-9 Multisystem effects of leukemia.

Figure 20-10 Protective isolation.

LEARNING OUTCOME 1

Describe the anatomy and physiology associated with hematologic system.

CONCEPTS FOR LECTURE

1. Hematology is the study of blood and blood-forming tissues.
2. Hematopoiesis is the production of blood cells in the bone marrow.
3. The primary oxygen-carrying cell in the body is the erythrocyte or red blood cell.
4. The primary cell in the body that helps to prevent infections is the leukocyte or white blood cell.
5. The primary cell in the body that assists with clotting is the thrombocyte or platelet.
6. The liver and spleen also play roles in the hematologic system.

POWERPOINT LECTURE SLIDES

(NOTE: The number on each PPT Lecture Slide directly corresponds with the Concepts for Lecture.)

1 Anatomy and Physiology of the Hematologic System
- Hematology
  - Study of blood and blood-forming tissues
  - Blood composed of plasma and blood cells
  - Ability to deliver oxygen and other nutrients
  - Regulation of fluids, electrolytes, and acid-bases
  - Protection of body through clotting, infection control

2 Anatomy and Physiology of the Hematologic System
- Hematopoiesis
  - Production of blood cells in bone marrow
  - Erythrocytes—red blood cells
  - Leukocytes—white blood cells
  - Thrombocytes—platelets

2a Anatomy and Physiology of the Hematologic System
- Figure 20-1

3 Anatomy and Physiology of the Hematologic System
- Erythrocytes
  - Carry oxygen and carbon dioxide
  - Regulate acid-base balance
  - Erythropoiesis—production of RBCs
  - Hemolysis—destruction of RBCs

4 Anatomy and Physiology of the Hematologic System
- Leukocytes
  - Granulocytes
    - Destroy bacteria, virus, atypical cells
  - Agranulocytes
    - Development of antibodies
    - Lymphocytes

5 Anatomy and Physiology of the Hematologic System
- Thrombocytes
  - Begin process of clumping or agglutination
  - Activate clotting factors for coagulation

6 Anatomy and Physiology of the Hematologic System
- Liver
  - Produces coagulants
- Spleen
  - Produces fetal RBCs, filters RBCs, and by-products
  - Stores lymphocytes, monocytes, platelets

SUGGESTIONS FOR CLASSROOM ACTIVITIES

- Divide students into groups. Assign each group a type of cell. Have them research where the cell is formed and the purposes of the cell. Present the information to the rest of the class.

SUGGESTIONS FOR CLINICAL ACTIVITIES

- None

LEARNING OUTCOME 2

Describe the anatomy and physiology associated with the lymphatic system.

CONCEPTS FOR LECTURE

1. The lymphatic system transports fluid and filters fluid between the interstitial spaces and the intravascular system and has a role in the body's immune system.

POWERPOINT LECTURE SLIDES

(NOTE: The number on each PPT Lecture Slide directly corresponds with the Concepts for Lecture.)

1 Anatomy and Physiology of the Lymphatic System
- Lymphatic system
  - Transports and filters lymph and fluids
  - Carries away debris from destroyed bacteria
  - Infection causes swelling of lymph nodes
  - Consists of lymph, lymph capillaries, ducts, nodes
  - Lymph contains leukocytes

1a Anatomy and Physiology of the Lymphatic System
- Figure 20-2

SUGGESTIONS FOR CLASSROOM ACTIVITIES

- Review the location of the lymph node throughout the body. Demonstrate how to palpate for enlarged lymph nodes.

SUGGESTIONS FOR CLINICAL ACTIVITIES

- None

LEARNING OUTCOME 3

Discuss the clinical manifestations of disorders of the hematologic and lymphatic systems.

CONCEPTS FOR LECTURE

1. To identify disorders of the hematologic and lymphatic systems, the nurse needs to know how to complete assessments on these systems.
2. Bleeding disorders are the result of decreased amount of blood clotting factors or decreased number of platelets.
3. Anemia is a decrease in the number of red blood cells and a decrease in hemoglobin or both; caused by blood loss, destruction of red blood cells, or decrease in production of red blood cells.
4. Hodgkin's lymphoma is a rare malignant disorder of the lymphatic system.
5. Leukemia is a cancer of blood-forming organs, characterized by an increase of abnormal white blood cells. There are two types of leukemia in children: acute lymphoblastic anemia and acute myeloid leukemia.

POWERPOINT LECTURE SLIDES

(NOTE: The number on each PPT Lecture Slide directly corresponds with the Concepts for Lecture.)

1 Assessment of the Hematologic and Lymphatic Systems
- History
  ○ Complaints of weakness, fatigue
  ○ Recent illness, infection, fever
  ○ Exposure to illness or infection
  ○ Bleeding or bruising, weight loss or gain
  ○ Family history of cancer, anemia, lymph disorders

1a Assessment of the Hematologic and Lymphatic Systems
- Physical
  ○ Observe for bruising
    – Note location, size, color
  ○ Palpate lymph nodes
    – Note size, mobility, consistency, tenderness, temperature

1b Assessment of the Hematologic and Lymphatic Systems
- Figure 20-3

2 Bleeding Disorders
- Hemophilia
  ○ Manifestations
    – Bleeding into soft tissue and joints
    – Prolonged bleeding with invasive procedures
    – Joint pain, tenderness, bleeding into joints
    – Bruising, nosebleeds, hematuria

2a Bleeding Disorders
- Idiopathic Thrombocytopenic Purpura (ITP)
  ○ Manifestations
    – Purpura, petechiae, hematuria, blood in stool
    – Nosebleeds, ecchymosis
    – Recent viral infection
    – May have spontaneous remission

3 Anemias
- Iron Deficiency Anemia
  ○ Manifestations
    – Pale, tired, irritable
    – Tachycardia, muscle weakness, systolic heart murmur
    – Growth retardation, mentally delayed
    – Deformed nail beds, pica

3a Anemias
- Sickle Cell Anemia
  ○ Manifestations
    – Infant asymptomatic until 3–4 months
    – Severe pain localized to vaso-occlusion area
    – Discoloration of skin, pallor, coolness

– Nausea, fever, swelling and painful joints
– Vomiting, anorexia, diarrhea

3b Sickle Cell Anemia
- Figure 20-5

3c Anemias
- Thalassemia
  - Manifestations
    - Hemosiderin deposits cause tanned appearance
    - Pallor, lethargy, activity intolerance, headache
    - Bone pain, pathologic fractures, skeletal deformities
    - Enlarged liver and spleen

4 Hodgkin's Lymphoma
- Manifestations
  - Nontender, firm, enlarged lymph nodes
  - Fever, night sweats, weight loss
  - Respiratory distress from mediastinal lymph nodes

4a Hodgkin's Lymphoma
- Figure 20-7

5 Leukemia
- Acute lymphoblastic leukemia (ALL)
- Acute myelogenous leukemia (AML)
  - Manifestations
    - Infections, especially respiratory
    - Signs of anemia
    - Bleeding gums, bruising

5a Leukemia
- Figure 20-9

SUGGESTIONS FOR CLASSROOM ACTIVITIES

- Develop case studies of children with hematologic or lymphatic disorders. Assign groups of students to complete the case study questions and then present the case study to the rest of the class.
- Review effects of sickle cell anemia on each body system and types of sickle cell crises. Refer to Table 20-3 and Box 20-3. Discuss appropriate treatment for the disorder.

SUGGESTIONS FOR CLINICAL ACTIVITIES

- Have students practice assessments of lymph nodes on each other in the clinical lab.

LEARNING OUTCOME 4

Discuss the medical management of disorders of the hematologic and lymphatic systems.

CONCEPTS FOR LECTURE

1. Hemophilia is a deficiency in specified blood clotting factors. It is a hereditary X-linked recessive disorder that affects mostly males.
2. Idiopathic thrombocytopenic purpura is a bleeding disorder that leads to a decrease in the number of platelets.

POWERPOINT LECTURE SLIDES

(NOTE: The number on each PPT Lecture Slide directly corresponds with the Concepts for Lecture.)

1 Hemophilia
- Diagnosis
  - History, physical exam
  - Decreased factor VIII or IX

3. Iron deficiency anemia results when the demand for stored iron is more than the body can supply. It is caused by blood loss or poor intake of iron.

   A common complication of iron supplementation is constipation. Fluids, exercise, and fiber are appropriate preventative measures for this complication.

4. Sickle cell anemia is abnormally shaped red blood cells that cannot travel through capillaries, resulting in decreased blood flow and decreased oxygen-carrying capacity.

5. Thalassemia is an inherited autosomal recessive disorder, caused by abnormal hemoglobin synthesis in which red blood cells are fragile and easily destroyed.

6. Hodgkin's lymphoma is characterized by enlarged lymph nodes usually in the cervical and supraclavicular areas.

7. Acute lymphoblastic leukemia is the overproduction of immature lymphocytes, which crowd out normal white blood cells, red blood cells, and platelets.

   Acute myelogenous leukemia occurs when cancer cells develop in the bone marrow and replace normal bone marrow. Immature white blood cells, red blood cells, and platelets circulate throughout the body.

- ○ Prolonged activated partial thromboplastin time
- ○ Normal prothrombin time, thrombin time, fibrinogen, platelets

[1a] Hemophilia
- Treatment
  - ○ Administer transfusion of clotting factors
  - ○ Administer desmopressin acetate or DDAVP
  - ○ Administer aminocaproic acid to stop bleeding

[2] Idiopathic Thrombocytopenic Purpura (ITP)
- Diagnosis
  - ○ History, physical findings
  - ○ Decreased platelets, decreased antiplatelet antibodies
  - ○ Presence of antinuclear antibodies
  - ○ Positive direct Coombs' test

[2a] Idiopathic Thrombocytopenia Purpura (ITP)
- Treatment
  - ○ Administer corticosteroid therapy
  - ○ Administer intravenous immune globulin
  - ○ Transfuse platelets if hemorrhaging
  - ○ Perform splenectomy

[3] Iron Deficiency Anemia
- Diagnosis
  - ○ History, physical examination
  - ○ Decreased hemoglobin, hematocrit, reticulocyte count
  - ○ Decreased serum ferritin, serum iron concentration
  - ○ Increased RBC count, total iron-binding capacity

[3a] Iron Deficiency Anemia
- Treatment
  - ○ Administration of oral supplemental iron preparations
  - ○ Arrange dietary counseling for iron intake
  - ○ Reevaluate laboratory studies in 2 months
  - ○ Decrease iron and reevaluate in 6 months

[4] Sickle Cell Anemia
- Diagnosis
  - ○ Hemoglobin electrophoresis for infants
  - ○ Sickledex test over 6 months
  - ○ If positive Sickledex, do hemoglobin electrophoresis
  - ○ Decreased hemoglobin
  - ○ Increased reticulocyte count

[4a] Sickle Cell Anemia
- Treatment
  - ○ Administer blood transfusion, clotting factors, albumin
  - ○ Administer parenteral analgesics
  - ○ Administer intravenous fluids
  - ○ Administer oxygen therapy
  - ○ Administer prophylactic antibiotics

5 Thalassemia
- Diagnosis
  - Genetic testing in pregnancy
  - History, symptoms, physical exam
  - Hemoglobin electrophoresis, CBC
  - Chest x-ray, MRI of liver

5a Thalassemia
- Treatment
  - Administer blood transfusions every 2 to 4 weeks
  - Administer iron-chelating agent
  - Perform splenectomy if spleen enlarged

6 Hodgkin's Lymphoma
- Diagnosis
  - Family history Hodgkin's disease
  - Elevated erythrocyte sedimentation rate, leukocyte counts
  - Lymph node biopsy, staging laparotomy
  - CT or MRI scans, lymphangiogram
  - Blood counts, bone marrow biopsy

6a Hodgkin's Lymphoma
- Treatment
  - Administer four or five antineoplastic agents
  - Observe for side effects of antineoplastic agents
  - Administer low-dose radiation

7 Leukemia
- Diagnosis
  - Elevated leukocytes
  - Abnormal lymphoblasts in bone marrow aspirate
  - Decreased red blood cell count
  - Decreased platelet count

7a Leukemia
- Treatment
  - Administer antibiotics, blood replacement, chemotherapy, radiation
  - Perform bone marrow transplant
  - Maintain sterile environment after transplant

SUGGESTIONS FOR CLASSROOM ACTIVITIES

- Have students discuss chemotherapy medications, dosages, and adverse effects of medications. Also discuss ways to minimize the adverse effects of the medications.
- Have students develop a teaching sheet for parents of children with hemophilia. Hand out the teaching sheet at health fairs or in the acute care setting. Refer to Box 20-1.

SUGGESTIONS FOR CLINICAL ACTIVITIES

- Have students view laboratory study results of their assigned clients. Discuss abnormal results in relation to the type of cell, where it is formed, and the reason for the abnormality.

LEARNING OUTCOME 5

Discuss nursing considerations related to disorders of the hematologic and lymphatic systems.

CONCEPTS FOR LECTURE

1. The priority nursing intervention when caring for a child with hemophilia is to prevent bleeding with the use of applying pressure, elevating the site, applying ice, monitoring vital signs, and obtaining venous access.

2. When caring for the child with iron deficiency anemia, the nurse must teach the child and the family about adequate dietary sources of iron.

   Liquid iron preparation causes staining of the teeth. The nurse can administer these preparations through a straw to prevent this complication.

3. Children who suffer from sickle cell crises experience pain. The nurse must be vigilant in assisting the child to properly manage their pain.

4. Preventing infection in children with leukemia is a priority nursing intervention.

5. Children, especially adolescents, must be assisted by the nurse in dealing with the side effects of antineoplastic drugs, which include bone marrow depression, nausea, vomiting, stomatitis, and hair loss.

POWERPOINT LECTURE SLIDES

(NOTE: The number on each PPT Lecture Slide directly corresponds with the Concepts for Lecture.)

1 Hemophilia
- Nursing Interventions
  - Prevent bleeding
    - Apply pressure to bleeding area
    - Elevate the site, apply ice to wound
    - Monitor vital signs
    - Start intravenous access to administer clotting factors

1a Hemophilia
- Nursing Interventions
  - Teach safety measures to prevent injury
  - Teach to avoid medications that alter clotting
  - Teach to wear medic-alert bracelet
  - Avoid rectal temperatures, rectal suppositories
  - Avoid unnecessary invasive procedures

2 Idiopathic Thrombocytopenic Purpura (ITP)
- Nursing Interventions
  - Control bleeding
  - Teach measures to decrease risk of bleeding
  - Teach signs and symptoms of occult bleeding

2a Iron Deficiency Anemia
- Nursing Interventions
  - Teach parents high-iron diet
  - Feed infants formula containing iron
  - Administer liquid iron preparations
    - Dilute and give through straw
    - Avoid constipation, overdose

3 Sickle Cell Anemia
- Nursing Interventions
  - Observe for pallor, fatigue, lethargy, irritability
  - Encourage diet high in calories, protein, fluids
  - Prevent infection, handwashing, avoid infected people
  - Administer immunizations, prophylactic antibiotics
  - Administer blood products, watch for reaction

3a Sickle Cell Anemia
- Nursing Interventions
  - Administer pharmacologic and nonpharmacologic pain relief
  - Ensure compliance with preventative measures
  - Help child family with coping measures
  - Refer to support groups

3b Thalassemia
- Nursing Interventions
  - Use strategies to minimize infection
  - Help child conserve energy
  - Teach family about disease and treatment

Hodgkin's Lymphoma
- Nursing Interventions
  - Give psychosocial support
  - Teach to avoid exposure to infection
  - Assist RN to administer intravenous antineoplastic agents
  - Assess for signs of infection, open lesions
  - Teach caretaker to prevent contamination of body fluids

 Leukemia
- Nursing Interventions
  - Assessment of bruising, bleeding, fever, infection
  - Monitor specific gravity, intake and output
  - Obtain daily weight
  - Monitor nausea, vomiting, constipation, mouth sores
  - Assess nutrition status, fluid balance

 Leukemia
- Nursing Interventions
  - Assist with side effects of medications
  - Assure rest periods, safe activities
  - Provide support and teaching
  - Organize interdisciplinary resources
  - Refer to support groups

SUGGESTIONS FOR CLASSROOM ACTIVITIES

- Have students research Web sites for new medications and treatments for cancer in children. Share the Web sites in class.

SUGGESTIONS FOR CLINICAL ACTIVITIES

- Assign students to provide nursing care for children with hematologic or lymphatic disorders in the acute-care setting. Have them develop a care plan or concept map on the care they administered.
- Have students assist the primary nurse with a blood transfusion. Review the procedure for administration and interventions for a blood transfusion reaction. Refer to Box 20-4.

CHAPTER 21
CARE OF THE CHILD WITH IMMUNE DISORDERS

RESOURCE LIBRARY

 CD-ROM

HIV/AIDS
Allergic rhinitis

COMPANION WEBSITE

Cell division
HIV/AIDS
Organ donor

IMAGE LIBRARY

Figure 21-1 Primary immune response.
Figure 21-2 The development and differentiation of lymphocytes shows how cell-mediated immunity works.
Figure 21-3 Oral thrush is a common finding in clients with HIV.
Figure 21-4 (A) Stretching exercises are an important part of physical therapy for a child who has juvenile rheumatoid arthritis. (B) Swimming is very helpful for maintaining joint function in children with JRA.

Figure 21-5 Butterfly rash of systemic lupus erythematosus.
Figure 21-6 (A) Inflammation of the skin caused by the metal salts in jewelry. (B) Inflammation of the lip caused by allergic reaction to peanuts.
Figure 21-7 Skin testing to determine the source of allergic reaction.
Figure 21-8 Parents and older children need instruction in use of the EpiPen, which should be carried with the child at all times.

LEARNING OUTCOME 1

Discuss the anatomy and physiology of the pediatric immunological system.

CONCEPTS FOR LECTURE

1. The primary role of the immune system is to recognize and eliminate foreign substances, which provides protection against many diseases.
2. There are two types of immunity: natural and acquired.
3. There are two types of acquired immunity: humoral and cell-mediated.
   Active immunity is the mechanism by which immunizations provide protection against childhood diseases.
4. Passive immunity is provided by administering immunoglobulins to protect against diseases to which the child has been exposed.

POWERPOINT LECTURE SLIDES

(NOTE: The number on each PPT Lecture Slide directly corresponds with the Concepts for Lecture.)

1 Anatomy and Physiology of the Immunological System
   - Immune Response
     ○ Antigens
       – Foreign substances
     ○ Antibodies
       – Proteins produced to attack antigens

2 Anatomy and Physiology of the Immunological System
   - Natural Immunity
     ○ Present at birth
     ○ Lasts three to six months
     ○ Intact skin, body pH hostile to antigens
     ○ Antibodies against antigens
     ○ Body processes of inflammation and phagocytosis

3 Anatomy and Physiology of the Immunological System
- Acquired Immunity
  - Develops over time by exposure to substances
  - Humoral immunity
    - Immunoglobulins
    - Primary immune response
    - Secondary immune response

3a Primary Immune Response
- Figure 21-1

3b Anatomy and Physiology of the Immunological System
- Acquired Immunity
  - Cell-Mediated Immunity
    - Thymus produces lymphocytes
    - Attack foreign substances
    - T lymphocytes, B lymphocytes, natural killer cells

3c Cell-Mediated Immunity
- Figure 21-2

4 Anatomy and Physiology of the Immunological System
- Active Immunity
  - Immunizations
  - Antigen given to produce antibodies
- Passive Immunity
  - Immunoglobulins
  - Protect when exposed to disease

SUGGESTIONS FOR CLASSROOM ACTIVITIES

- Compare the types of immunity. Have the students give examples of each type of immunity.

SUGGESTIONS FOR CLINICAL ACTIVITIES

- Arrange for students to administer immunizations in a pediatrician's office or in the acute care setting.

LEARNING OUTCOME 2

Describe immunological disorders to include HIV, AIDS, juvenile rheumatoid arthritis, and allergies.

CONCEPTS FOR LECTURE

1. Congenital immune disorders may affect humoral and cellular immunity or immunoglobulins.
2. The infant can contract HIV via the placenta during pregnancy, by exposure at birth, or through breast milk. The adolescent can be exposed to the virus by sexual contact and intravenous drug use.
3. Juvenile rheumatoid arthritis is a chronic autoimmune disorder that causes joint and surrounding tissue inflammation.
4. Systemic lupus erythematosus is an autoimmune connective tissue and blood vessel disease that causes inflammation in any organ of the body.

POWERPOINT LECTURE SLIDES

(NOTE: The number on each PPT Lecture Slide directly corresponds with the Concepts for Lecture.)

1 Congenital Immune Disorders
- Severe Combined Immunodeficiency Disease (SCID)
  - Absent humoral and cellular immunity
  - Lack of functioning T and B cells
  - Genetic mutations cause impaired lymphoid development

1a Congenital Immune Disorders
- Common Variable Immunodeficiency
  - Acquired hypogammaglobulinemia
  - Low level circulating immunoglobulins
  - Occurs equally in male and female adolescents

5. Allergies are altered reactions to antigens or allergens. Latex allergy is an IgE-mediated response to repeated exposure to latex.

2 HIV and AIDS
- Human Immunodeficiency Virus
  - Retrovirus that causes AIDS
  - Perinatal transmission, during birth, breast milk
  - Transmitted through unprotected sexual activity
  - Transmitted through intravenous drug use

2a HIV and AIDS
- Acquired Immunodeficiency Syndrome
  - Defect in cell-mediated immunity
  - Difficulty fighting infections

3 Juvenile Rheumatoid Arthritis
- Autoimmune disorder causing joint inflammation
  - Body perceives own cells as foreign
  - Body attacks itself
  - Periods of remission are common

4 Systemic Lupus Erythematosus
- Autoimmune disease of connective tissue, blood vessels
  - Inflammation in any organ
  - Increased incidence in African American, Asian, Hispanic children

5 Allergies
- Altered reaction to an antigen or allergen
  - Reactions to allergen occur with repeated exposure

5a Allergies
- Latex allergy
  - IgE-mediated response to repeated latex exposure
  - Type I—local or systemic
  - Type IV—delayed hypersensitivity
  - Allergies to bananas, avocados, potatoes, tropical fruits
  - Allergies to gloves, drains, adhesives, catheters

SUGGESTIONS FOR CLASSROOM ACTIVITIES

- Assign students to view animations on the CD-ROM on HIV, AIDS, and cell structure.
- Ask students whether they have any allergies or have had an anaphylactic reaction. Have them discuss the medications they use or have used for the allergic reaction.

SUGGESTIONS FOR CLINICAL ACTIVITIES

- Have students discuss how they feel about taking care of HIV/AIDS clients. Discuss the needs of these clients and the use of Standard Precautions when providing nursing care.

LEARNING OUTCOME 3

Discuss clinical manifestations, diagnostic procedures, medical management, and nursing interventions related to immunological disorders.

CONCEPTS FOR LECTURE

1. To perform an assessment of the immunological system, the nurse needs to understand how the body protects itself against diseases.
2. Congenital immune disorders decrease the infant's ability to fight off infections.
3. The child who develops AIDS is immunocompromised. The nurse must be diligent in assisting the child and family in preventing infections.

   The nurse should teach the client that risk for perinatal transmission is significantly reduced if the mother receives zidovudine therapy during pregnancy and if the infant is delivered by cesarean section.
4. Both juvenile rheumatoid arthritis and systemic lupus erythematosus cause inflammation and therefore discomfort and pain in affected children. The nurse must assist the child in maintaining mobility and preventing pain.
5. Corticosteroid therapy is commonly prescribed for treatment of systemic lupus erythematosus. There are numerous side effects to monitor for when administering corticosteroids.
6. Careful history taking is required to assist the diagnosis of allergies. Common allergies in children include pet fur, cockroaches, cow's milk, dust, egg whites, medications, mites, mold, pollen, peanuts, seafood, shellfish, soy, tree nuts, and wheat.
7. Anaphylactic shock is a systemic reaction to an allergen that occurs within minutes or up to 2 hours after exposure. Anaphylaxis symptoms, if not treated promptly, can lead to respiratory distress and death.
8. Immunotherapy is the prevention and treatment of disease with medications.

POWERPOINT LECTURE SLIDES

(NOTE: The number on each PPT Lecture Slide directly corresponds with the Concepts for Lecture.)

1 Assessment of the Immunological System
- History
  - Recent illnesses or infections
  - Allergy symptoms
  - Stiffness or pain in joints
  - Appetite
  - Immunization record

1a Assessment of the Immunological System
- Physical
  - Obtain height and weight, vital signs
  - Inspect oral cavity for thrush
  - Inspect skin for lesions
  - Assess range of motion in joints
  - Palpate lymph nodes

2 Severe Combined Immunodeficiency Disease (SCID)
- Manifestations
  - Susceptible to infections
- Treatment
  - Intravenous immunoglobulin, prophylactic antibiotics
  - Hematopoietic stem cell transplant
  - Enzyme replacement therapy

2a Common Variable Immunodeficiency
- Manifestations
  - Susceptible to infections
- Treatment
  - Regular administration of immunoglobulins
  - Regular administration of antibiotics

3 HIV and AIDS
- Manifestations
  - Chronic otitis media, fever, skin irritation
  - Failure to thrive, lack of weight gain
  - Chronic diarrhea, hepatosplenomegaly
  - Lymphadenopathy, oral candidiasis
  - Karposi's sarcoma

3a HIV and AIDS
- Figure 21-3

3b HIV and AIDS
- Diagnosis
  - Polymerase chain reaction test (PCR)
  - Enzyme-linked immunosorbent assay (ELISA)
  - OraQuick Advance HIV 1/2 Antibody Test

3c HIV and AIDS
- Treatment
  - Administer antiretroviral agents
  - Perform cesarean delivery of infant

- Prophylactic antibiotics and immune globulin for newborns
- Administer antifungal medications for oral candidiasis

3d HIV and AIDS
- Nursing Interventions
  - Reduce infection, reverse isolation
  - Assess physical and mental functioning
  - Promote growth and development
  - Use proper sterile technique
  - Avoid invasive procedures if possible

3e HIV and AIDS
- Nursing Interventions
  - Use and teach proper handwashing
  - Teach to avoid individuals with infections
  - Administer immunizations
  - Promote respirations with deep breathing exercises
  - Promote nutrition with proteins, vitamins, antioxidants

4 Juvenile Rheumatoid Arthritis
- Manifestations
  - Fever, rash, lymphadenopathy, splenomegaly, hepatomegaly
  - Limp or favor one extremity
  - Pain, stiffness, swelling of joints
  - Loss of movement of joints

4a Juvenile Rheumatoid Arthritis
- Diagnosis
  - Clinical symptoms
  - Positive rheumatoid factor
  - Human leukocyte antigen B27
  - Antinuclear antibody

4b Juvenile Rheumatoid Arthritis
- Treatment
  - Relieve pain and joint inflammation
    - Administer salicylates and NSAIDS
  - Arrange physical therapy to prevent contractures
    - Range-of-motion exercises, hydrotherapy
    - Muscle strengthening, warm compresses
  - Provide adequate nutrition

4c Juvenile Rheumatoid Arthritis
- Figure 21-4

4d Juvenile Rheumatoid Arthritis
- Nursing Interventions
  - Administer medication, teach side effects
  - Arrange for physical therapy to increase mobility
  - Arrange for school attendance
  - Help child develop a positive self-image
  - Referrals for home care

5 Systemic Lupus Erythematosus
- Manifestations
  - Erythematous butterfly rash on face, mouth ulcers
  - Photosensitivity, swollen and painful joints
  - Alopecia, Raynaud's phenomenon, anemia, headache

5a Systemic Lupus Erythematosus
- Manifestations
  - Memory loss, weight loss, fatigue, nephritis
  - Low-grade fever, seizures, mood changes
  - Pericarditis, myocardial infarction, pleuritis
  - Periods of exacerbation and remission

5b Systemic Lupus Erythematosus
- Diagnosis
  - Physical findings
  - Positive antinuclear antibodies, antiphospholipid antibodies
  - Anti–double-stranded DNA antibodies
  - Decreased RBCs, WBCs, platelets
  - Blood, protein, cast cells in urine

5c Systemic Lupus Erythematosus
- Diagnosis
  - Kidney biopsy, x-rays, ECG
  - Echogram, EEG
  - MRI, CT scans

5d Systemic Lupus Erythematosus
- Treatment
  - Administer NSAIDS—Naprosyn, Advil, Tolectin
  - Administer antimalarials—Plaquenil (hydroxychloroquine)
  - Administer corticosteroids
    - Monitor for side effects
  - Administer immunosuppressants—Imuran, Cytoxan

5e Systemic Lupus Erythematosus
- Nursing Interventions
  - Teach medication administration, report side effects
  - Teach infection prevention, symptoms to report
  - Administer immunizatons
  - Explore feelings and body image disturbances

5f Systemic Lupus Erythematosus
- Nursing Interventions
  - Teach to protect skin from sun exposure
    - Wear sunscreen, appropriate clothing
  - Assess diet
    - Teach to eat fruits and vegetables
    - Low in salt and sugar

6 Allergies
- Manifestations
  - Mild, severe, threatening
  - Type I—localized or systemic

○ Type II—tissue specific
○ Type III—immune complex
○ Type IV—delayed

 Allergies
- Figure 21-6

 Allergies
- Diagnosis
  ○ History
  ○ Intradermal testing to identify antigens
  ○ Remove one food at a time

 Allergies
- Treatment
  ○ Administer oral antihistamines
  ○ Desensitization

Allergies
- Figure 21-7

 Allergies
- Nursing Interventions
  ○ Assess for hypersensitivity reactions or infusion reactions
  ○ Teach how to avoid allergens
  ○ Teach how to administer epinephrine or EpiPen
  ○ Teach care of EpiPen for anaphylactic reaction
  ○ Arrange for EpiPen at home, school, day care

 Allergies
- Figure 21-8

Immunotherapy
- Prevention and treatment of disease
- Administration of allergens, immunostimulants, immunosuppressants
- Administration of interferon, immune globulin IM or IV

Suggestions for Classroom Activities

- Develop case studies of children with various immunological disorders. Assign groups of students to complete the case study questions and then present the case study to the rest of the class.
- Invite a pediatric oncology nurse to speak to the class about nursing care to children with cancer. Discuss how to achieve growth and developmental progress with frequent hospitalizations.
- Invite a dietician to talk to the students about diets for immunosuppressant children, especially with cancer and HIV or AIDS. Discuss how to feed children with nausea and vomiting from chemotherapy treatments.
- Prioritize nursing interventions for a child who has a hypersensitivity reaction. Refer to Box 21-4.

Suggestions for Clinical Activities

- Assign students to provide nursing care for children with immunological disorders in the acute care setting. Have them develop a care plan or concept map on the care they administered.
- Review laboratory studies of children with immunological diseases. Have students identify the laboratory studies with the disease process that causes the disorder.

LEARNING OUTCOME 4

Describe the care of children requiring organ transplants.

CONCEPTS FOR LECTURE

1. Kidneys, hearts, bone marrow, tissues, corneas, and other organs can be transplanted in children.
2. Donors for organs can come from either living and deceased individuals or animals.
3. The nurse can assist in preparing the child for organ transplantation and providing postoperative care to prevent rejection of the organ.

POWERPOINT LECTURE SLIDES

(NOTE: The number on each PPT Lecture Slide directly corresponds with the Concepts for Lecture.)

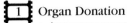 Organ Donation
- Autogenous graft
  - Graft transplanted from one site to another
  - Graft from same recipient
- Xenograft
  - Graft from animal to human

1a Organ Donation
- Major organ transplants
  - From brain dead individuals
  - Confirmed by clinical signs and medical testing
    - Cerebral blood flow studies
    - EEG

1b Organ Donation
- Organ Screening
  - Screen for compatibility, malignancy, diabetes mellitus
  - Screen for drug abuse, hypertension, HIV
  - Screen for hepatitis B or C, syphilis, TB, septicemia
- Donor consent
  - Consent from client or family member

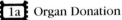 Organ Donation
- Living Donors
  - Need psychological support
  - Understand associated risks
  - Follow-up care

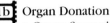 Organ Transplant
- Nursing Interventions
  - Preoperative care
    - Evaluate physical and emotional readiness
    - Teach administration of immunosuppressant medications
    - Control environment to protect organ from microorganisms

3a Organ Transplant
- Nursing Interventions
  - Postoperative care
    - Provide emotional and physical care
    - Evaluate maintenance of function of organ
    - Monitor for signs of rejection, infection
    - Administer immunosuppressant medications

SUGGESTIONS FOR CLASSROOM ACTIVITIES

- Discuss types of organs that can be transplanted and the signs and symptoms to monitor for in an organ rejection.
- Assign students to research a medication used for immunosuppressant therapy. Have students look at use of the medication, dosage, and adverse effects of the immunosuppressant medication. Have them share the information with each other.
- Discuss cultural and religious beliefs regarding organ donation. Discuss the legal and ethical issues involved in organ transplantation. Refer to Box 21-3.

SUGGESTIONS FOR CLINICAL ACTIVITIES

- If possible, arrange for students to visit an organ transplant unit in an acute-care setting or arrange for a nurse from an organ transplant unit to talk to students about care of a child with an organ transplant.

CHAPTER 22
CARE OF THE CHILD
WITH GASTROINTESTINAL DISORDERS

RESOURCE LIBRARY

 CD-ROM

Digestive system
Gavage feeding

 COMPANION WEBSITE

Liver
Probiotics

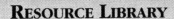 **IMAGE LIBRARY**

Figure 22-1 Organs of the alimentary canal and related accessory organs.
Figure 22-2 Salivary glands.
Figure 22-3 (A) Bilateral cleft lip. (B) Repaired bilateral cleft lip.
Figure 22-4 Esophageal atresia and tracheoesophageal fistula.
Figure 22-5 Gastrostomy tube feeding into stomach.
Figure 22-6 Imperforate anus.
Figure 22-7 (A) McBurney's point is the common location of pain in children and adolescents with appendicitis. (B) Appendectomy.

Figure 22-8 Nursing strategies to address altered perception of body image and increase feelings of independence are important when working with an adolescent who has an ostomy.
Figure 22-9 Healthy-appearing stoma.
Figure 22-10 Multisystem effects of malnutrition.
Figure 22-11 Pathophysiology of hepatitis.
Figure 22-12 Pyloric stenosis results in symptoms of projectile vomiting and visible peristalsis.
Figure 22-13 Selective causes of mechanical obstruction.

LEARNING OUTCOME 1

Describe the basic structures and functioning of the GI tract and accessory structures.

CONCEPTS FOR LECTURE

1. To understand treatment of gastrointestinal disorders, the LPN/LVN must have an understanding of the anatomy and physiology of the gastrointestinal system.

   The primary organs are hollow-like structures through which food is digested and solid waste is eliminated.

   Deciduous teeth erupt beginning around 6 months of age and continue until 2 years of age until all 20 are in place.

   Deciduous teeth are replaced by 32 permanent teeth beginning around 6 years of age and continuing until 17 to 24 years of age.

   Salivary glands empty secretions into the oral cavity to begin digestion.

2. Hydrochloric acid and digestive enzymes are released into the stomach to break down food into a semiliquid substance called chyme.

   In the small intestines, the duodenum continues chemical digestion with intestinal enzymes, and the jejunum and ileum absorb the nutrients.

POWERPOINT LECTURE SLIDES

(NOTE: The number on each PPT Lecture Slide directly corresponds with the Concepts for Lecture.)

1 Anatomy and Physiology of the GI Tract
- Primary Organs
  - Hollow tubelike structures
    - Lined with mucous membranes
    - Peristalsis
    - Food is digested
    - Solid waste is eliminated

1a Anatomy and Physiology of the GI Tract
- Figure 22-1

1b Anatomy and Physiology of the GI Tract
- Primary Organs
  - Oral cavity
    - Hard and soft palate, uvula
    - Tongue, lingual fermium, papillae
    - Cheeks, gingival
    - Teeth—deciduous, permanent

The large intestine removes water from the chyme, leaving the solid waste or feces, which are expelled through the anus.

The accessory organs of the gastrointestinal system are the liver and pancreas, which aid in the digestion process.

The liver stores blood; produces clotting factors; stores proteins, fats, glucose, iron, vitamins; and detoxifies drugs, hormones, and other substances.

Chemical digestion is the breakdown of food into small particles that can be absorbed into the blood.

1c Anatomy and Physiology of the GI Tract
- Primary Organs
  - Salivary glands
    - Parotid gland
    - Submandibular gland
    - Sublingual gland

1d Anatomy and Physiology of the GI Tract
- Figure 22-2

1e Anatomy and Physiology of the GI Tract
- Primary Organs
  - Esophagus
    - Cardiac sphincter
  - Stomach
    - Hydrochloric acid, digestive enzymes, mucus released
    - Chyme—semi-liquid digested food

1f Anatomy and Physiology of the GI Tract
- Primary Organs
  - Small intestine
    - Duodenum
    - Jejunum
    - Ileum
    - Ileocecal valve—joins ileum and cecum

1g Anatomy and Physiology of the GI Tract
- Primary Organs
  - Large intestine or colon
    - Cecum, appendix
    - Ascending, transverse, descending, sigmoid colon
    - Water removed from chyme, leaving feces
    - Anus

1h Anatomy and Physiology of the GI Tract
- Accessory Organs
  - Liver
    - Produces and excretes bile, detoxifies chemicals
    - Catabolism, anabolism, breaks down RBCs
    - Production of blood clotting factors, plasma proteins
    - Recycles needed chemicals, regulates blood glucose

1i Anatomy and Physiology of the GI Tract
- Accessory Organs
  - Pancreas
    - Releases pancreatic juice into pancreatic duct
    - Produces glycogen and insulin
    - Regulates blood glucose

2 Anatomy and Physiology of the GI Tract
- Chemical Digestion
  - Begins in mouth
    - Amylase starts food breakdown
  - Enters stomach
    - Hydrochloric acid and enzymes produce chyme
  - Duodenum changes pH, bile excreted

2a Anatomy and Physiology of the GI Tract
- Chemical Digestion
  - Pancreatic enzymes further change chyme
  - Absorbed into blood
    - Glucose, galactose
    - Amino acids, fatty acids, glycerol

SUGGESTIONS FOR CLASSROOM ACTIVITIES

- Assign students to view the animation of the digestion system tour on the textbook CD-ROM.
- Assign students to complete the interactivities: match the digestive system and match the intestinal wall on the textbook CD-ROM.

SUGGESTIONS FOR CLINICAL ACTIVITIES

- In the clinical laboratory, have students review the anatomy of the gastrointestinal system on a model of the gastrointestinal system. Discuss the physiology of the primary and accessory organs of the gastrointestinal system.

LEARNING OUTCOME 2

Describe major gastrointestinal disorders in clear, simple terms.

CONCEPTS FOR LECTURE

1. Gastrointestinal disorders in children include congenital malformations, malabsorption conditions, and problems with motility.

    Gastrointestinal disorders are potentially life-threatening due to fluid and electrolyte imbalance and malnutrition.

    Congenital defects of the gastrointestinal system are the most common of the congenital defects but are not usually life-threatening.
2. Children with gastrointestinal inflammatory diseases should be placed on enteric precautions.
3. Intestinal parasite outbreaks occur in areas where water is not treated, poor sanitation exists, food is not properly cooked, or children play in contaminated dirt or sandboxes.
4. Malabsorption disorders result from lack of nutrients in diet, inability of small intestine to absorb nutrients, or liver disorders that result in lack of bile for digestion and alter metabolism of nutrients.
5. Nutrition disorders may have physical or environmental causes.
6. Hepatic disorders may cause destruction of the liver, necessitating a liver transplant.
7. Motility disorders prevent gastrointestinal contents from moving through the system in a normal manner.
8. Most poisonings of toxic substances occur in the home.

POWERPOINT LECTURE SLIDES

(NOTE: The number on each PPT Lecture Slide directly corresponds with the Concepts for Lecture.)

1 Congenital Gastrointestinal Defects
- Cleft Lip
  - Upper lip fails to join medially
  - Bilateral or unilateral
- Cleft Palate
  - Medial nasal and maxillary processes fail to join
  - Complete or partial

1a Congenital Gastrointestinal Defects
- Tracheoesophageal Fistula
  - Connection between trachea and esophagus
  - Oral intake enters trachea through fistula
- Esophageal Atresia
  - Esophagus ends in blind pouch
  - Ends before entering stomach

1b Tracheoesophageal Fistula and Esophageal Atresia
- Figure 22-4

1c Congenital Gastrointestinal Defects
- Imperforate Anus
  - Thin membrane covering anus
  - Malformation of flat anus or deep dimple

 2 Gastrointestinal Inflammation
- Gastroenteritis
  - Inflammation of stomach
  - Caused by bacteria, virus, toxins, allergies
  - Results in mild to severe dehydration

 2a Gastrointestinal Inflammation
- Appendicitis
  - Inflammation of vermiform appendix
  - Common in boys between 10 and 16
  - Blockage of lumen of appendix

○ Followed by infection and inflammation
○ Risk of rupture and peritonitis

2b Appendicitis
- Figure 22-7

2c Gastrointestinal Inflammation
- Inflammatory bowel disease
  ○ Crohn's disease
    – Inflammation of entire gastrointestinal tract
    – Involves all layers of bowel wall
  ○ Ulcerative colitis
    – Inflammation with mucosa slough of large intestine

3 Intestinal Parasites
- Caused by untreated water, poor sanitation
- Caused by not properly cooked food
- Caused by play in contaminated dirt, sandbox

4 Malabsorption Disorders
- Celiac disease
  ○ Chronic malabsorption syndrome
  ○ Unable to digest gluten
  ○ Results in increase in glutamine, steatorrhea
  ○ Damages intestinal villi
  ○ Decreases absorption of nutrients

4a Malabsorption Disorders
- Lactose Intolerance
  ○ Failure to produce lactase
  ○ Congenital or acquired disorder

5 Nutrition Disorders
- Kwashiorkor
  ○ Deficiency in protein
  ○ Results in muscle wasting and malnutrition
  ○ Protein deficiency with adequate calories

5a Nutrition Disorders
- Rickets
  ○ Vitamin D deficiency
  ○ Improper absorption of calcium and phosphorus
  ○ Improper utilization of calcium and phosphorus
  ○ Failure of bones to develop

5b Nutrition Disorders
- Scurvy
  ○ Lack of vitamin C in diet
  ○ Lack of citrus fruits, raw leafy vegetables

5c Nutrition Disorders
- Failure to Thrive
  ○ Failure to gain weight
  ○ Loss of weight
  ○ Unknown cause—physical or environmental

6 Hepatic Disorders
- Biliary Atresia
  ○ Failure of bile ducts to form properly
  ○ Obstruction of bile ducts

○ Back-up of bile destroys liver
○ Requires liver transplant

6a Hepatic Disorders
• Hepatitis
  ○ Inflammation of the liver
  ○ Caused by a viral infection
  ○ There are five types of hepatitis
    – Hepatitis A through hepatitis E
  ○ Fulminating hepatitis—total destruction of liver

6b Hepatic Disorders
• Hepatitis
  ○ Virus attacks parenchymal cells of liver
  ○ Local degeneration and necrosis of tissue
  ○ Inflammatory process is stimulated
  ○ Swelling and accumulation of WBC block bile
  ○ Bile backs up and damages liver

6c Hepatitis
• Figure 22-11

6d Hepatic Disorders
• Phenylketonuria
  ○ Autosomal recessive inherited disorder
  ○ Deficiency of liver enzyme, phenylalanine hydroxylase
  ○ Inability to breakdown phenylalanine into tyrosine

7 Motility Disorders
• Gastroesophageal reflux disease
  ○ Relaxation of the cardiac sphincter
  ○ Gastric contents return to esophagus

7a Motility Disorders
• Pyloric stenosis
  ○ Obstruction of pyloric canal
  ○ Caused by thickening of pyloric sphincter
  ○ Narrowing of passageway between stomach and duodenum
  ○ Mucous membranes become inflamed and swollen
  ○ Further narrowing causes total obstruction

7b Pyloric Stenosis
• Figure 22-12

7c Motility Disorders
• Colic
  ○ Acute abdominal pain
  ○ Caused by spasmodic contractions of intestines
  ○ Occurs during first three months of life

7d Motility Disorders
• Intussusception
  ○ Mechanical obstruction of small bowel
  ○ One portion telescopes into another portion
  ○ Walls of intestines rub together
    – Inflammation, swelling, obstruction
    – Ischemia, necrosis, perforation, hemorrhage

7e Intussusception
- Figure 22-13

7f Motility Disorders
- Hernia
  ○ Protrusion of stomach or intestine
  ○ Through malformation or opening in muscle
  ○ Three common locations
    – Diaphragmatic, umbilical, inguinal

7g Motility Disorders
- Meckel's Diverticulum
  ○ Outpouch in ileum
  ○ Contains gastric or pancreatic tissue
    – Secretes acid and enzymes
    – Cause irritation and ulceration

7h Motility Disorders
- Hirschsprung's Disease
  ○ Autonomic parasympathetic ganglia absent
  ○ Inadequate motility
  ○ Mechanical bowel obstruction of large intestine

8 Poisonings
- Ingestion of toxic substances
- Ingestion of poisonous household plants
- Lead poisoning
  ○ Toxic amount of lead in blood
  ○ Interferes with normal cell function
  ○ Deposits in bones and teeth

SUGGESTIONS FOR CLASSROOM ACTIVITIES

- Assign students to view the CD-ROM animation: gastroesophageal reflux disease
- Develop a crossword puzzle with answers to definitions in the puzzle.

SUGGESTIONS FOR CLINICAL ACTIVITIES

- Have students speak to children in the school system or at a health fair about the dangers of poisonings and how to treat poisonings. Refer to Table 22-5.

LEARNING OUTCOME 3

Discuss clinical manifestations, diagnostic procedures, and medical management related to gastrointestinal disorders.

CONCEPTS FOR LECTURE

1. Deep palpation of the abdomen is not the responsibility of the LPN, although it is important to understand.
2. Congenital malformation of the gastrointestinal system may require multiple surgeries to correct, and therefore, nutrition may be provided by IV administration of TPN.
3. The goal of nutritional therapy with gastrointestinal inflammatory diseases is to provide adequate calories and nutrients for growth without aggravating the inflammation and diarrhea.

POWERPOINT LECTURE SLIDES

(NOTE: The number on each PPT Lecture Slide directly corresponds with the Concepts for Lecture.)

1 Assessment of the Gastrointestinal System
- History
  ○ Question about appetite, vomiting, diarrhea, constipation
  ○ Foods eaten within 24 hours of symptoms
  ○ Family history of similar symptoms

1a Assessment of the Gastrointestinal System
- Physical
  ○ Inspect abdomen for symmetry, round, flat

4. All family members and others in direct contact with a child with a parasitic infection should be treated.
5. Most malabsorption disorders require lifelong treatment.
6. Nutrition deficiencies may occur even in a diet with adequate calories.
7. Hepatic disorders affect the ability to detoxify substances and to metabolize medications at the usual rate. Medication dosages may need to be adjusted.
8. Motility disorders need surgical treatment if medical treatment is not effective.

   Gastroesophageal reflux is more common in premature infants and children with neurological impairment. Treatment depends on the severity of the disorder.
9. Emergency treatment for poisonings is based on the goal of preventing further absorption of the poison and reversing its effects.

- ○ Auscultate abdomen for bowel sounds
- ○ Palpate abdomen for softness, firmness, tenderness
- ○ Visualize and assess anal area

[2] Cleft lip and Cleft Palate
- • Treatment
  - ○ Perform surgical correction lip with Logan clamp
  - ○ May perform revision of suture line
  - ○ Perform surgical correction palate in stages
  - ○ Begin at 4 months, complete by 2 years

[2a] Tracheoesophageal Atresia and Esophageal Atresia
- • Manifestations
  - ○ Copious amounts thin mucus after birth
  - ○ Stomach distended with trapped air
  - ○ Regurgitation with feedings, aspirate into lungs
  - ○ Severe respiratory distress, aspiration pneumonia

[2b] Tracheoesophageal Atresia and Esophageal Atresia
- • Diagnosis
  - ○ Attempt to pass 5 or 8 French catheter
  - ○ X-ray, ultrasound, echocardiogram
- • Treatment
  - ○ Perform surgical repair
  - ○ Administer gastrostomy feedings

[2c] Tracheoesophageal Atresia and Esophageal Atresia
- • Figure 22-5

[2d] Imperforate Anus
- • Diagnosis
  - ○ Meconium not passed within 24 hours of birth
  - ○ Meconium passed in urine
- • Treatment
  - ○ Perform surgical correction
  - ○ Administer intravenous fluids and nutrition

[2e] Imperforate Anus
- • Figure 22-6

[3] Gastroenteritis
- • Manifestations
  - ○ Nausea, vomiting, diarrhea, fever
  - ○ Dehydration, bleeding
- • Diagnosis
  - ○ History, clinical findings
  - ○ Stool cultures

[3a] Gastroenteritis
- • Treatment
  - ○ Administer intravenous fluids, electrolytes, antibiotics
  - ○ Place on enteric precautions
  - ○ Progress diet to full liquid, soft foods

[3b] Appendicitis
- • Manifestations
  - ○ Right lower quadrant pain, rebound tenderness
  - ○ Fever, nausea

- ○ Side-lying position with knees flexed
- ○ Rupture is sudden relief of pain

`3c` Appendicitis
- Diagnosis
  - ○ Elevated white blood cell count
  - ○ CT with contrast, abdominal x-rays

`3d` Appendicitis
- Treatment
  - ○ Preoperative care
    - – Obtain surgical consent, start intravenous fluids
    - – Administer sedation
  - ○ Perform surgery to remove appendix

`3e` Appendicitis
- Treatment
  - ○ Postoperative care
    - – Teach parents home care
  - ○ Ruptured appendix
    - – Treat peritonitis, septic shock
    - – Monitor for obstruction, electrolyte imbalance

`3f` Crohn's Disease
- Manifestations
  - ○ Onset gradual
  - ○ Abdominal cramps with diarrhea
  - ○ Subsides and recurs
  - ○ Anorexia, weight loss, general malaise

`3g` Ulcerative Colitis
- Manifestations
  - ○ Abdominal cramps, diarrhea
  - ○ Lower abdominal pain with bowel movement
  - ○ Stool mixed with mucus and blood
  - ○ Weight loss, delayed growth

`3h` Crohn's Disease and Ulcerative Colitis
- Diagnosis
  - ○ Stool specimens
  - ○ Biopsy during colonoscopy
  - ○ Lab studies for anemia, electrolyte imbalance

`3i` Crohn's Disease and Ulcerative Colitis
- Treatment
  - ○ Administer corticosteroids, antibiotics, antidiarrheals
  - ○ Administer immunosuppressants for severe Crohn's
  - ○ Provide adequate calories and nutrients
    - – Administer total parenteral nutrition
  - ○ Perform temporary colostomy or ileostomy

`3j` Crohn's Disease and Ulcerative Colitis
- Figure 22-8

`4` Intestinal Parasites
- Manifestations
  - ○ Abdominal cramps, diarrhea, weight loss

○ Anal irritation and itching
○ Intestinal obstruction
○ Liver and lung involvement

 Intestinal Parasites
• Diagnosis
  ○ Stool specimen
• Treatment
  ○ Administration of medication to all family
  ○ Collect follow-up stool specimen
  ○ Teach prevention techniques

 Celiac Disease
• Manifestations
  ○ Chronic diarrhea, vomiting, failure to grow
  ○ Large, foul-smelling, greasy, frothy stool
• Diagnosis
  ○ Symptoms
  ○ Fat is stool, intestinal biopsy

 Celiac Disease
• Treatment
  ○ Eliminate gluten from diet
  ○ Administer vitamin supplements
  ○ Monitor growth patterns

 Lactose Intolerance
• Manifestations
  ○ Diarrhea when milk consumed
• Treatment
  ○ Implement lactose-free diet
  ○ Administer soy formulas to infants
  ○ Administer enzyme tablets for milk products

 Kwashiorkor
• Manifestations
  ○ Failure to grow, muscle wasting, abdominal edema
  ○ Anorexia, diarrhea, vomiting
  ○ Hair becomes thin, brittle, lightens in color
  ○ Skin breaks down and becomes infected
  ○ Irritable, mentally dull

 Kwashiorkor
• Figure 22-10

Kwashiorkor
• Treatment
  ○ Use of powdered protein on foods
  ○ Increase protein in diet

Rickets
• Manifestations
  ○ Bowed legs, knock-knees, beading along ribs
  ○ Improper formation of teeth
• Treatment
  ○ Administer vitamins and vitamin D fortified food
  ○ Exercise in sunlight

6e Scurvy
- Treatment
  - Teach to cook vegetables at low heat
  - Administer vitamin C tablets

6f Failure to Thrive
- Manifestations
  - Irritable, weak
  - Vomiting, diarrhea, anorexia, pica
  - Apathetic, listless, limpness

6g Failure to Thrive
- Treatment
  - Hospitalize for evaluation
  - Treat malabsorption, heart, liver disorders
  - Arrange multidisciplinary approach to treatment
  - Provide care by one nurse

7 Biliary Atresia
- Manifestations
  - Jaundice, abdominal distention, hepatomegaly
  - Easily bruised, pruritis, splenomegaly, weak
  - Stools off-white or clay colored, putty consistency
  - Tea-colored urine from bilirubin excretion
  - Unable to digest fat, fat-soluble vitamins

7a Biliary Atresia
- Diagnosis
  - Elevated bilirubin, serum aminotransferase, alkaline phosphatase
  - Elevated ammonia levels, prolonged prothrombin time
  - Ultrasound to rule out cause

7b Biliary Atresia
- Treatment
  - Perform surgery
    - Hepatoportoenterostomy or Kasai procedure
  - Perform liver transplant

7c Hepatitis
- Diagnosis
  - Elevated bilirubin, ALT, alkaline phosphatase
  - Serology studies positive for antibodies to virus

7d Phenylketonuria
- Manifestations
  - Musty odor of body and urine
  - Vomiting, irritability, seizures
  - Hyperactivity, rash, mental retardation
- Diagnosis
  - Heel stick blood test screening

7e Phenylketonuria
- Treatment
  - Administer special formulas
  - Teach diet low in phenylalanine for life

8 Gastroesophageal Reflux Disease
- Diagnosis
  - Vomiting, appear hungry, irritable
  - Eat but lose weight
  - Aspiration, pneumonia, apnea

 8a Gastroesophageal Reflux Disease
- Treatment
  - Mild cases
    - Add rice cereal to thicken feedings
    - Position upright 30 degrees after feeding
    - Avoid acidic juices
    - Administer medication to reduce stomach acid

 8b Gastroesophageal Reflux Disease
- Treatment
  - Severe cases
    - Perform Nissen fundoplication
    - Administer gastrostomy feedings for 6 weeks

 8c Pyloric Stenosis
- Manifestations
  - Vomiting after feedings, projectile vomiting
  - Dehydration, weight loss
  - Passes fewer and smaller stools
  - Small round mass in right upper quadrant
  - Visible peristaltic waves, irritable, then lethargic

 8d Pyloric Stenosis
- Diagnosis
  - Abdominal ultrasound, x-ray
- Treatment
  - Perform surgical correction
    - Pyloroplasty

 8e Colic
- Diagnosis
  - Cry loudly, pull arms and legs up
  - Become red in face
  - Expel flatus or belch frequently
  - Spit up mucus, undigested milk or formula

8f Colic
- Treatment
  - Pick up infant, burp gently
  - Give warm water to drink
  - Rock and soothe infant in calm manner

 8g Intussusception
- Manifestations
  - Sudden severe abdominal pain, vomiting
  - Passage of brown stool
  - Periods of comfort with recurrence of pain
  - Stools resemble currant jelly
  - Palpable abdominal mass

8h Intussusception
- Diagnosis
  - History, barium enema

- Treatment
  - Administer barium to reduce intestine into place
  - Perform surgery to reduce, remove damage tissue

 Hernia
- Diagnosis
  - Soft swelling below umbilicus or in groin
  - Enlarges with coughing, crying, straining
- Treatment
  - May resolve spontaneously by 3–4 years
  - Perform surgery to close muscle

8j Meckel's Diverticulum
- Manifestations
  - Painless bleeding, dark or bright red stools
  - Abdominal pain, volvulus or intussusception
- Diagnosis
  - History
  - If untreated, perforation, peritonitis

8k Meckel's Diverticulum
- Treatment
  - Perform surgical removal of diverticulum
  - Perform removal of damaged tissue

8l Hirschsprung's Disease
- Manifestations
  - Infants
    - Failure to pass meconium, meconium emesis
    - Refusal to suck, abdominal distention
  - Older children
    - Constipation alternating with diarrhea, abdominal distention

8m Hirschsprung's Disease
- Diagnosis
  - History, radiographic contrast, biopsy
- Treatment
  - Encourage high fiber diet, adequate fluids
  - Administer stool softeners, isotonic enemas
  - Perform surgery, colostomy

9 Lead Poisonings
- Manifestations
  - Cognitive deficit, learning disabilities, hearing impairment
  - Growth delays, fetal malformations, premature birth
- Diagnosis
  - Blood test for Pb-B

9a Lead Poisonings
- Administer chelation therapy with chemicals

9b Other Poisonings
- Treatment
  - Call local Poison Control Center immediately
  - Bring emesis with child to emergency department
  - Treat with SIRES method
  - Perform ABCs and CPR priority treatment
  - Administer intravenous fluids, antidotes, activated charcoal

- Divide students into five groups. Assign each group a different type of hepatitis. Have them research the causes, modes of transmission, clinical manifestations, and preventative measures to teach clients. Have each group present their findings in class. Refer to Table 22-3.
- Develop case studies of infants or children with gastrointestinal disorders. Assign groups of students to complete the case study questions and then present the case study to the rest of the class.
- Arrange for an emergency department nurse to speak with students about the emergency treatment for poisonings.

- Have students practice abdominal assessments on models in the clinical laboratory to help them become more proficient with assessing assigned clients.
- Have students view laboratory and diagnostic studies on clients with gastrointestinal disorders in the acute care setting. Discuss abnormal results to identify the causative factors.

LEARNING OUTCOME 4

Explain appropriate nursing interventions for children with gastrointestinal disorders.

CONCEPTS FOR LECTURE

1. The role of the LPN/LVN in caring for children with gastrointestinal disorders is one of assisting with data collection and monitoring the effectiveness of treatments.

   In gastrointestinal disorders, nursing care focuses on meeting the infant's and child's needs for fluids and nutrition, promoting comfort, preventing infection, eliminating solid waste, and supporting the parents.

   Frequent hand washing may help to prevent intestinal parasite infestations.

   When failure-to-thrive is the result of environmental factors, the nurse must be alert in observing child/parent interaction to identify any areas of concern in the relationship.

   Nurses and other health care workers could come in contact with blood or body fluids containing hepatitis virus. Standard Precautions should be used at all times.

   Families need to be taught to administer nutrition by tube feeding or IV when long-term treatment is required.

   Nursing implications in health promotion include early detection and treatment of gastrointestinal disorders and community teaching regarding poison risks, environmental assessment, and screening individuals at risk.

POWERPOINT LECTURE SLIDES

(NOTE: The number on each PPT Lecture Slide directly corresponds with the Concepts for Lecture.)

1. Cleft Lip and Cleft Palate
   - Preoperative Nursing Interventions
     - Providing nutrition
     - Instruct parents in use of special feeders
     - Provide emotional support and encouragement
     - Arrange speech therapy

1a. Cleft Lip and Cleft Palate
   - Postoperative Nursing Interventions
     - Administer fluids through dropper or syringe
     - Position in supine or side-lying position
     - Apply soft elbow restraints
     - Administer antibiotic ointment, pain medications

1b. Cleft Lip and Cleft Palate
   - Postoperative Nursing Interventions
     - Teach parents care to prevent trauma, infection
     - Refer to speech therapy
     - Offer psychological support
     - Role model positive response to newborn

1c. Tracheoesophageal Fistula and Esophageal Atresia
   - Nursing Interventions
     - Administer preoperative care
     - Administer postoperative care
     - No oral feedings for 7 to 14 days
     - Instruct parents in home care

1d. Appendicitis
   - Nursing Interventions
     - Monitor for infection, small bowel obstruction
     - Place nasogastric tube for bowel obstruction
     - Administer intravenous fluids, antibiotics
     - Advance diet when bowel sounds return

1e Appendicitis
- Nursing Interventions
  - Teach parents home care
    - Administration of pain medication, antibiotics
    - Care of incision, follow-up visits
    - Normal activity in few days
    - No vigorous activity until approved by MD

1f Crohn's Disease and Ulcerative Colitis
- Nursing Interventions
  - Teach medication administration
  - Monitor nutritional status, TPN administration
  - Provide emotional support
  - Provide appropriate referrals
  - Demonstration of central venous catheters, ostomy care

1g Celiac Disease
- Nursing Considerations
  - Teach gluten-free diet, nutrition consult
  - Teach to read labels
  - Provide emotional support
  - Refer to support groups

1h Biliary Atresia
- Nursing Interventions
  - Provide emotional support and teaching
  - Tepid baths to relieve itching
  - Pat skin dry
  - Preoperative care

1i Biliary Atresia
- Postoperative care
  - Teach parents incision care
  - Teach parents to administer pain medication
  - Teach parents to administer immunosuppressant medications
  - Teach signs of tissue rejection

1j Hepatitis
- Nursing Interventions
  - Use Standard Precautions at all times
  - Receive 3 doses of hepatitis B immunization
  - Teach appropriate handwashing
  - Teach prevention methods
  - Administer medications carefully, monitor side effects

1k Pyloric Stenosis
- Nursing Interventions
  - Keep infant NPO, administer intravenous fluids
  - Monitor intake and output
  - Postoperative care
    - Advance diet clear fluid to formula
    - Administer pain medication, avoid pressure on incision

1l Pyloric Stenosis
- Nursing Interventions
  - Teach parents signs of incision infection

○ Teach no tub bath until healed

○ Encourage swaddling, holding, rocking

 Intussusception

- Nursing Interventions
  ○ Preoperative care
    – Keep NPO, insert nasogastric tube
  ○ Postoperative care
    – Administer intravenous fluids, analgesics
    – Teach parents medications, infection, diet

 Hernia

- Nursing Interventions
  ○ Instruct parents not to push on hernia
  ○ Instruct not to apply tape, straps
  ○ Instruct not to apply coins

 Hirschsprung's Disease

- Nursing Interventions
  ○ Observe meconium passage in infant
  ○ Monitor growth patterns, nutritional intake
  ○ Monitor bowel habits
  ○ Teach parents to give saline enemas, medications
  ○ Teach colostomy care, watch for malabsorption

 Lead Poisoning

- Nursing Interventions
  ○ Teach community poisoning risks
  ○ Perform environmental assessments
  ○ Screen individuals at risk
  ○ Teach parents risks, administration of chelation therapy
  ○ Teach to avoid all sources of lead

SUGGESTIONS FOR CLASSROOM ACTIVITIES

- Assign students to view CD-ROM videos: gastric lavage and inserting NG tube.
- Assign students to view CD-ROM animation: enema.

SUGGESTIONS FOR CLINICAL ACTIVITIES

- Assign students to provide nursing care on clients with gastrointestinal disorders. Have them develop a nursing care plan or concept map on nursing care provided.
- Review standard precautions with students before providing nursing care to children with infectious gastrointestinal disorders.

CHAPTER 23
CARE OF THE CHILD WITH GENITOURINARY DISORDERS

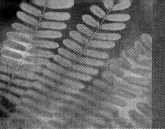

RESOURCE LIBRARY

CD-ROM
Renal corpuscle

COMPANION WEBSITE
UTI
Pelvic exam

IMAGE LIBRARY

Figure 23-1 The kidneys are located between the twelfth thoracic (T12) and the third lumbar (L3) vertebrae.

Figure 23-2 (A) Epispadias; the urethra is on the dorsal surface of the penis. (B) Hypospadias; the urethra is on the ventral surface of the penis.

Figure 23-3 This child has bladder exstrophy, noted by extrusion of the posterior bladder wall through the lower abdominal wall.

Figure 23-4 The double-diapering technique protects the urinary stent after surgery for hypospadias or epispadias repair.

Figure 23-5 The common sites of obstruction in the upper and lower urinary tract.

Figure 23-6 In acute postinfectious glomerulonephritis, an immune response to group A beta-hemolytic *Streptococcus* causes inflammation and damage to the glomerular membrane.

Figure 23-7 Young boy with edema characteristic of nephrotic syndrome or renal failure.

Figure 23-8 Multisystem effects of uremia.

Figure 23-9 This child is undergoing hemodialysis.

Figure 23-10 Hydrocele is a nontender, fluid-filled mass within the tunica vaginalis.

Figure 23-11 Testicular torsion occurs most frequently in adolescents.

LEARNING OUTCOME 1

Discuss anatomy and physiology of the pediatric urinary and reproductive systems.

CONCEPTS FOR LECTURE

1. The genitourinary system consists of structures of the urinary system and the reproductive system.
2. The primary functions of the urinary system include waste excretion; homeostasis, fluid, electrolyte, and acid-base balance; regulation of blood pressure; regulation of calcium metabolism; and stimulation of erythrocyte development.
3. At birth, the kidneys take over the functions performed by the placenta.

    The kidneys continue to develop until adolescence.

    It is important for the nurse to know the normal bladder capacity for the child according to age group.
4. The reproductive system consists of internal and external organs that will, when mature, assist the individual in achieving conception and assist the female in maintaining and achieving childbirth.

    The male and female reproductive systems function to produce, protect, and transport sperm or ova; regulate hormone production; and provide sexual pleasure.

POWERPOINT LECTURE SLIDES

(NOTE: The number on each PPT Lecture Slide directly corresponds with the Concepts for Lecture.)

 1 Anatomy and Physiology of the Urinary System
- Structures of the urinary system
  - Kidneys, ureters, bladder, urethra
  - Renal arteries and veins

1a Anatomy and Physiology of the Urinary System
- Figure 23-1

2 Anatomy and Physiology of the Urinary System
- Functions of the urinary system
  - Waste excretion, homeostasis
  - Fluid, electrolyte, acid-base balance
  - Regulation of blood pressure, calcium metabolism
  - Stimulation of erythrocyte development

3 Anatomy and Physiology of the Urinary System
- Urine production begins 3rd month of pregnancy
- Kidneys assist in maintenance of amniotic fluid

- Kidneys develop until adolescence
- Filtration refined by age 2 years
- Output increases as child ages
- Bladder capacity/oz—add age plus 2

4 Anatomy and Physiology of the Reproductive System
- Structures of the male reproductive system
  ○ Penis, scrotum, testes, prostate, epididymis
- Structures of the female reproductive system
  ○ Ovaries, fallopian tubes, uterus, cervix, vagina, vulva
- Tanner's stages of sexual development

4a Anatomy and Physiology of the Reproductive System
- Puberty
  ○ Maturation process of reproductive system
- Males
  ○ Onset between 10 and 15
- Females
  ○ Onset between ages 8 and 13

SUGGESTIONS FOR CLASSROOM ACTIVITIES

- Using illustrations of the urinary system, discuss how urine is made and the importance of urinary excretion.
- When reviewing the anatomy of the reproductive system, discuss the Tanner's system of sexual development.

SUGGESTIONS FOR CLINICAL ACTIVITIES

- Using male and female models of the urinary and reproductive systems, point out the anatomy of these systems and discuss the physiology of each part.

LEARNING OUTCOME 2

Describe urinary and reproductive disorders, including urinary tract infections, acute and chronic renal failure, Wilms' tumor, hypospadias, phimosis, cryptorchidism, ambiguous genitalia, and menstrual disorders.

CONCEPTS FOR LECTURE

1. Disorders of the urinary system that affect the child include congenital anomalies, infections, and tumors.

   While the reproductive system is immature until puberty, many congenital anomalies of the urinary system also affect the reproductive system.
2. In the infant, urinary tract infections are more common in males primarily due to structural defects. In the young child, urinary tract infections are usually caused by bacteria.
3. Urinary inflammatory disorders may be caused by an immune response to a bacterial infection.
4. Renal failure is the inability of the kidneys to remove liquid waste from the blood.
5. A gene that promotes normal kidney function is missing in a child with Wilms' tumor.
6. Enuresis is urinary incontinence in a child who has achieved continence.

POWERPOINT LECTURE SLIDES

(NOTE: The number on each PPT Lecture Slide directly corresponds with the Concepts for Lecture.)

1 Congenital Urinary Defects
- Urethral Malposition
  ○ Hypospadias
    – Urethral opening on ventral surface penis
  ○ Chordee
    – Ventral curvature of penis

1a Congenital Urinary Defects
- Figure 23-2

1b Congenital Urinary Defects
- Urethral Malposition
  ○ Epispadias
    – Urethral opening on dorsal surface penis
  ○ Bladder exstrophy
    – Protrusion of posterior wall of bladder

7. Ambiguous genitalia is a rare condition in which it is difficult to determine the sex of the child.
8. Disorders of the male reproductive system may be present at birth.
9. Female circumcision is a type of surgical procedure on young girls for cultural purposes rather than medical purposes.

    As puberty begins, adolescent girls may develop menstrual disorders.

1c Congenital Urinary Defects
- Figure 23-3

1d Obstructive Uropathy
- Altered structure or function of urinary system
  - Obstruction of urinary flow
  - Congenital
    - Polycystic kidney
  - Acquired
    - Tumors, kidney stones, crystal formation

1e Obstructive Uropathy
- Figure 23-5

2 Urinary Tract Infections
- Bacterial infections
  - Cystitis, pyelonephritis
  - Acute, chronic, persistent
- Vesicoureteral reflux
  - Urinary stasis

3 Urinary Inflammatory Disorders
- Acute Postinfectious Glomerulonephritis
  - Inflammation of glomeruli
  - Body's immune response to bacterial infection
    - Immune complexes deposited in glomeruli
    - Obstruct capillary blood flow
    - Can lead to acute or chronic renal failure

3a Acute Postinfectious Glomerulonephritis
- Figure 23-6

3b Urinary Inflammatory Disorders
- Nephrotic Syndrome
  - Primary
    - Affects kidneys, follows infection
  - Secondary
    - Follows multisystem disorder
  - Affects males, ages 2 to 7 years

3c Urinary Inflammatory Disorders
- Nephrotic Syndrome
  - Altered glomeruli permeability
  - Albumin shift changes osmotic pressure of blood
  - Kidney reabsorbs sodium water, edema results
  - Liver makes lipoproteins
  - Immunoglobulins are excreted

4 Acute and Chronic Renal Failure
- Inability of kidneys to remove liquid waste
- Causes
  - Lack of circulation to kidney
  - Damage to glomeruli
  - Blockage that prevents kidney from draining

4a Acute and Chronic Renal Failure
- Acute
  - Sudden onset diminished kidney function
- Chronic
  - Progressive, irreversible loss kidney function

- End-stage renal disease
  - Kidney function < 10%, dialysis or transplant

5 Wilms' Tumor or Nephroblastoma
- Metastatic, cancerous tumor of kidney
- Genetic link

6 Eneuresis
- Urinary incontinence after urinary continence obtained
- Noctural or diurnal incontinence

7 Ambiguous Genitalia
- Difficult to determine sex of child
- Pseudohermaphroditism
- Urinary and intestinal systems may be involved

8 Male Disorders
- Hydrocele
  - Accumulation of fluid in the scrotum
  - Fluid trapped in the tunica vaginalis

8a Male Disorders
- Phimosis
  - Inability to retract the foreskin
  - Due to tightened prepuce
  - Complications of balanoposthitis and paraphimosis

8b Male Disorders
- Cryptorchidism
  - Undescended testicle into scrotum
  - Due to lower testosterone levels or structural defect

8c Male Disorders
- Testicular torsion
  - Spermatic cord becomes twisted

9 Female Disorders
- Imperforate Hymen
  - Intact mucous membrane at introitus of vagina
  - Does not allow passage of vaginal secretions

9a Female Disorders
- Female Circumcision
  - Three types of circumcision
    - Sunna—excision of clitoris
    - Excision of clitoris and labia minora
    - Infabulation—excision and labia majora scraped
  - Cultural practice in some countries

9b Female Disorders
- Menstrual Disorders
  - Dysmenorrhea—painful menstruation
    - Due to release of prostaglandin
  - Metrorrhagia—bleeding between cycles
  - Amenorrhea—absence of menses
  - Premenstrual syndrome—hormone imbalance prior to menses

9c Female Disorders
- Vaginitis
  - Inflammation of the vagina
  - Caused by infection, infestation, insertion of object
  - Caused by chemical irritation, sexual abuse

SUGGESTIONS FOR CLASSROOM ACTIVITIES

- Develop a jeopardy game to have students identify disease processes of the urinary and reproductive systems. Develop the game on the computer so that when a student clicks on the disease process, the definition will appear.
- Present a video on the nursing care of a child with renal or reproductive disorders.

SUGGESTIONS FOR CLINICAL ACTIVITIES

- Assign each student a renal or reproductive disorder. Have them present a 5- to 10-minute presentation on the disorder.

LEARNING OUTCOME 3

Discuss clinical manifestations, diagnostic procedures, medical management related to urinary and reproductive disorders.

CONCEPTS FOR LECTURE

1. To identify disorders of the urinary and reproductive systems, the nurse needs to know how to complete assessments on these systems.
2. The newborn who does not void within 24 hours after birth may be assessed for congenital anomalies.
3. Children with urinary infections should be monitored for changes in body temperature, elevated white blood cells, and poor urine output.
4. Acute postinfectious glomerulonephritis is the most common type of kidney inflammation.
5. The child with renal failure should be assessed for signs of fluid overload, including weight gain, pitting edema, pulmonary edema, and ascites.
6. Wilms' tumor is a highly metastatic cancer of the kidney.
7. Stressors in a child's life may contribute to enuresis. It is important to determine how the child was toilet trained and whether there is a family history.
8. While the reproductive system is immature until puberty, many congenital anomalies of the urinary system also affect the reproductive system.

   Acute pain is often associated with disorders of the reproductive system. Assessment for verbal and nonverbal symptoms of pain is done by using age-appropriate pain scales.

POWERPOINT LECTURE SLIDES

(NOTE: The number on each PPT Lecture Slide directly corresponds with the Concepts for Lecture.)

1 Assessment of the Urinary System
- History
  - Determine patterns of urination, toilet training
  - Complaints of pain, burning, frequency, urgency
  - Involuntary urination situations
  - Recent weight gain
  - Past urinary disorders, family history

1a Assessment of the Urinary System
- Physical
  - Weigh child, inspect adequate hydration
  - Inspect extremities for edema
  - Observe for bladder distention
  - Determine if infant is able to urinate

2 Urethral Malposition
- Manifestations
  - Urethral opening anywhere along shaft of penis
  - Dimple or pit along shaft of penis
- Diagnosis
  - Physical findings, genetic testing
  - Ultrasound

2a Urethral Malposition
- Treatment
  - Perform surgical correction
  - No circumcision until repair done
  - Insert urethral stent following surgery

2b Obstructive Uropathy
- Manifestations
  - Urinary tract infections
  - Loss of renal function, hydronephrosis
- Diagnosis
  - Ultrasound, cystoscopy

2c Obstructive Uropathy
- Treatment
  - Place urethral or suprapubic catheter
  - Perform surgical intervention
    - Pyeloplasty
    - Valve ablation

3 Urinary Tract Infections
- Manifestations
  - Fever, nausea and vomiting, anorexia
  - Strong-smelling urine, abdominal pain, dysuria
  - Hematuria, incontinence or hesitancy
  - Crying during urination

3a Urinary Tract Infections
- Diagnosis
  - Hematuria, WBCs and nitrates in urine
  - Urine culture
- Treatment
  - Administer antibiotics
  - Administer oral or intravenous fluids

4 Acute Postinfectious Glomerulonephritis
- Manifestations
  - Sudden onset flank pain, irritability, malaise
  - Fever, gross or microscopic hematuria
  - Dysuria, edema, hypertension, oliguria
- Diagnosis
  - Urinalysis, serum studies
  - Electrocardiogram

4a Acute Postinfectious Glomerulonephritis
- Treatment
  - Provide supportive care, bed rest
  - Administer antihypertensives
  - Plan fluid restriction
  - Document intake and output
  - Test and treat family for strep

5 Nephrotic Syndrome
- Manifestations
  - Edema, dramatic weight gain, periorbital edema
  - Ascites, scrotum and extremity edema
  - Blood pressure increases, irritability
  - Foamy urine, appear malnourished

5a Nephrotic Syndrome
- Figure 23-7

5b Nephrotic Syndrome
- Diagnosis
  - Urinalysis for proteinuria, hematuria
  - Hypoalbuminemia, hyperlipidemia

- Treatment
  - Administer oral corticosteroids, diuretic therapy
  - Administer potassium supplements, cyclophosphamide

 5c Acute and Chronic Failure
- Manifestations
  - Acute
    – Oliguria, pale skin, headache, nausea, fatigue
    – Edema, tachycardia, hypertension
  - Chronic
    – Decreased mental alertness, anemia, growth retardation

 5d End-Stage Renal Disease
- Figure 23-8

 5e Acute and Chronic Failure
- Diagnosis
  - Oliguria
  - Increased serum creatinine, BUN, serum potassium
  - Decreased arterial bicarbonate
  - Increased or decreased sodium
  - Kidney function tests, glomerular filtration rate

 5f Acute and Chronic Renal Failure
- Treatment
  - Acute
    – Administer intravenous fluids, albumin
    – Administer diuretics, Kayexalate, restrict fluids

 5g Acute and Chronic Renal Failure
- Treatment
  - Chronic
    – Strict dietary management, vitamin and mineral supplements
    – Administer phosphate-binding agents, growth hormones
    – Administer hematopoietic growth factors, iron supplements
    – Administer antihypertensive drugs, dialysis, kidney transplant

 5h Acute and Chronic Renal Failure
- Treatment
  - Dialysis
    – Mechanical process of removing wastes from blood
    – Peritoneal, hemodialysis, continuous renal replacement therapy
    – Disequilibrium syndrome complication

 5i Hemodialysis
- Figure 23-9

6 Wilms' Tumor or Nephroblastoma
- Manifestations
  - Abdominal mass, firm with several lobes
  - Hematuria, hypertension, abdominal pain
- Diagnosis
  - Ultrasound, MRI

6a Wilms' Tumor or Nephroblastoma
- Treatment
  - Perform surgery to remove kidney, lymph nodes
  - Chemotherapy
  - Radiation

7 Eneuresis
- Diagnosis
  - Child history, family history
  - Urinalysis, urine culture
  - Bladder capacity studies, uroflow measurement
  - Ultrasound

7a Eneuresis
- Treatment
  - Administer antidiuretics, anticholinergics, tricyclic antidepressants
  - Monitor fluid intake
  - Use bed alarm, voiding schedule
  - Use positive reinforcement and rewards

8 Assessment of the Reproductive System
- History
  - Family history reproductive disorders
  - Redness, swelling, discharge from genitals
  - Burning or itching of genitals
  - Lumps or masses on genitals
  - Sexual abuse

8a Assessment of the Reproductive System
- Physical
  - Inspect external genitalia
    - Color, size, hair distribution, lumps, masses
    - Drainage, symmetry of organs
  - In males, note placement of urinary meatus
    - Circumcised

8b Ambiguous Genitalia
- Diagnosis
  - Chromosome analysis
- Treatment
  - Perform surgical reconstruction in stages
  - Evaluate loss of reproductive function

8c Hydrocele
- Manifestations
  - Palpate round, smooth, nontender mass
- Diagnosis
  - Transillumination

8d Hydrocele
- Treatment
  - Resolves spontaneously in first 2 years
  - Assist family to understand disorder

Phimosis
- Treatment
  - Perform circumcision
  - Administer pain medication
  - Reduce anxiety

 Cryptorchidism
- Diagnosis
  - Physical examination, Ballard screening at birth
  - Ultrasound, CT scan, MRI
- Treatment
  - Administration of human chorionic gonadotrophin
  - Perform orchiopexy to reposition testicle

 Testicular Torsion
- Manifestations
  - Intense scrotal pain
  - Nausea and vomiting
  - Testicular ischemia
- Treatment
  - Perform surgical correction within 4 hours

 Imperforate Hymen
- Manifestations
  - Uterine pressure
  - Abdominal discomfort and distention
- Treatment
  - Perform surgery to remove hymen
  - Provide reassurance about future sexuality

 Female Circumcision
- Treatment
  - Monitor for complications
    - Hemorrhage, pain, infection
  - Treat psychological complications
    - Anxiety, depression, frigidity, painful intercourse

 Dysmenorrhea
- Treatment
  - Administer prostaglandin inhibitors
  - Encourage low sodium diet
  - Apply heat to lower abdomen and back
  - Encourage rest and exercise

8k Vaginitis
- Manifestations
  - Pruritis, pain, vaginal discharge
  - Vaginal bleeding, foul odor to discharge
- Diagnosis
  - Examination of genitalia
  - Vaginal discharge specimen

8l Vaginitis
- Treatment
  - Administer Nystatin for *Candida albicans*
  - Administer metronidazole for trichomoniasis

LEARNING OUTCOME 4

Explain appropriate nursing interventions for children with urinary and reproductive disorders.

CONCEPTS FOR LECTURE

1. When caring for children with urinary disorders other than renal failure, the nurse should seek to maintain renal function and fluid balance.
2. The nurse should be able to recognize symptoms of urinary infection. In the infant and young child, dysuria may be displayed as crying during urination.
3. Due to the fragility of Wilms' tumor, health care providers need to avoid palpating the child's abdomen.
4. Nursing assessment for children with reproductive disorders includes monitoring for signs and symptoms of infection.

    The nurse must be very sensitive to the anxiety and embarrassment related to reproductive system disorders and take care to communicate in a professional manner.
5. The nurse can help the young girl avoid vaginitis by teaching her to wipe her perineum from front to back, therefore avoiding infestation of the vagina with harmful bacteria from the rectum.

    The nurse determines the child's and family's level of knowledge and understanding related to health conditions and the prescribed treatments.

POWERPOINT LECTURE SLIDES

(NOTE: The number on each PPT Lecture Slide directly corresponds with the Concepts for Lecture.)

 Urethral Malposition
- Nursing Interventions
  - Postoperative care
    - Observe for edema, dysuria, bleeding, infection
    - Maintain hydration
    - Document intake and output
    - Double diaper if stent present

 Urethral Malposition
- Nursing Interventions
  - Postoperative care
    - Blood tinged urine normal
    - Monitor for bladder spasms
    - Administer anticholinergics, antibiotics, analgesics
    - Observe for infection

 Urethral Malposition
- Figure 23-4

 Obstructive Uropathy
- Nursing Interventions
  - Preoperative care
    - Assist in diagnostic process
    - Ensure family understanding of condition, treatment

 Obstructive Uropathy
- Nursing Interventions
  - Postoperative care
    - Observe for urinary retention
    - Observe for fluid and electrolyte imbalance
    - Teach family care of urinary devices
    - Teach family when to report complications

2. Urinary Tract Infections
- Nursing Interventions
  - Clean infant perineum thoroughly
  - Teach to wipe front to back
  - Wash child's perineum daily
  - Discourage use of bubble baths, hot tubs

2a. Acute Postinfectious Glomerulonephritis
- Nursing Interventions
  - Maintain bed rest, reposition frequently
  - Maintain adequate nutritional intake
  - Encourage child to eat
  - Explain to parents laboratory studies

2b. Nephrotic Syndrome
- Nursing Interventions
  - Weigh daily, monitor blood pressure
  - Administer intravenous fluids, albumin, diuretics, steroids
  - Encourage regular diet with low sodium
  - Use infection prevention methods
  - Teach parents home care

2c. Acute and Chronic Renal Failure
- Nursing Interventions
  - Assess for fluid overload, small, frequent feedings
  - Monitor intake and output, blood values
  - Administer medications, prevent infection
  - Evaluate for undue stress, provide support
  - Teach family diet, activity, medication administration

3. Wilms' Tumor or Nephroblastoma
- Nursing Interventions
  - Avoid palpating abdomen, perform preoperative care
  - Postoperative care
    - Manage pain and fluid balance,
    - Monitor blood pressure
    - Administer chemotherapy, monitor side effects

4. Cryptorchidism
- Nursing Interventions
  - Teach testicular self-examination

4a. Female Circumcision
- Nursing Interventions
  - Learn about practice of female circumcision
  - Treat child with dignity and respect
  - Encourage child to talk about feelings
  - Educate about complications

5. Vaginitis
- Nursing Interventions
  - Teach to wipe perineum front to back
  - Discourage use of bubble baths, hygiene products
  - Encourage daily cleansing of perineum

5a Vaginitis
- Nursing Interventions
  - Instruct in frequent changes of tampons
  - Instruct in frequent changes of sanitary napkins
  - Change wet clothes promptly
  - Teach to wear cotton underwear

SUGGESTIONS FOR CLASSROOM ACTIVITIES	SUGGESTIONS FOR CLINICAL ACTIVITIES
• Discuss intake and output, include how to collect urine with babies and young children and how to collect 24-hour urine collections. • Have students research Web sites on reproductive issues to assist parents with talking to their children about these issues.	• Assign students to provide nursing care to children with urinary and reproductive disorders. Have them develop a nursing care plan or concept map that includes the interventions they performed. • Arrange for students to work with a school nurse to provide a sex education class. Bring an assortment of contraceptives to demonstrate.

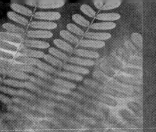

CHAPTER 24
CARE OF THE CHILD WITH INTEGUMENTARY DISORDERS

RESOURCE LIBRARY

CD-ROM
Eczema

COMPANION WEBSITE
Tattoos
Aloe vera therapy
Skin cancer

IMAGE LIBRARY

Figure 24-1 Anatomic view of skin and accessory structures.
Figure 24-2 Adult versus child integumentary system.
Figure 24-3 Vascular skin lesions.
Figure 24-4 (A) Capillary (strawberry) hemangioma. (B) Port-wine stain.
Figure 24-5 Diaper dermatitis.
Figure 24-6 Chronic eczema.
Figure 24-7 Acne lesion.
Figure 24-8 Head lice nits in the hair.
Figure 24-9 Diffuse scabies in an infant.
Figure 24-10 Warts on a child's hand.
Figure 24-11 Bullous impetigo.
Figure 24-12 Cellulitis. Markings on leg show fullest extent of infection.

Figure 24-13 (A) Tinea capitis. (B) Tine corporis.
Figure 24-14 (A) Thermal (scald) burns are the most common burn injury in infancy. (B) Burns of the hands or feet that are distributed like gloves or stockings are associated with child abuse. (C) Electrical burn caused by biting an electric cord.
Figure 24-15 Classifications of burns in children.
Figure 24-16 Serious burns are most often treated in the ICU or in a specialized burn center.
Figure 24-17 (A) Benign juvenile melanoma on the nose of a child; this is a superficial skin tumor that is most common in children. (B) Malignant melanoma.

LEARNING OUTCOME 1

Review the basic structure and function of skin and describe differences between the skin of a child and an adult.

CONCEPTS FOR LECTURE

1. The integumentary system is the largest organ system in the body, which includes the skin and associated structures.
2. Main functions of the skin include protecting the body from pathogens, temperature regulation, preventing dehydration, providing sensory receptors, and aiding in production of vitamin D.
3. Many changes occur in the skin from birth through adolescence as the child grows.

POWERPOINT LECTURE SLIDES

(NOTE: The number on each PPT Lecture Slide directly corresponds with the Concepts for Lecture.)

1 Structure and Function of the Integumentary System
- Skin
- Associated structures
  - Hair, nails, sebaceous and sweat glands
  - Blood vessels, nerve endings, sensory organs

1a Structure and Function of the Integumentary System
- Figure 24-1

1b Structure and Function of the Integumentary System
- Skin structure
  - Defense against infection
  - Two layers
    - Epidermis containing melanin
    - Dermis contains associated structures

2 Structure and Function of the Integumentary System
- Skin function
  - Protect body from pathogens
  - Temperature regulation
  - Prevent dehydration

○ Provide sensory receptors
○ Aid in production of vitamin D

2a Structure and Function of the Integumentary System
- Hair
  ○ Arrector pili—pulls hair upright
  ○ Keeps dust and insects from entering
  ○ Reflects nutritional status
  ○ Color provided by melanocytes

2b Structure and Function of the Integumentary System
- Nails
  ○ Consist of keratinized epidermal cells
  ○ Firm, transparent, pink over body
  ○ Brittle indicates poor nutrition status

2c Structure and Function of the Integumentary System
- Sebaceous Glands
  ○ Located in dermis, secrete sebum
  ○ Lubricating effect from sebum
  ○ Prevents growth of bacteria
  ○ Stimulated by sex hormones

2d Structure and Function of the Integumentary System
- Sweat (Sudoriferous) Glands
  ○ Eccrine glands
    – Maintain body temperature
    – Dissipates heat as sweat
  ○ Apocrine glands
    – Produce sweat

2e Structure and Function of the Integumentary System
- Subcutaneous layer
  ○ Includes elastic, fibrous, adipose tissue
  ○ Cushions internal organs
  ○ Stores fat for energy
  ○ Insulates body
  ○ Connects skin to surface of muscles

3 Growth and Development of Integumentary System
- Newborn skin
  ○ Thin, high in water content
  ○ Absorbs chemicals readily
  ○ Friction causes blisters, little melanin
  ○ Little subcutaneous fat contributes to heat loss
  ○ Regulates temperature through eccrine glands

3a Growth and Development of Integumentary System
- Child's skin
  ○ Thickens, more tightly bound layers
  ○ Eccrine glands increase function
  ○ Apocrine glands function at puberty
  ○ Increased melanin
  ○ Prone to skin infections, pH more acidic

3b Growth and Development of Integumentary System
- Figure 24-2

SUGGESTIONS FOR CLASSROOM ACTIVITIES

- Show a model of different layers of the integumentary system. Discuss the physiology of each layer.
- Compare differences between the skin of a child with the skin of an adult.
- Develop a matching quiz using the definitions of skin lesions in Box 24-1.
- Assign students to complete the CD-ROM interactivity: Match the Skin Layer and view the animations: Cell Structure Fly-through, Integumentary Repair

SUGGESTIONS FOR CLINICAL ACTIVITIES

- Have students practice doing skin inspections on each other.

LEARNING OUTCOME 2

Discuss common congenital disorders of skin, their treatment, and nursing care.

CONCEPTS FOR LECTURE

1. Skin disorders are common among pediatric clients. All birthmarks should be examined for color, size, location, texture, and elevation.
2. Contact dermatitis can stem from allergens or repeated exposure to irritants.
3. Breastfed infants are not as prone to diaper dermatitis.
4. Seborrheic dermatitis may be a result of changes in sebaceous glands.
5. Eczema is a chronic inflammatory disorder that has been associated with an immune dysfunction of the skin.
6. Acne is a common skin condition affecting adolescents.
7. Pediculosis and scabies are infestation with parasites that live on the human host.
8. Any break in skin integrity provides an opportunity for infection to take hold.
9. Dermatophytes are fungi that affect the surface of the skin, hair, and nails.
10. Oral candidiasis is usually found in a child with a depressed immune system.

POWERPOINT LECTURE SLIDES

(NOTE: The number on each PPT Lecture Slide directly corresponds with the Concepts for Lecture.)

1 Congenital Lesions
- Capillary (Strawberry) Hemangioma
  - Benign cutaneous tumor
  - Involves capillaries in dermis
  - Appears few weeks after birth
  - Begins to decrease by 2–3 years

1a Congenital Lesions
- Port-Wine Stains
  - Permanent vascular stains
  - Involve vascular bed in dermis
  - On face and head
  - Darken and thickens with growth of child

1b Skin Disorders
- Miliaria (prickly heat)
  - Blocked eccrine gland
  - Causes back-up pressure of sweat
  - Occurs in high temperature and humidity

1c Skin Disorders
- Intertrigo
  - Skin irritation
  - Opposing skin creates friction
  - Sweat retained between skin folds
  - Obese children more prone

2 Inflammatory Disorders
- Contact Dermatitis
  - Inflammation of dermis or skin
  - Caused by allergen
  - Caused by repeated exposure to irritant
  - Latex—allergy and irritant

3 Inflammatory Disorders
- Diaper Dermatitis
  - Irritation from urine and/or stool
  - Formula and solid foods change pH level
  - Can become infected with *Candida albicans*

3a Diaper Dermatitis
- Figure 24-5

 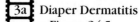

4 Inflammatory Disorders
- Seborrheic Dermatitis (cradle cap)
  - Changes in sebaceous glands
  - Dandruff begins with puberty

5 Inflammatory Disorders
- Eczema
  - Chronic inflammatory skin disorder
  - Associated with immune dysfunction of skin
  - Linked to allergies, asthma, hay fever
  - Self-esteem issues with skin changes
  - More common in winter

5a Eczema
- Figure 24-6

6 Inflammatory Disorders
- Acne Vulgaris
  - Sebum production increases
  - Hair follicles become blocked
  - Comedones develop
  - Bacteria invades and inflammation results

6a Acne
- Figure 24-7

7 Parasitic Infestations
- Pediculosis
  - Infestation with lice
  - Female louse lay eggs (nits)
  - Nits hatch within 8 to 10 days

7a Parasitic Infestations
- Figure 24-8

7b Parasitic Infections
- Scabies
  - Infestation caused by mites
  - On hands, feet, folds of skin
  - Mite burrows into epidermis, lays eggs
  - Eggs hatch in 2 to 4 days
  - Mature and grow on skin surface

7c Scabies
- Figure 24-9

8 Skin Infections
- Warts
  - Benign tumors in epithelial cells
  - Caused by human papillomavirus
  - Transmitted person to person
  - Transmitted from one site to another

8a Warts
- Figure 24-10

8b Skin Infections
- Impetigo
  - Superficial skin infection
  - Caused by streptococci or staphylococci
  - Highly contagious
  - More common in summer

8c Skin Infections
- Cellulitis
  - Bacterial infection of dermis, subcutaneous tissue
  - Rapid onset
  - Due to infection or injury
  - May result in septicemia, septic arthritis, meningitis

8d Cellulitis
- Figure 24-12

8e Skin Infections
- Herpes Simplex Type I
  - Viral infection
  - Passed from one person to another
  - May lie dormant until triggered to activate

8f Fungal Infections
- Dermatophytes (Ringworm or Tinea)
  - Fungi affecting surface of skin, hair, nails
  - Transfer human to human
  - Transfer animal to human
  - Type depends on body location

9 Dermatophytes
- Figure 24-13

10 Fungal Infections
- Oral Candidiasis (Thrush)
  - Yeast-like fungal infection
  - Caused by *Candida albicans*
  - Affects newborn from infected mother
  - Affects children receiving antibiotics, corticosteroids
  - Affects children with immune disorder

SUGGESTIONS FOR CLASSROOM ACTIVITIES

- Assign students to view the CD-ROM animations: Pressure ulcers, Eczema.
- Develop flash cards of symptoms or pictures of inflammatory and other skin conditions. Hold up the flash cards and have students identify the condition and discuss the appropriate nursing interventions for the condition.

SUGGESTIONS FOR CLINICAL ACTIVITIES

- Divide students into groups. Have them compare and contrast the different skin disorders they may see in the clinical setting.
- Arrange for students to observe assessments at a dermatologist's office. Have them write a paper on what skin disorders they observed and the treatments that were administered.

LEARNING OUTCOME 3

Discuss common infections and infestations of skin in children as well as treatment and nursing care.

CONCEPTS FOR LECTURE

1. Assessment of the skin can be a window into systemic problems involving oxygenation, circulation, nutrition, and hydration.
2. The LPN/LVN provides support and education to the family about congenital lesions.
3. Irritants cause cells to release histamine, resulting in redness, swelling, and itching

POWERPOINT LECTURE SLIDES

(NOTE: The number on each PPT Lecture Slide directly corresponds with the Concepts for Lecture.)

1 Assessment of the Integumentary System
- History
  - Past health history of skin disorders
  - Family history of skin disorders
  - Inquire about allergies, current medications
  - Inquire about skin care habits

4. Important priorities for the LPN/LVN are promoting healthy skin care and providing methods to prevent skin infections while decreasing pain and discomfort.

    Skin infections should be assessed for signs of erythema, vesicles or pustules, edema, fever, malaise, and texture of skin lesions.

    Focus of nursing care is on preventing the spread of infection and eradicating the infestation.

5. Eczema flare-ups are more common during the winter when the air is dry.

6. Acne treatment may be topical or systemic, depending on the severity of the condition.

    Psychological and social development may be altered if skin disorders lead to disfigurement.

7. Nursing care for head lice focuses on methods to kill the parasite and alleviate itching.

    Pediculosis and scabies can be eradicated with washing clothes, towels, and bed linens with hot water and heated drying.

8. Hand washing can help prevent the spread of infection of highly contagious skin infections such as impetigo.

9. Cellulitis is a rapid-onset infection that requires medical attention to prevent septicemia.

10. Dermatophytes may be transmitted from human to human or from animals to humans.

11. Oral candidiasis appears as white plaque in the mouth that bleeds easily.

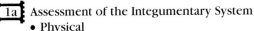

1a Assessment of the Integumentary System
- Physical
  - Inspect skin for color pigment changes
  - Inspect for birthmarks
  - Palpate to assess moisture, texture, turgor, temperature
  - Identify lesions, tattoos, piercings
  - Inspect for malignant lesions using ABCDE

1b Assessment of the Integumentary System
- Figure 24-3

2 Capillary Hemangioma
- Manifestations
  - Bright red area of skin
  - Elevates with growth
  - Rough surface, rubbery feel
  - Well-defined margins, on face and head

2a Capillary Hemangioma
- Diagnosis
  - Inspection and palpation
- Treatment
  - Administer oral prednisone, laser therapy
  - Administer subcutaneous injection of alfa-2a
  - Administer subcutaneous injection of interferon alfa-2b

2b Port-Wine Stains
- Manifestations
  - Pink to reddish purple stain
  - Becomes thick with verrucose nodular surface
- Diagnosis
  - Inspection and palpation
  - Rule out structural malformations

2c Port-Wine Stains
- Treatment
  - Use cosmetics if small, laser if large
- Nursing Interventions
  - Give support and encouragement
  - Teach care after laser therapy
    - Use water to clean, topical antibiotic

3 Miliaria
- Manifestations
  - Minute vesicles with papules
  - Erythema, itching
- Diagnosis
  - Inspection and palpation

3a Miliaria
- Treatment
  - Provide cool environment, allow good ventilation
  - Administer cool baths and dusting powders
- Nursing Interventions
  - Advise parents to monitor room temperature
  - Avoid being outside if too humid

3b Intertrigo
- Manifestations
  - Inflammation, erythema of skin
  - Skin appears warm and moist
  - *Candida* infections
- Diagnosis
  - Inspection and palpation

3c Intertrigo
- Treatment
  - Apply nonmedicated powder, encourage weight loss
  - Apply 1% hydrocortisone cream
- Nursing Interventions
  - Keep affected area clean and dry
  - Expose skin to air and light

4 Contact Dermatitis
- Manifestations
  - Reddened papules with allergy
    - Ooze, crust, itch, edematous
  - Irritants
    - Redness, edema, scaling of skin
    - Disappear when irritant removed

4a Contact Dermatitis
- Diagnosis
  - History of exposure, physical examination
  - Allergy skin testing
- Treatment
  - Use proper cleansing with mild soap
  - Apply hydrocortisone topical ointment

4b Contact Dermatitis
- Nursing Interventions
  - Collect data to identify irritants
  - Administer medication to relieve itching
  - Advise family to avoid irritants
  - Teach signs of infection

4c Diaper Dermatitis
- Manifestations
  - Red, edematous, blistered skin
  - Occurs in diaper area
- Diagnosis
  - Inspection and palpation of lesions

4d Diaper Dermatitis
- Treatment
  - Apply 0.25% to 1% hydrocortisone cream
  - Apply sealant to protect against moisture
  - Cleanse with mild soap and water
  - Allow to air dry
  - Apply hydrocortisone and antifungal for *Candida*

4e Diaper Dermatitis
- Nursing Interventions
  - Educate parents on prevention
  - Use superabsorbent diapers
  - Change soiled diapers immediately, thoroughly cleanse

○ Avoid using diaper wipes
○ Apply barrier creams or sealants, hydrocortisone

 Seborrheic Dermatitis
- Manifestations
  ○ Oily, yellow scaly patches
  ○ On scalp and forehead
  ○ Mildly erythematous underneath
- Diagnosis
  ○ Inspection and palpation

 Seborrheic Dermatitis
- Treatment
  ○ Daily shampoo with mild nonmedicated shampoo
  ○ Emollients to loosen crusts
  ○ Remove with soft bristle hairbrush or fingertips
  ○ Adolescents use medicated dandruff shampoo

 Seborrheic Dermatitis
- Nursing Interventions
  ○ Teach proper cleansing
  ○ Apply emollient for 20 minutes
  ○ Vigorous brushing with soft hair brush
  ○ Encourage adolescents to seek treatment

 Eczema
- Manifestations
  ○ Infant
    – Erythematous areas with papulovesicular lesions
    – Irritable, restless, pruritis
  ○ Child
    – Erythematous, dry, scaly skin
    – Papules that rupture and weep, pruritis

 Eczema
- Diagnosis
  ○ History
  ○ Inspection and palpation of papules, vesicles
  ○ Skin testing for food allergies

Eczema
- Treatment
  ○ Relieve pruritis with hydration and lubrication
  ○ Administer emollients, antihistamines
  ○ Administer topical and oral corticosteroids, antibiotics

Eczema
- Nursing Interventions
  ○ Identify and remove allergens or irritants
  ○ Use moisturizing lotions or creams, lubricants
  ○ Apply wet compresses soaked in aluminum acetate
  ○ Shower after swimming in chlorine water
  ○ Wear loose clothing, soft fabrics

5d Eczema
- Nursing Interventions
  - Use mild detergents to wash clothes
  - Cut fingernails short
  - Administer antihistamines for itching
  - Educate parents in signs of infection
  - Encourage expression of feelings

6 Acne Vulgaris
- Manifestations
  - Formation of comedones, pustules, papules
- Diagnosis
  - Identification of lesions
  - Inspect and palpate lesions

6a Acne Vulgaris
- Treatment
  - Administer topical medications
  - Administer systemic antibiotics
  - Administer isotretinoin if severe

6b Acne Vulgaris
- Nursing Interventions
  - Teach skin care, avoid oil-based cosmetics
  - Maintain prescribed medical treatments
  - Encourage use of sunscreen
  - Avoid picking or squeezing lesions

7 Pediculosis
- Manifestations
  - Intense itching over scalp
  - Visible nits on one side of hair shaft
- Diagnosis
  - Inspection with bright light, magnifying glass

7a Pediculosis
- Treatment
  - Apply a pediculicide shampoo
  - Comb with fine-toothed comb dipped in vinegar
  - Apply second treatment in 7 days

7b Pediculosis
- Nursing Interventions
  - Demonstrate how to inspect for lice
  - Instruct in administration of shampoo
  - Instruct in combing out nits with vinegar
  - Instruct in care of clothing, bedding
  - Educate in prevention

7c Scabies
- Manifestations
  - Erythematous papules, vesicles, pustules, pruritis
- Diagnosis
  - History and physical examination
  - Skin scrapings for mites, eggs, feces

7d Scabies
- Treatment
  - Administer premethrin cream
  - Teach good hygiene practices

    ○ Wash clothing, linens, towels at 140°F

    ○ Dry clothing, linens, towels in high heat

 Scabies
- Nursing Interventions
  - Leave cream on 8 to 12 hours
  - Treat all household members
  - Place unwashable items in plastic bag
  - Use nonjudgmental care

 Warts
- Manifestations
  - Rough, scaly papules and nodules
  - Painless on hands
  - Painful on bottom of feet
- Diagnosis
  - Inspection of papules and nodules

 Warts
- Treatment
  - Use chemical substances or peeling agents
  - Perform cryotherapy, laser therapy, duct tape
- Nursing Interventions
  - Explain medical therapy may take months
  - Reduce frequency is painful

 Impetigo
- Manifestations
  - Vesicles or pustules, edema, redness
  - After rupture, covered with honey-yellow crust
- Diagnosis
  - Inspection and palpation of lesions
  - Bacterial cultures

 Impetigo
- Treatment
  - Soak crusted lesion in warm water
  - Scrub with medicated soap
  - Apply topical bactericidal ointment for 1 week
  - Administer systemic antibiotic

 Impetigo
- Nursing Interventions
  - Teach family not to share towels, clothes
  - Instruct to wash and remove crusts
  - Instruct in application of bacterial ointment

9 Cellulitis
- Manifestations
  - Red, tender, warm, red streaks
  - Fever, headache, pain, chills, malaise, lymphangitis
- Diagnosis
  - Complete blood count
  - Wound and blood cultures

9a Cellulitis
- Treatment
  - Administer oral antibiotics
  - If severe, intravenous antibiotics

Cellulitis
- Nursing Interventions
  - Teach antibiotic administration
  - Rest and elevate affected area
  - Apply warm compresses
  - Teach handwashing
  - Teach sign of infection or sepsis

 Herpes Simplex Type I
- Manifestations
  - Tingling or burning sensation at site
  - Single vesicle or cluster of vesicles
  - Red inflamed skin
  - Vesicles dry and heal in 8 to 10 days

 Herpes Simplex Type I
- Diagnosis
  - Inspection of lesion, culture lesion
- Treatment
  - Administer acyclovir (Zovirax)
- Nursing Interventions
  - Instruct to prevent spreading of lesions

 Dermatophytes
- Manifestations
  - Tinea capitus
    - Hair loss, papules scaly and red
  - Tinea corporis
    - Circular red patch with raised border

 Dermatophytes
- Tinea pedis
  - Red, deep scaly fissures between toes
  - Painful, itchy
- Tinea cruris
  - Red, scaly skin in groin
  - Raised papules, vesicles form circular rash

 Dermatophytes
- Diagnosis
  - Skin scraping of lesion
- Treatment
  - Use antifungal topical ointment, powder, spray
- Nursing Interventions
  - Instruct in prevention measures, medication

 Oral Candidiasis
- Manifestations
  - White plaques on tongue, palate, buccal
  - Plaques bleed easily, painful
- Diagnosis
  - Inspection of oral mucosa, fungal culture
  - Skin scraping of lesion

11a Oral Candidiasis
- Treatment
  - Use of oral and topical antifungal medications
  - If systemic, administer intravenous amphotericin B
- Nursing Interventions
  - Swab medication or swish and swallow
  - Teach methods to decrease re-infection

LEARNING OUTCOME 4

Discuss various types of skin trauma in children as well as treatment and nursing care.

CONCEPTS FOR LECTURE

1. There are four types of burns: thermal, chemical, electrical, and radiation burns. Any unusual burn occurring in a pattern could suggest child abuse.
2. Burns are assessed for burn depth and amount of burn area. Treatment depends on the seriousness of the burn.
3. Nursing care focuses on fluid replacement, pain control, and prevention of infection.
4. Low levels of melanin, thin epidermal layer, and long periods of time in sun place children at higher risk for sunburns.
5. Melanoma arises from melanocytes, which are the cells damaged by overexposure to the sun's ultraviolet rays over a prolonged period of time.
6. Nursing care for frostbite focuses on rewarming the affected area while protecting the skin from further injury.
7. Nursing care for bites focuses on assessing local and systemic reactions to bites and teaching about how to prevent further instances of trauma.

POWERPOINT LECTURE SLIDES

(NOTE: The number on each PPT Lecture Slide directly corresponds with the Concepts for Lecture.)

 Burns
- Types of burns
  - Thermal—flame, hot objects
  - Chemical—strong acids or alkaline
  - Electrical—Contact with exposed electrical wires
  - Radiation—exposure to sunlight
- Unusual burn patterns indicate child abuse

 Burns
- Figure 24-14

2a Burns
- Manifestations
  - Partial thickness burns
    - Red, blisters, blanches, painful, may regenerate
  - Full thickness burns
    - Brown, form eschar, decreased sensation to pain
    - Requires skin grafting

2b Burns
- Figure 24-15

2c Burns
- Diagnosis
  - Assess thickness of burn
  - Assess percentage of body surface area
  - Use Lund and Browder chart

2d Burns
- Treatment
  - Stop burning process by removing cause
  - Monitor airway, breathing, circulation
  - Replace fluid loss, manage pain control
  - Prevent infection, promote nutrition, salvage tissue

 Burns
- Nursing Interventions
  - Replace volume with intravenous hydration
  - Begin enteral feedings within 6 hours
  - Assess pain level and medicate

○ Demonstrate proper wound care
○ Provide psychological support, referrals

3a Burns
• Figure 24-16

4 Sunburn
• Manifestations
○ Red, tender if minor
○ Edema, vesiculation, bullae, blistering if prolonged
○ Headache, fatigue, chills, malaise

4a Sunburn
• Treatment
○ Increase oral fluids, apply cool compresses
○ Apply topical corticosteroid
• Nursing Interventions
○ Teach prevention, use of sunscreen
○ Avoid sun exposure between 10AM and 4PM

5 Melanoma
• Manifestations
○ Lesions or moles with color variations
○ Irregular border, diameter > 6mm
○ May become ulcerated and bleed
• Diagnosis
○ Inspection, palpation, and biopsy of lesion

5a Melanoma
• Figure 24-17

5b Melanoma
• Treatment
○ Perform surgical removal of lesion
• Nursing Interventions
○ Teach warning signs of melanoma
○ Teach prevention techniques
○ Discourage use of tanning beds

6 Frostbite
• Manifestations
○ Appears pale and white, decreased sensation
○ If deep, appears cyanotic with mottling
○ Then red and edematous
○ Blisters or bullae appear
○ If severs, tissue necrosis

6a Frostbite
• Diagnosis
○ Inspection and palpation of skin
• Treatment
○ Place in warm environment, remove wet clothes
○ Submerge in 100.4 to 104.0°F water
○ Cleanse with saline; cover with sterile dressing

6b Frostbite
• Nursing Interventions
○ Monitor for increase in circulation, sensation
○ Assess need for pain medication

○ Maintain sterile dressings, antibiotic therapy
○ Encourage proper nutrition
○ Educate to layer clothing, monitor numbness

 Bites
• Manifestations
  ○ Animal bites
    – Redness, edema, lacerations, drainage, cellulites
  ○ Insect bites
    – Redness, itching, pain, hives, papules, edema
    – Wheezing, urinary, laryngeal or angioedema, anaphylaxis

 Bites
• Manifestations
  ○ Snake bite
    – Burning, redness, ecchymosis, edema, dizziness, hypotension
    – Tachycardia, sweating, nausea, and vomiting
• Diagnosis
  ○ Inspection and palpation of skin

 Bites
• Treatment
  ○ Irrigate wound, remove dead tissue
  ○ Perform surgical removal or closure of wound
  ○ Administer antibiotics
  ○ Administer human rabies immune globulin
  ○ Administer human diploid cell rabies vaccine

 Bites
• Nursing Interventions
  ○ Identify source of bite
  ○ Demonstrate how to clean and dress wound
  ○ Discuss prevention methods with parents
  ○ Discuss use of insect repellents with DEET

SUGGESTIONS FOR CLASSROOM ACTIVITIES

• Assign students to view the video on the CD-ROM on Skin Cancer.
• Have students research procedures for tattooing and body piercing. Have them develop a teaching sheet for care of tattoos and body piercings for children and parents.
• Compare clinical manifestations and nursing interventions of different types of bites.
• Develop case studies of children with various types and depths of burn injuries. Discuss how to use the Lund and Browder chart to determine the burned body surface area. Discuss nursing interventions for the different types of burns.

SUGGESTIONS FOR CLINICAL ACTIVITIES

• Arrange for students to visit a burn unit or arrange for a burn nurse to speak to the students about the nursing care for the child with burns.
• Have students develop a teaching sheet for parents about the dangers of sunburns and tanning beds and how to prevent skin damage. Have them hand out the teaching sheet to parents in the acute clinical setting.

CHAPTER 25
CARE OF THE CHILD WITH ENDOCRINE DISORDERS

RESOURCE LIBRARY

CD-ROM
Endocrine system
Diabetes
Nutrition

IMAGE LIBRARY

Figure 25-1 Major organs and glands of the endocrine system.
Figure 25-2 Negative feedback mechanism with blood glucose and insulin.
Figure 25-3 Multisystem effects of hypothyroidism and hyperthyroidism.

COMPANION WEBSITE
Tay–Sachs

Figure 25-4 Classic symptoms of diabetes mellitus.
Figure 25-5 Multisystem effects of diabetes mellitus.
Figure 25-6 Locations for rotating administration of insulin.

LEARNING OUTCOME 1

Identify the location of each endocrine gland, the hormones produced, and the function of each.

CONCEPTS FOR LECTURE

1. The endocrine system performs the function of communication and slow, long-lasting control of various other body systems.

   Hormones are proteins that are the main regulators of growth and development, metabolism, and reproduction.

   Prostaglandins are hormones produced by various tissues throughout the body.

   The pineal gland produces melatonin, which regulates body cycles such as sleep/wake cycles.

   The pituitary gland is called the master gland as it exerts control over other glands.

   The thyroid gland secretes hormones that stimulate cellular metabolism.

   The parathyroid glands release hormones to maintain blood calcium levels.

   The thymus gland has a role in the development and function of the body's immune system.

   The adrenal glands are two separate glands that secrete different hormones.

   The pancreas is the only organ that is both an exocrine and an endocrine gland.

POWERPOINT LECTURE SLIDES

(NOTE: The number on each PPT Lecture Slide directly corresponds with the Concepts for Lecture.)

1 Anatomy and Physiology of the Endocrine System
- Hormones
  - Proteins produced by endocrine glands
  - Secreted into blood
  - Transported to target organs
  - Regulated by negative feedback mechanism
  - Regulate growth and development, metabolism, reproduction

1a Anatomy and Physiology of the Endocrine System
- Prostaglandins
  - Hormones produced by various tissues
  - Affect respirations, blood pressure
  - Affect gastrointestinal secretions, reproduction

1b Anatomy and Physiology of the Endocrine System
- Pineal Gland
  - Located in third ventricle inside brain
  - Produces melatonin
  - Regulates body cycles, inhibits gonadotropic hormones

1c Anatomy and Physiology of the Endocrine System
- Pituitary Gland
  - Suspended from hypothalamus of brain
  - Anterior pituitary
    - Secretes growth hormone, prolactin, trophic hormones
  - Posterior pituitary
    - Secretes antidiuretic hormone and oxytocin

1d Anatomy and Physiology of the Endocrine System
- Thyroid Gland
  - Located in neck below larynx
  - Stimulated by thyroid stimulating hormone
  - Secretes and stores thyroxine, triiodothyronine, calcitonin

1e Anatomy and Physiology of the Endocrine System
- Parathyroid Glands
  - Four glands located behind the thyroid gland
  - Secrete parathyroid hormone

1f Anatomy and Physiology of the Endocrine System
- Thymus Gland
  - Located in the mediastinum
  - Atrophies in puberty
  - Secretes thymosin

1g Anatomy and Physiology of the Endocrine System
- Adrenal Glands
  - Located on top of kidneys
  - Adrenal cortex
    - Secretes mineralocorticoids and glucocorticoids, androgens
  - Adrenal medulla
    - Secretes epinephrine and norepinephrine

1h Anatomy and Physiology of the Endocrine System
- Pancreas
  - Located in left upper quadrant abdomen
  - Exocrine and endocrine gland
  - Produces digestive hormones
  - Alpha cells secrete glucagon
  - Beta cells secrete insulin

SUGGESTIONS FOR CLASSROOM ACTIVITIES

- Using illustrations of the endocrine glands, discuss the purpose of each endocrine gland. Refer to Table 25-1 Review of Endocrine Glands.
- Discuss the types of hormones released by each endocrine gland. Review the influence of each hormone on the functioning of the body.

SUGGESTIONS FOR CLINICAL ACTIVITIES

- Using a full-body model, point out the anatomy of the endocrine system and discuss the physiology of each endocrine gland.

LEARNING OUTCOME 2

Discuss the interrelationship of the normally functioning endocrine system.

CONCEPTS FOR LECTURE

1. Hormones are regulated by a negative feedback system to control the amount of circulating hormones within a normal range.
2. Positive feedback systems occur in response to major events.
3. The anterior pituitary gland secretes hormones that stimulate other hormones to be released.
4. The posterior pituitary secretes an antidiuretic hormone in response to hydration to prevent dehydration from occurring.
5. The thyroid gland secretes calcitonin, and the parathyroid gland secretes parathyroid hormone. The two hormones work together to maintain normal calcium levels in the body.

    Alpha cells in the pancreas secrete glucagon. Beta cells in the pancreas secrete insulin. Glucagon and insulin work together to maintain blood glucose in a normal range.

POWERPOINT LECTURE SLIDES

(NOTE: The number on each PPT Lecture Slide directly corresponds with the Concepts for Lecture.)

1 Functioning of the Endocrine System
- Negative Feedback System
  - High levels of hormones inhibit hormone production
  - Low levels of hormones trigger hormone production

2 Functioning of the Endocrine System
- Positive Feedback System
  - Increase in one substance causes increased response
  - Major event occurs; causes decreased substance

3 Functioning of the Endocrine System
- Anterior pituitary gland
  - Growth hormone slows glucose breakdown
    - High glucose levels stimulate pancreas
    - Pancreas releases insulin to lower glucose
  - Thyroid-stimulating hormone
    - Stimulates thyroid gland to release hormones

3a Functioning of the Endocrine System
- Anterior pituitary gland
  - Adrenocorticotropic hormone
    - Stimulated adrenal cortex to release hormones
  - Follicle-stimulating hormone, luteinizing hormone
    - Stimulate ovary to ripen and release ova

4 Functioning of the Endocrine System
- Posterior pituitary gland
  - Antidiuretic hormone
    - Accelerates reabsorption of water
    - Results in decreased urinary output
    - Prevents dehydration

5 Functioning of the Endocrine System
- Calcitonin by thyroid and parathyroid hormones
  - Together maintain calcium levels in body
- Pancreas
  - Insulin and glucagon work together
    - Maintain blood glucose level in normal range

SUGGESTIONS FOR CLASSROOM ACTIVITIES

- Discuss how negative and positive feedback systems affect the endocrine glands. Give examples of how each system works.
- Present a video on the nursing care of a child with endocrine disorders.

SUGGESTIONS FOR CLINICAL ACTIVITIES

- Assign each student to research an endocrine disorder. Have them prepare and give a 5- to 10-minute presentation on the disorder, including new medications and treatments.

CONCEPTS FOR LECTURE

1. Endocrine disorders display symptoms similar to those of other body systems, making diagnosis difficult at times.

   Endocrine disorders require long-term treatment and monitoring.

   Endocrine disorders are potentially life-threatening due to lack of regulation of other body systems.

   Inborn errors of metabolism are missing or defective enzymes to metabolize certain foods. Special diet must be adhered to in an attempt to prevent complications.

2. Pituitary disorders may be caused by brain infections, infarction of the pituitary gland, cranial injury, hypothalamic or pituitary tumors, or psychosocial deprivation.

   Response to growth hormone, sex hormones, and antidiuretic hormone are controlled by the pituitary glands. Treatment is prescribed based on monitoring these blood levels.

3. Thyroid hormones are necessary for cellular metabolism, mental functioning, and growth.

   Thyroid disorders must be diagnosed and treated early by monitoring the TSH, T3, and T4 levels and also calcium and phosphate levels.

4. Adrenal gland disorders affect the release of corticosteroids, aldosterone, and catecholamines, which affect glucose levels, electrolyte balance, blood pressure, and the fight-or-flight response.

   Treatment of adrenal disorders is aimed at keeping glucose, electrolyte, and blood pressure levels within a normal range for the child.

5. The islets of Langerhans of the pancreas affect glucose, protein, and fat metabolism. Disorders range from resistance to insulin to deficient production of insulin.

   A main treatment goal of all types of diabetes mellitus is to prevent complications.

6. Metabolic syndrome is an example of the complex nature of endocrine disorders. It affects not only blood glucose levels but also cortisol, thyroid, and sex hormones, cardiac disease, and liver function.

   Treatment of metabolic syndrome is aimed at weight loss and frequent monitoring of blood levels.

POWERPOINT LECTURE SLIDES

(NOTE: The number on each PPT Lecture Slide directly corresponds with the Concepts for Lecture.)

1 Inborn Errors of Metabolism
- Galactosemia
  - Autosomal recessive disorder of carbohydrate metabolism
  - Deficiency in galactose-1-phosphate uridyltransferase
    - Enzyme for converting galactose into glucose
  - Damage to kidneys, liver, brain, eyes

1a Galactosemia
- Manifestations
  - Vomiting, diarrhea, hypoglycemia, enlarged liver
  - If not treated, jaundice, ascites, cataracts
  - Mental retardation, seizures, lethargy, coma, death

1b Galactosemia
- Diagnosis
  - Newborn screening
- Treatment
  - Order lactose-free or galactose-free diet

1c Inborn Errors of Metabolism
- Maple Syrup Sugar Disease
  - Autosomal recessive disease
  - Missing or defective enzyme
    - Prevents breakdown of amino acids
    - Leucine, isolucine, valine amino acids
    - Increased leucine causes neurologic damage, death

1d Maple Syrup Sugar Disease
- Manifestations
  - Lethargic, variable muscle tone, irritable
  - High-pitched cry, sweet-smelling skin
- Diagnosis
  - Laboratory findings

1e Maple Syrup Sugar Disease
- Treatment
  - Order diet rich in other proteins
  - Prescribe special low-protein foods
  - Daily urine testing for ketones

1f Inborn Errors of Metabolism
- Tay-Sachs Disease
  - Caused by inherited autosomal recessive disorder
  - Abnormal gene which lacks hexosaminidase enzyme
  - Inability to breaks down fatty material
  - Excess fatty material causes nerve damage
  - Both parents must carry abnormal gene

1g Tay-Sachs Disease
- Manifestations
  - Muscle weakness progresses to paralysis
  - Deaf, blind, neurologic damage, death
- Diagnosis
  - Genetic testing
  - Chorionic villus sampling if pregnant

1h Tay-Sachs Disease
- Treatment
  - No effective treatment

2 Pituitary Disorders
- Growth Hormone Deficiency
  - Manifestations
    - Height growth < 3rd percentile by 1 year
    - Overweight
    - Hypoglycemic seizures, hyponatremia, jaundice
    - Pale optic disc, male genital problems

2a Growth Hormone Deficiency
- Manifestations
  - Youthful facial features, higher-pitched voice
  - Delayed skeletal and sexual maturity
- Diagnosis
  - Lack of height growth
  - Blood testing for growth hormone

2b Growth Hormone Deficiency
- Treatment
  - Administer growth hormone subcutaneous injections
  - Administer 3 to 7 times/week at least 1 year

2c Pituitary Disorders
- Growth Hormone Excess
  - Manifestations
    - Tall stature, rapid growth
    - If precocious puberty, suspect hypothalamic tumor

2d Growth Hormone Excess
- Diagnosis
  - History, laboratory studies, radiological studies
- Treatment
  - High doses sex hormones to stop growth

2e Pituitary Disorders
- Precocious Puberty
  - Manifestations
    - Secondary sex characteristics develop early
    - Advanced bone age, short stature
    - Rapid growth, rapid closure epiphyseal plates
    - Mood swings, emotional lability

2f Precocious Puberty
- Diagnosis
  - Monitor sex steroids—FSH and LH
  - Determine pituitary dysfunction

- Treatment
  - Administer hormones to suppress FSH, LH

 Pituitary Disorders
- Diabetes Insipidus
  - Two types of diabetes insipidus
    - Inadequate pituitary production of ADH
    - Lack of response to ADH—nephrogenic

 Diabetes Insipidus
- Manifestations
  - Polyuria, polydipsia, specific gravity < 1.010, hypernatremia
- Diagnosis
  - Serum electrolytes, serum and urine osmolality
  - Plasma arginine vasopressin level with fluid deprivation

 Diabetes Insipidus
- Treatment
  - For ADH insufficiency
    - Administration of desmopressin acetate (DDAVP)
    - Titrate DDAVP to lower urine output
    - Ensure adequate caloric intake

 Diabetes Insipidus
- Treatment
  - For nephrogenic diabetes insipidus
    - Administration of diuretics
    - Increase fluid intake
    - Order salt- and protein-restricted diet

 Thyroid Disorders
- Hypothyroidism
  - Can be congenital, autosomal recessive gene mutation
  - Deficiency in TSH, inflammation of thyroid gland

 Hypothyroidism
- Manifestations
  - Tongue and lips thicken, dull expression
  - Jaundice, hypotonia, bradycardia, lethargy, feeding problems
  - Cool extremities, precocious puberty, irregular menses
  - Hair loss, slowing of growth
  - Increased weight, goiter

 Hypothyroidism
- Diagnosis
  - Newborn screen of TSH, T4
  - Elevated TSH—caused by pituitary gland
- Treatment
  - Administer levothyroxin
  - Refer to pediatric endocrinologist

Hyperthyroidism
- Associated with Grave's disease
  - Autoimmune disorder
  - Antibodies attack thyroid gland
  - Overproduction of hormones occurs
- Congenital hyperthyroidism
  - Mother with Grave's disease

3d Hyperthyroidism
- Manifestations
  - Goiter, exophthalmos, nervousness, restlessness, irritability
  - Weight loss with increased appetite
  - Heat intolerance, muscle weakness
  - Decreased ability to concentrate, easily fatigued
  - Difficulty relaxing and sleeping

 Hyperthyroidism
- Diagnosis
  - Serum TSH, T3, T4, thyroid scan
- Treatment
  - Administer antithyroid medication
  - Administer radiation with radioactive iodine
  - Perform thyroidectomy, lifelong replacement therapy

 Adrenal Disorders
- Cushing's syndrome
  - Hyperfunction of adrenal cortex
  - Increased levels of glucocorticosteroids
  - Caused by tumor, increased secretion ACTH, hyperplasia
  - May have symptoms with corticosteroid medications

 Cushing's Syndrome
- Manifestations
  - Gradual, excessive weight gain, slow growth
  - "Moon face," "buffalo hump,"
  - Delayed puberty, mental changes

4b Cushing's Syndrome
- Diagnosis
  - Clinical symptoms
  - Sodium, potassium, calcium, phosphorus, glucose labs
  - Adrenal suppression tests

 Cushing's Syndrome
- Treatment
  - Provide symptomatic treatment for hydrocortisone administration
  - Perform surgical intervention if tumor
  - Prognosis poor if malignant tumor

4d Adrenal Disorders
- Congenital Adrenal Hyperplasia
  - Autosomal recessive disorder
  - Deficient enzyme for cortisol, aldosterone production
  - Blocked aldosterone causes loss of salt
  - Decreased cortisol stimulates increased ACTH

4e Congenital Adrenal Hyperplasia
- Manifestations
  - Ambiguous genitalia in newborn
  - Precocious genitalia in children
  - Epiphyseal plates close early, small stature

4f Congenital Adrenal Hyperplasia
- Diagnosis
  - Elevated serum 17-hydroxyprogesterone
  - Chromosome studies to confirm gender
  - Electrolytes performed often

4g Congenital Adrenal Hyperplasia
- Treatment
  - Administration of glucocorticoid medication
  - Administration of mineralocorticoid or salt intake
  - Reconstructive surgery of genitals

4h Adrenal Disorders
- Adrenal Insufficiency (Addison's Disease)
  - Decrease in glucocorticoids and mineralocorticoids
  - Caused by trauma to adrenal glands

4i Adrenal Insufficiency
- Manifestations
  - Weakness, fever, abdominal pain, hypoglycemia
  - Dehydration, shock, may crave salt

4j Adrenal Insufficiency
- Diagnosis
  - Low levels of serum cortisol
  - Low levels of urinary 17-hydroxycorticoid
  - Low levels sodium and glucose
  - High level potassium

4k Adrenal Insufficiency
- Treatment
  - Administration of deficient hormones

4l Adrenal Disorders
- Pheochromocytoma
  - Adrenal tumor
  - Releases epinephrine and norepinephrine
  - Occurs between 6 and 14 years of age

4m Pheochromocytoma
- Manifestations
  - Severe hypertension, blurred vision, headache
  - Palpitations, weakness, polyuria, polydipsia
  - Symptoms come and go

Pheochromocytoma
- Diagnosis
  - 24-hour urine for urinary catecholamines, VMA
  - MRI to localize tumor
- Treatment
  - Administer beta-alpha-adrenergic blocking agents
  - Perform surgical removal adrenal gland
  - Repeat 24-hour urine after surgery

 Pancreatic Islet Disorders
- Diabetes Mellitus
  - Disorder of carbohydrate, protein, fat metabolism
  - Two types of diabetes mellitus
    - Type I or insulin-dependent diabetes mellitus
    - Type II or non–insulin–dependent diabetes mellitus

 Type I Diabetes Mellitus
- Autoimmune response damages islets of Langerhans
- Antigens generate the production of antibodies
- Antibodies further destroy islets of Langerhans
- Level of insulin falls, blood glucose rises
- Decrease in cell metabolism
- Cells convert protein and fat into glucose

 Type I Diabetes Mellitus
- Manifestations
  - Polyuria, polydipsia, polyphagia, hyperglycemia, weight loss
  - Fatigue, headache, poor wound healing, infection
  - Vaginitis by *Candida* in adolescent girls

 Type I Diabetes Mellitus
- Diagnosis
  - Nonfasting blood glucose > 200 mg/dL
  - Follow-up fasting blood glucose > 126 mg/dL
  - C-peptide test

 Type I Diabetes Mellitus
- Treatment
  - Administer insulin by injection or pump
  - Prescribe meal plan
    - 50–60% carbohydrate, 10–20% protein, 20–30% fat
  - Prescribe exercise plan

Pancreatic Islet Disorders
- Diabetic Ketoacidosis
  - Insufficient amount of insulin
  - Caused by infection, illness, omission of insulin

Diabetic Ketoacidsis
- Manifestations
  - Polyuria, polydipsia, polyphagia
  - Fruity or acetone breath, Kussmaul's respirations
  - Dehydration, decreased level of consciousness
  - Flushed dry skin, electrolyte imbalance, arrhythmias
  - Shock, death

 Diabetic Ketoacidosis
- Treatment
  - Begin intravenous infusion of isotonic fluid
  - Administer insulin intravenously
  - Add dextrose to IV when blood glucose 200–300mg/dL
  - Administer potassium intravenously
  - Monitor electrolytes and replace appropriately

 Type II Diabetes Mellitus
- Body produces insulin
- Unable to use insulin effectively
- Insulin resistance is precursor
- Over time, insulin production decreases
  - Hyperglycemia results

 Type II Diabetes Mellitus
- Manifestations
  - Polydipsia, polyuria, polyphagia
  - Tired, develop infections frequently
- Diagnosis
  - Fasting blood glucose testing

 Type II Diabetes Mellitus
- Treatment
  - Ensure balanced diet
    - Low calories for weight loss
  - Monitor blood glucose
  - Administer oral hypoglycemic agents, insulin
  - Plan exercise program

 Pancreatic Islet Disorder
- Metabolic Syndrome
- Group of related metabolic disorders
  - Central obesity, insulin resistance
  - Complications of type II diabetes
  - Athrogenic dyslipidemia
  - Prethrombotic state, hypertension
  - Preinflammatory state

6 Metabolic Syndrome
- Diagnosis
  - Clinical findings
    - Waist measurement—female > 40 in.
    - Waist measurement—male > 35 in.
    - Elevated blood pressure, fatigue, chronic infections
    - Polycystic ovarian disease, depression, irritable bowel

6a Metabolic Syndrome
- Diagnosis
  - Laboratory studies
    - High blood glucose and cortisol, low thyroid
    - Low HDL cholesterol, decreased liver function
    - Elevated estrogen in women
    - Low testosterone in men

6b Metabolic Syndrome
- Treatment
  - Lose weight, increase activity
  - Maintain blood glucose within normal range
  - Encourage diet with decreased calories
  - Encourage diet with increased protein and fiber
  - Administer medications as indicated

SUGGESTIONS FOR CLASSROOM ACTIVITIES

- Discuss nutrition and meal plans for various endocrine disorders, including the carbohydrate diet for diabetes, calorie-reduction diets, and increased protein and fiber diets. Refer to Box 25-3 Low-Salt, Low-Protein Diet for diabetes insipidus. Bring play foods to class and have students put together appropriate meals.
- Develop case studies of children with various endocrine disorders. Assign groups of students to complete the case study questions for a case study, and then present the case study to the rest of the class.

SUGGESTIONS FOR CLINICAL ACTIVITIES

- Have students view laboratory and diagnostic study results of clients with endocrine disorders. Discuss abnormal results in relation to the function of the endocrine system.
- Arrange for students to make rounds with a diabetic educator. Have them write a paper on the duties of the diabetic educator and the topics taught by the educator.

LEARNING OUTCOME 4

Explain appropriate nursing interventions for children with endocrine disorders.

CONCEPTS FOR LECTURE

1. By recognizing and reporting symptoms, the LPN/LVN may assist in identification of an endocrine disorder.

   Families may need to be taught to monitor the child's condition and administer treatments including medication.

   Many treatments of endocrine disorders are expensive and may not be covered by insurance. The nurse may need to provide resource information.

   Nutrition counseling is required for administration of proper diets to children with inborn errors of metabolism.

2. Assist the family to receive genetic counseling and grief counseling when the child has Tay-Sachs disease.

3. The nurse should support parents and children and help to explain body changes with pituitary disorders.

4. Diabetes insipidus can be reversed with treatment, but hypovolemic shock and death can occur if not treated promptly.

5. In hypothyroid conditions, teach the importance of lifelong therapy of thyroid replacement medications.

POWERPOINT LECTURE SLIDES

(NOTE: The number on each PPT Lecture Slide directly corresponds with the Concepts for Lecture.)

1 Galactosemia
- Nursing Interventions
  - Teach parents prescribed diet
  - Refer to nutritionist for counseling
  - Teach to screen foods and medications
  - Refer for genetic counseling

1a Maple Syrup Sugar Disease
- Nursing Interventions
  - Teach parents to maintain prescribed diet
  - Develop plan to prevent ketoacidosis
  - Refer to nutritionist
  - Refer to support groups

2 Tay-Sachs Disease
- Nursing Interventions
  - Relieve symptoms, make child comfortable
  - Prepare child and family for death
  - Refer for genetic counseling

6. With hyperthyroid surgery, monitor for swelling of the throat and how to communicate when the child cannot speak due to the swelling.
7. With the child having an adrenal disorder, it is necessary for the nurse to monitor electrolytes and blood pressure levels. Teach parents to perform blood pressure readings correctly.
8. Disorders of the pancreas require much client and parent teaching to maintain blood glucose levels within a normal range for the child.

    It is important for the nurse to teach how to monitor blood glucose levels and to teach proper administration of insulin.
9. The main emphasis for nursing care of the child with metabolic syndrome is to monitor weight loss and activity to stop and to prevent obesity.

3 Growth Hormone Deficiency
- Nursing Interventions
  - Monitor growth, provide support
  - Teach parents to give injections

3a Growth Hormone Excess
- Nursing Interventions
  - Teach parents about condition
  - Provide emotional support to child and family

3b Precocious Puberty
- Nursing Interventions
  - Provide support to child and parents
  - Teach about early body changes
  - Teach to dress for chronologic age
  - Teach parents to talk about sexuality
  - Refer for counseling

4 Diabetes Insipidus
- Nursing Interventions
  - Teach parents how to manage disease
  - Teach medication administration
  - Teach to recognize signs of complications
  - Teach to seek medical attention when ill
  - Communicate diagnosis to health care providers

5 Hypothyroidism
- Nursing Interventions
  - Teach parents about condition
  - Teach parents to administer medication
  - Teach signs of inadequate hormone replacement
  - Stress need for lifelong thyroid replacement

6 Hyperthyroidism
- Nursing Interventions
  - Teach child and parents about disorder
  - Teach about type of treatment
  - Complete preoperative care, give support
  - Administer postoperative care
    - Maintain airway, prevent blood loss

7 Cushing's Syndrome
- Nursing Interventions
  - Monitor lab values
  - Teach about pathology of disorder, treatment
  - Instruct to wear medical alert bracelet

7a Congenital Adrenal Hyperplasia
- Nursing Interventions
  - Teach symptoms of electrolyte imbalance
  - Provide emotional support
  - Refer for counseling and genetic counseling

7b Pheochromocytoma
- Nursing Interventions
  - Teach parents to monitor blood pressure
  - Perform preoperative and postoperative care
  - Instruct in urine screening for life

Diabetes Ketoacidosis
- Nursing Interventions
  ○ Stabilize child's condition
    – Use skilled assessments
    – Administer isotonic intravenous fluids
    – Monitor blood glucose, electrolytes, acid-base balance
    – Administer electrolyte replacements

8a Diabetes Ketoacidosis
- Nursing Interventions
  ○ Ensure balanced nutrition
  ○ Administer insulin intravenously
  ○ Teach family to manage condition at home
  ○ Prevent long-term complications

 8b Type II Diabetes Mellitus
- Nursing Interventions
  ○ Teach signs, symptoms of hypohyperglycemia
  ○ Teach complications of diabetes
  ○ Teach treatment as for type I diabetes
  ○ Teach administration of oral hypoglycemic agents
  ○ Monitor and report side effects of medication

 9 Metabolic Syndrome
- Nursing Interventions
  ○ Teach proper diet
  ○ Plan exercise program
  ○ Monitor weight and weight loss
  ○ Monitor blood glucose levels
  ○ Teach about syndrome, stress reduction

SUGGESTIONS FOR CLASSROOM ACTIVITIES

- Show pictures of children with endocrine disorders. Have students identify the disorder and discuss appropriate nursing interventions for the disorder.
- Have students develop a poster or teaching tool comparing the signs and symptoms of hypoglycemia and hyperglycemia. Refer to Table 25-3 Symptoms of Hyperglycemia and Hypoglycemia. Use this to present an in-service for nursing staff.

SUGGESTIONS FOR CLINICAL ACTIVITIES

- Assign students to provide nursing care to children with endocrine disorders. Have them develop a nursing care plan or concept map, including the interventions they performed.
- Arrange for students to interview a school nurse to understand the nursing care required for the student with an endocrine disorder such as diabetes.
- In postconference, review the steps of preoperative and postoperative care for children having surgery to remove endocrine glands.

LEARNING OUTCOME 5

Discuss teaching topics for children with diabetes and their parents.

CONCEPTS FOR LECTURE

1. Although the complete teaching plan is the responsibility of the registered nurse, the LPN/LVN may be asked to provide instruction on the management of diabetes mellitus in the home.
2. The young child can be taught to assemble insulin equipment, assist with blood glucose testing, and help with selection of nutritious snacks.

POWERPOINT LECTURE SLIDES

(NOTE: The number on each PPT Lecture Slide directly corresponds with the Concepts for Lecture.)

 Diabetes Mellitus Teaching Topics
- Perform blood glucose testing
- Ensure balanced nutrition with regular meals and snacks
- Plan regular daily activity/exercise

The older child can be taught to perform blood glucose testing, administer insulin, and complete daily records.

- Administer insulin by subcutaneous injection or pump
- Understand insulin peak, onset, duration
- Know signs/symptoms of hypo- and hyperglycemia

1a Insulin injection sites
- Figure 25-6

2 Diabetes Mellitus Teaching Topics
- Prevent complications of diabetes mellitus
- Health promotion to prevent injury
- Health promotion to prevent infection
- Understand sick day management
- Teach child to manage health needs
- Provide emotional support

2a Complications of Diabetes Mellitus
- Figure 25-5

SUGGESTIONS FOR CLASSROOM ACTIVITIES

- Assign students to view the animation on Diabetes on the CD-ROM with the textbook.
- Arrange for students to display a poster presentation on diabetes, emphasizing diet and proper administration of insulin, at a health fair or as health in-service at a middle or high school.

SUGGESTIONS FOR CLINICAL ACTIVITIES

- Have students develop a teaching tool for diabetic children, including insulin administration, diet, activity, sick day management, and complications. Have them use this tool in the acute care setting. Refer to Box 25-6 for sick day management.

CHAPTER 26
CARE OF THE CHILD
WITH A COMMUNICABLE DISEASE

RESOURCE LIBRARY

 CD-ROM

Throat culture

COMPANION WEBSITE

Avian flu
Disaster kit

IMAGE LIBRARY

Figure 26-1 Chain of infection.
Figure 26-2 Common infectious diseases of childhood.
Figure 26-3 Erythema migrans ("target" sign in Lyme disease).

Figure 26-4 Rocky Mountain spotted fever.
Figure 26-5 Cupping (A) and coining (B) are non-Western healing practices of some cultural groups that must be distinguished from child abuse.

LEARNING OUTCOME 1

Discuss the chain of infection.

CONCEPTS FOR LECTURE

1. Communicable diseases are diseases transmitted directly from person to person or indirectly to a person from a contaminated object.
2. For a communicable disease to be transmitted from person to person, there must be a pathogen, reservoir, portal of exit, portal of entry, and a susceptible host.
3. Harmful organisms are transmitted by direct and indirect methods.
4. Stages of the infectious process include the incubation period, the prodromal period, illness or the stage where clinical symptoms appear, and the convalescent period.

POWERPOINT LECTURE SLIDES

(NOTE: The number on each PPT Lecture Slide directly corresponds with the Concepts for Lecture.)

1 Communicable Diseases
- Diseases transmitted from one person to another
  - Direct contact with body fluids
  - Indirect contact with contaminated object

2 Chain of Infection
- Pathogen
  - Harmful organism
- Reservoir
  - Site of growth and reproduction of organism
- Portal of Exit
  - Method harmful organism leaves reservoir

2a Chain of Infection
- Transmission
  - Travel from portal of exit
  - Travel to portal of entry
- Portal of Entry
  - Method harmful organism enters new host

2b Chain of Infection
- Susceptible Host
  - Individual at risk for contracting disease
    - Young child, ill child, immunocompromised child

2c Chain of Infection
- Figure 26-1

3 Transmission of Harmful Organisms
- Direct Methods
  - Direct contact with body fluids, skin
  - Direct contact with mucous membranes

3a Transmission of Harmful Organisms
- Indirect Methods or Droplet Method
  - Sneezing, coughing, kissing, breathing, talking
    - Organisms attach to dust particles
  - Airborne transmission—organisms suspended in air
  - Fomites—inanimate objects transmit organisms
    - Comb or hairbrush, clothes, linens, eating utensils

4 Stages of Infectious Process
- Incubation Period
  - Time between entry into reservoir
  - And onset of clinical signs and symptoms
  - Pathogen multiplies in number

4a Stages of Infectious Process
- Prodromal Period
  - Prior to onset of clinical symptoms
  - Exhibit nonspecific symptoms
    - Lethargy, low-grade temperature
  - Contagious during this period

4b Stages of Infectious Period
- Illness
  - Clinical symptoms are exhibited
- Convalescent Period
  - Time between beginning of resolving symptoms and restoration of wellness

SUGGESTIONS FOR CLASSROOM ACTIVITIES

- Develop a matching quiz with terminology on the left side and definitions on the right side. Use the quiz as a review for an examination.
- Divide students into six groups. Assign each group a concept in the chain of infection. Have them give illustrations of each concept and discuss how to break the chain.

SUGGESTIONS FOR CLINICAL ACTIVITIES

- None

LEARNING OUTCOME 2

Explain the specific risk factors for communicable disease in children.

CONCEPTS FOR LECTURE

1. The healthy child is able to fight many infections due to active and passive immunity.
2. The child is particularly susceptible to communicable diseases due to many factors.

POWERPOINT LECTURE SLIDES

(NOTE: The number on each PPT Lecture Slide directly corresponds with the Concepts for Lecture.)

1 Immunity to Diseases
- Active Immunity
  - Organism enters body and becomes antigen
  - Body produces antibody to stop antigen

By 1 year of age, the child has adult levels of immunoglobulin M antibodies as a defense mechanism to help fight off infections.

Infants, toddlers, and preschoolers do not have the cognitive ability to understand the danger of passing bacteria from the hand to the mouth and the importance of hand washing.

Children are exposed to many varieties of harmful bacteria in school, day care, church nurseries, mothers' morning out groups, family gatherings, hospitals, and travel.

Children under the age of 2 years and those who are immunocompromised or in a weakened state are at an increased risk of nosocomial infections during hospitalization.

- White blood cells can destroy the antigen
- Memory B cells and T cells identify antigens
- Memory B/T cells reactivate with future exposure

1a Immunity to Diseases
- Passive Immunity
  - Passing of antibodies
  - From person who produced antibodies
  - Lasts short time
    - Mother to infant through placenta

2 Risk Factors for Communicable Diseases
- Immature immune system
- Lower number neutrophils
- Exposure to varieties of harmful bacteria
- Developmental level or cognitive ability
- Sharing toys and foods
- Sneezing, close contact when talking

2a Risk Factors for Communicable Diseases
- Nosocomial infection with hospitalization
- Travel to different parts of world
- Travel to different parts of own country
- Acts of bioterrorism
- Inconsistent hand washing
- Medical asepsis to reduce harmful bacteria

SUGGESTIONS FOR CLASSROOM ACTIVITIES

- Compare the difference between active immunity and passive immunity. Give examples of each.
- Have students discuss ways to prevent nosocomial infections.

SUGGESTIONS FOR CLINICAL ACTIVITIES

- Have students wash their hands with soap that leaves a glow under a black light to determine how well they wash their hands.
- Have students observe hand washing by hospital staff and discuss in postconference whether hand washing is done properly or not.

LEARNING OUTCOME 3

Describe methods of communicable disease prevention in children.

CONCEPTS FOR LECTURE

1. Nursing care for children with communicable diseases includes a variety of standards and precautions designed to prevent transmission of the disease or protect the child from additional harmful bacteria.

   The nurse must be able to implement these precautions: universal, standard, airborne, droplet, contact, and reverse isolation.

   The single most effective way to prevent the spread of communicable diseases is through hand washing.

2. Immunizations are an essential tool to protect children against communicable diseases.

3. An important nursing role is client and family teaching regarding methods of communicable disease prevention and disaster planning.

POWERPOINT LECTURE SLIDES

(NOTE: The number on each PPT Lecture Slide directly corresponds with the Concepts for Lecture.)

1 Communicable Disease Prevention
- Universal Precautions
  - Blood and body fluids of all clients
  - Potentially infectious for HIV, HBV
  - Other bloodborne pathogens

1a Communicable Disease Prevention
- Standard Precautions
  - Universal precautions and body substance isolation
  - Applies to all hospitalized clients
  - Includes hand washing, protective clothing

○ Includes equipment care, linen care
○ Private room for airborne or droplet transmission

 Communicable Disease Prevention
- Transmission-based Precautions
  ○ Standard plus airborne, droplet, contact precautions
  ○ Airborne precautions
    – Private room with negative air pressure
    – Door kept closed, chicken pox, measles
    – Wear particulate air filter respirator mask

 Communicable Disease Prevention
- Transmission-based Precautions
  ○ Droplet precautions
    – Private room with open door
    – Wear surgical mask within 3 feet
    – Child wears mask to leave room

 Communicable Disease Prevention
- Transmission-based Precautions
  ○ Contact precautions
    – Private room
    – Wear gloves upon entering room
    – Wear gown for body fluid contact
    – Remove gown and gloves to leave room

 Communicable Disease Prevention
- Transmission-based Precautions
  ○ Reverse isolation
    – For immunocompromised child
    – Wear gown, gloves, mask to enter room
    – Disinfect all equipment brought into room

 Immunizations
- Process of inducing resistance to disease
  ○ Vaccine
    – Killed, live, recombinant, conjugated microorganisms
    – Administered parenterally to induce immunity
    – Toxoid—type of vaccine
  ○ Immunization schedule for children

 Immunizations
- Immunotherapy
  ○ To prevent and treat diseases
  ○ Administration of allergens
  ○ Administration of immunostimulants, immunosuppressants
  ○ Administration of interferon, immune globulins

 Communicable Disease Prevention Teaching
- Discard tissues in trash immediately
- Wash hands after contact with body fluids
- Wash hands after toileting
- Wash hands after sneezing into hands
- Sneeze into elbow instead of hands
- Wash hands after coughing into hands

3a Communicable Disease Prevention Teaching
  • Wash and disinfect toys regularly
  • During communicability period, do not share toys
  • Avoid nail biting, thumb sucking
  • Avoid sharing drinks and eating utensils
  • Avoid putting items on floor into mouth
  • Monitor young child's behavior

3b Teaching Emergency Preparedness
  • Have specified disaster plan
  • Involve children in disaster plan
  • Involve children in creating disaster kit

SUGGESTIONS FOR CLASSROOM ACTIVITIES

• Have students view the animations on the textbook CD-ROM: Hand hygiene with soap and water, Glove application and removal.
• Review types of vaccines, recommended immunization schedules and nursing concerns about immunizations. Refer to Table 26-1 and Table 26-2.
• Arrange for a speaker from the Red Cross or another disaster preparedness agency to speak to students about disaster preparedness and planning a disaster kit.

SUGGESTIONS FOR CLINICAL ACTIVITIES

• Arrange for students to administer immunizations in a pediatrician's office or at a health clinic.
• Have students identify the use of precautions for infection control in the acute care setting. Discuss the proper use of gloves, gowns, and masks.
• Develop a teaching tool for creating a disaster kit. Hand out the teaching tool at a health fair, in schools, and in the acute care setting.

LEARNING OUTCOME 4

Discuss clinical manifestations, diagnostic procedures, and medical management related to childhood communicable diseases.

CONCEPTS FOR LECTURE

1. Communicable diseases are acute infections. It is important for the nurse to understand routes of transmission, the incubation periods, and clinical manifestations of communicable diseases.

    Comfort measures for children with communicable diseases include pain relief measures and measures to relieve pruritus.

2. Lyme disease and Rocky Mountain spotted fever are transmitted through tick bites. Tick removal and treatment need to be implemented promptly.

    Lyme disease has three stages of clinical manifestations. Supportive therapy is needed to treat the manifestations.

    The child with Rocky Mountain spotted fever needs to be monitored for bleeding and signs of shock.

3. Rabies is transmitted through the bite of an infected animal. Treatment needs to be implemented prior to completing studies on the animal. If animal is found to be rabies free, the vaccines may be stopped.

    The child with rabies may develop hydrophobia. The sight of liquid causes a reflex contraction accompanied by painful contractures in the muscles used for swallowing.

POWERPOINT LECTURE SLIDES

(NOTE: The number on each PPT Lecture Slide directly corresponds with the Concepts for Lecture.)

1 Common Communicable Diseases
  • Communicable diseases are acute infections
  • Have a limited duration time
  • Treatable in most cases
  • Route of transmission important
  • Incubation period important

1a Common Communicable Diseases
  • Diagnosis
    ○ Clinical manifestations
    ○ History of exposure to diseased child

1b Common Communicable Diseases
  • Treatment
    ○ Give supportive therapy
    ○ Teach parents prevention
    ○ Assist physician in providing medical treatment
    ○ Refer to Table 26-3

2 Infectious Diseases from Insects or Animals
  • Lyme Disease
    ○ Caused by *Borrelia burgdorferi*
    ○ Transmitted through tick bite
    ○ Incubation period 3 to 32 days

2a Lyme Disease
- Manifestations
  - Stage 1
    - Erythema migrans, malaise, headache, stiff neck
    - Low-grade fever, muscle or joint aches
    - Erythema migrans resolved in 4 weeks

2b Lyme Disease
- Manifestations
  - Stage 2
    - Pain and swelling of joints
    - Facial palsy, meningitis, AV block
  - Stage 3
    - Advanced musculoskeletal pain, deafness, encephalopathy

 2c Lyme Disease
- Diagnosis
  - ELISA or Western blot test
- Treatment
  - Administer antibiotics
  - Avoid fatigue
  - Administer pharmacologic and nonpharmacologic pain relief

 2d Infectious Diseases from Insects or Animals
- Rocky Mountain Spotted Fever
  - Caused by *Rickettsia rickettsii*
  - Transmitted through tick bite
  - Incubation period 2 to 12 days

 2e Rocky Mountain Spotted Fever
- Manifestations
  - Moderate to high fever, malaise
  - Abdominal and muscle pain, nausea, vomiting
  - Severe headache, conjunctival infection
  - Maculopapular rash that blanches, petechiae

 2f Rocky Mountain Spotted Fever
- Manifestations
  - GI bleeding, DIC, pulmonary complications
  - Encephalitis, neurologic dysfunction
  - Cardiac and renal complications

2g Rocky Mountain Spotted Fever
- Figure 26-4

2h Rocky Mountain Spotted Fever
- Diagnosis
  - Indirect immunofluorescent antibody assay
  - Enzyme immunoassay, indirect hemagglutination test
- Treatment
  - Administration of antibiotics
  - Observe for abnormal bleeding, shock

 3 Infectious Diseases from Insects or Animals
- Rabies
  - Caused by *Rhabdoviridae*
  - Transmitted by bite from infected animal
  - Incubation period is 1 to 7 weeks

3a Rabies
- Manifestations
  - Asymptomatic during incubation period
  - Pain at site of bite, headache, fever
  - Anorexia, malaise, hydrophobia, hallucinations
  - Disorientation, manic episodes, seizures
  - Stupor, coma, death

3b Rabies
- Diagnosis
  - Fluorescent antibody staining of dead animal's brain tissue

3c Rabies
- Treatment
  - Irrigate and wash bite thoroughly, suture
  - Administer human rabies immune globulin
  - Administer human diploid cell rabies vaccine
    - Five doses—days 0, 3, 7, 14, 28
  - Hospitalize with contact precautions

SUGGESTIONS FOR CLASSROOM ACTIVITIES

- Arrange for a school nurse to speak to students about their policies for handling an outbreak of communicable diseases in the schools.
- Develop case studies of children with various communicable diseases. Assign groups of students to complete the case study questions for a case study, and then present the case study to the rest of the class.
- Ask students about any communicable diseases they have had. How old were they, and what symptoms did they exhibit?

SUGGESTIONS FOR CLINICAL ACTIVITIES

- Arrange for students to spend time at the health department to find out the epidemiological studies they track for infectious diseases.

LEARNING OUTCOME 5

Explain appropriate nursing interventions for children with childhood communicable diseases.

CONCEPTS FOR LECTURE

1. The nurse has an important role in recognizing communicable disease symptoms and assisting the family in obtaining appropriate care.

   Priority nursing care includes managing fever, preventing respiratory distress, promoting skin integrity, and promoting comfort.

   The nurse uses skills in communication to teach children and parents how to manage care at home and how to prevent spread of infection.

   Children living in tick-prone areas need added protection from tick bites, which may cause Lyme disease and Rocky Mountain spotted fever. This protection includes insect repellent, long-sleeved shirts, long pants, and a hat when in tick-prone areas and vaccination with LYMErix for older children.

POWERPOINT LECTURE SLIDES

(NOTE: The number on each PPT Lecture Slide directly corresponds with the Concepts for Lecture.)

1 Lyme Disease
- Nursing Interventions
  - Teach proper method of tick removal
    - Use tweezers to grasp tick
    - Pull gently, do not squeeze body
  - Inspect whether entire tick removed
  - Recommend 3 dose vaccination LYMErix

1a Rocky Mountain Spotted Fever
- Nursing Interventions
  - Avoid fatigue by encouraging rest
  - Avoid strenuous physical activity
  - Administer pain relief measures
  - Implement preventative measures
    - Wear protective clothing, use insect repellent

1b Rabies
- Nursing Interventions
  - Observe for side effects of vaccine
  - Keep fluids away if hydrophobia present
  - Provide emotional support
  - Administer sedation to avoid exhaustion
  - Teach to stay away from stray animals

SUGGESTIONS FOR CLASSROOM ACTIVITIES

- Show pictures of children with communicable diseases. Have students identify the disease and discuss treatment and nursing interventions.

SUGGESTIONS FOR CLINICAL ACTIVITIES

- Assign students to provide nursing care to children with communicable diseases. Have them develop a nursing care plan or concept map, including the interventions they performed.
- Arrange for students to observe sick baby/child examinations in a pediatrician's office. Have them write a paper on their observations.

CHAPTER 27
CARE OF THE CHILD WITH PSYCHOSOCIAL DISORDERS

RESOURCE LIBRARY

 CD-ROM

What is autism?
Eating Disorders, Anorexia, and Bulimia
Identifying child abuse (Sexual)

COMPANION WEBSITE

Newborn safety

IMAGE LIBRARY

Figure 27-1 Child with autistic disorder.
Figure 27-2 Body image is the sum of a person's conscious and unconscious attitudes about his or her body.
Figure 27-3 The timing of physical abuse can be assessed by the color of bruises in soft tissue.

Figure 27-4 Alcoholism runs in families because of a combination of genetic and environmental factors.
Figure 27-5 Fetal alcohol syndrome is the result of a woman consuming alcohol during pregnancy, and it can have many severe effects on children.
Figure 27-6 The psychologist uses play therapy to help this girl re-enact a car crash.

LEARNING OUTCOME 1

Describe an appropriate psychosocial assessment of the child.

CONCEPTS FOR LECTURE

1. Psychosocial health includes mental, emotional, social, and spiritual stability.
    Alterations in psychosocial health affect the child as well as the entire family.

POWERPOINT LECTURE SLIDES

(NOTE: The number on each PPT Lecture Slide directly corresponds with the Concepts for Lecture.)

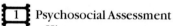 Psychosocial Assessment
- History
    - Past emotional or psychiatric problems
    - Family history of emotional or psychiatric problems
    - Child's growth and development
    - Performance in school, other activities
    - Relationships with others

[1a] Psychosocial Assessment
- History
    - Emotional response to illness and crises
    - Ask to define hope and faith
    - Determine self-concept
    - Use of alcohol and street drugs
    - Ask about eating disorders, sexual abuse

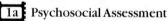 Psychosocial Assessment
- Physical
    - General appearance—dress, hygiene, grooming
    - Inspect dental enamel of teeth
    - Describe facial expression and affect
    - Observe body posture and gait
    - Describe speech patterns

LEARNING OUTCOME 2

Describe psychosocial disorders, including autism, Asperger's syndrome, attention deficit disorder, Giles de la Tourette syndrome, anxiety, depression, anorexia nervosa and bulimia, child abuse (physical and emotional), and substance abuse.

CONCEPTS FOR LECTURE

1. The *Diagnostic and Statistical Manual of Mental Disorders—Fourth Edition* (DSM-IV) serves as the main diagnostic reference of mental health professionals in the United States

2. Children with autism have difficulty with verbal and nonverbal communication, social interactions, and leisure or play activities.

3. The child with ADD has difficulty finishing tasks, is easily distracted, and may move from topic to topic, have difficulty working with others, and have difficulty maintaining relationships.

    The child with ADHD has difficulty finishing tasks, fidgets, may become loud and disrupt others, and has difficulty maintaining relationships.

4. Anxiety is subjective feelings of worry, helplessness, insecurity, and apprehension.

5. Giles de la Tourette syndrome is a syndrome of involuntary movements and verbalizations, which increase in stressful situations.

6. Depression is a persistent feeling of sadness or hopelessness.

7. Bipolar disorder is a disorder characterized by mood swings between mania and depression.

8. Anorexia nervosa is a serious disorder and may require hospitalization for teens that have lost significant weight, have severe electrolyte imbalances, or need constant psychological intervention.

9. Bulimia is an eating disorder characterized by binge eating and purging.

10. Physical abuse of a child is inflicting pain and injury in a deliberate manner. Bullying and shaken baby syndrome are types of physical abuse.

    Emotional abuse of a child includes attacks on a child's self-esteem and efforts to control, frighten, and embarrass the child.

    Physical neglect is the deliberate withholding of physical care or resources to the child.

11. Nonorganic failure to thrive is a disorder characterized by inadequate growth in height and weight.

12. Sexual abuse is defined as sexual acts imposed on children or teens who cannot protect themselves due to their incomplete emotional or cognitive development.

POWERPOINT LECTURE SLIDES

(NOTE: The number on each PPT Lecture Slide directly corresponds with the Concepts for Lecture.)

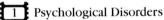 **1** Psychological Disorders
- *Diagnostic and Statistical Manual of Mental Disorders*
- Published by American Psychiatric Association
- Main diagnostic reference of mental health professionals
- Includes diagnostic criteria for disorders
- Uses for research purposes
- Used by insurance companies for payment charges

2 Psychosocial Disorders
- Autism and Asperger's Syndrome
  - Autism
    - Neurological disorder affecting brain function
    - Difficulty with social interaction and communication
  - Asperger's Syndrome
    - Similar to autism, preoccupation with something

3 Psychosocial Disorders
- Attention Deficit Disorder (ADD)
  - Central nervous system disorder
  - Inappropriate behaviors related to attention
- Attention Deficit/Hyperactivity Disorder (ADHD)
  - Inattention, hyperactivity, impulsiveness

4 Psychosocial Disorders
- Anxiety
  - Emotional feeling
  - Not related to actual past
  - Not related to upcoming event
  - Exists consistently
  - Out of proportion to reality

4a Anxiety
- Generalized anxiety disorder
  - Excessive worry about future
- Separation anxiety disorder
  - Fear of separation from individuals or location
- Obsessive-compulsive disorder
  - Ritualistic thoughts or actions

13. Children and teens are vulnerable to the hazards of substance abuse due to their incomplete physical developmental levels.

   Fetal alcohol syndrome can occur if a pregnant woman consumes alcohol during pregnancy.

5 Psychosocial Disorders
- Giles de la Tourette Syndrome
  - Possibly genetic syndrome
  - Involuntary movements
  - Verbal noises
  - Related to stressful periods

6 Psychosocial Disorders
- Depression
  - Persistent feeling of sadness or helplessness
  - Increasing in older adolescents

7 Psychosocial Disorders
- Bipolar Disorder
  - Called manic depression
  - Mood swings between mania and depression

8 Psychosocial Disorders
- Anorexia Nervosa
  - Eating disorder
  - Weight loss, emaciation, fear of gaining weight
  - Body weight < 85% expected weight
  - Decreased caloric intake, preoccupation with food
  - Strenuous exercise program

8a Psychosocial Disorders
- Anorexia Nervosa
  - Prepare elaborate meals for others
  - Cut up food and push around plate
  - Cry frequently, feel depressed and lonely
  - Consider suicide, fear of becoming fat
  - May have anxiety, obsessive compulsive disorder

9 Psychosocial Disorders
- Bulimia
  - Eating disorder of binge eating and purging
  - Induced vomiting and diarrhea

9a Anorexia Nervosa and Bulimia
- Figure 27-2

10 Child Abuse
- Crime punishable in all states
- Due to parental frustration, anger, stress
- Learned pattern of discipline and child rearing
- Unrealistic expectations of child
- Often abuse alcohol and other substances
- Children with birth defects or prematurity

10a Child Abuse
- Physical abuse
  - Inflicting pain and injury deliberately
  - Hitting, burning, biting, choking, shaking, throwing
  - Use hands, head, teeth, knees, feet
  - Use weapons
  - Administer excessive doses of or withhold medications

Child Abuse
- Physical abuse
  - Shaken Baby Syndrome
    - Jarring motion of head causes brain injuries
  - Bullying
    - Teasing, threatening, hitting, shoving, kicking, pushing
    - At school, community activities, religious activities

 Child Abuse
- Emotional abuse and neglect
  - Attacks on a child's self-esteem
  - Words to control and frighten child
  - Shamed, ridiculed, embarrassed
  - Withhold physical care or resources
  - Cold and insensitive to child's need

 Child Abuse
- Nonorganic failure to thrive
  - Inadequate growth in height and weight
  - Parents who are depressed, abuse substances
  - Parents who are mentally retarded, psychotic
  - Parents who are poor, low education level

 Child Abuse
- Sexual abuse
  - Sexual acts imposed on children
  - Lack of emotional or cognitive development
  - Most perpetrators are male

 Substance Abuse
- Use of tobacco, alcohol, illegal drugs
- Over-the-counter chemicals, household chemicals
- Adolescents struggling for identity, independence
- Exposure to addictive substances through peers, parents
- May work, steal, prostitute to purchase

Substance Abuse
- Fetal Alcohol syndrome
  - Pregnant woman consumes alcohol
  - Greater the consumption, greater the risk
  - No alcohol is safe during pregnancy

SUGGESTIONS FOR CLASSROOM ACTIVITIES

- Assign students to view the animations on the textbook CD-ROM: What is autism? Obsessive-Compulsive Behavior.
- Provide the fourth edition of the *Diagnostic and Statistical Manual of Mental Disorders* for the students to see. Discuss how the manual is used in clinical practice.
- Because bulimics can eat 10,000 to 12,000 calories a day, have the students develop a 24-hour meal plan with this many calories. Discuss interventions to help the child or adolescent with bulimia.

SUGGESTIONS FOR CLINICAL ACTIVITIES

- Arrange for students observe in an alternative classroom for children with developmental and learning difficulties. Have them discuss interventions used with the children to assist with their learning.

LEARNING OUTCOME 3

Describe associated manifestations of psychological disorders to include overeating and obesity and suicide.

CONCEPTS FOR LECTURE

1. Suicide is the second leading cause of death for 15- to 19-year-olds. Early detection is key to preventing suicide.
2. Many children have learned a pattern of overeating and obesity from their families and use overeating to compensate for insecurities. Sedentary lifestyle contributes to the risk of obesity.

POWERPOINT LECTURE SLIDES

(NOTE: The number on each PPT Lecture Slide directly corresponds with the Concepts for Lecture.)

 Associated Manifestations of Psychological Disorders
- Suicide
  - Second leading cause of death 15 to 19 years
  - Early detection is key to preventing
  - Lack of parental support with increased stressors
  - Easy access to firearms and drugs

1a Suicide
- Manifestations
  - Behavior changes, depression, doing poor in school
  - Withdrawn or isolated, overly impulsive
  - Uninterested in activities once enjoyed
  - Cries frequently, gives away treasured items
  - Verbalizes suicidal thoughts

1b Suicide
- Treatment
  - Administer antidepressants
  - Refer for individual and family counseling

1c Suicide
- Nursing Interventions
  - Use therapeutic communication to question client
  - Explore plan for suicide
  - Do not leave unattended
  - Refer depressed teen
  - Teach coping skills

2 Associated Manifestations of Psychological Disorders
- Overeating and Obesity
  - Obesity
    - Excessive weight and accumulation of body fat
    - BMI $\geq 95^{th}$ percentile
  - Overeating
    - Learned pattern from family

2a Overeating and Obesity
- Manifestations
  - Poor body image, depression
  - Low self-esteem, insecure
  - Lack of parental attention
  - Feelings of stress, anxiety, depression
  - Sedentary lifestyle

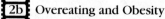 Overeating and Obesity
- Treatment
  - Refer to nutritionist
  - Perform bariatric surgery

2c Overeating and Obesity
- Nursing Interventions
  - Accurate height and weight
  - Measure blood pressure
  - Obtain serum cholesterol, triglycerides, glucose, hemoglobin A1
  - Assist family with nutrition needs
  - Promote self-esteem, exercise

SUGGESTIONS FOR CLASSROOM ACTIVITIES

- Assign students to view the animations on the textbook CD-ROM: Eating Disorders, Anorexia, and Bulimia.
- Have students research the Internet for articles on adolescent suicide and suicide prevention. Have the students share the main information from the articles.
- Assist students to develop a care plan for weight loss and exercise for a child who has obesity.

SUGGESTIONS FOR CLINICAL ACTIVITIES

- Arrange for students to visit a child/adolescent mental health unit or invite a child psychologist to speak to the students about suicide prevention and treatments for eating disorders.

LEARNING OUTCOME 4

Discuss clinical manifestations, diagnostic procedures, medical management, and nursing interventions related to psychosocial disorders.

CONCEPTS FOR LECTURE

1. Ensuring the safety of a child with autism is a priority nursing action due to the child's repetitive behaviors, such as head banging and the lack of fear of dangerous situations.
2. The nurse must assist the child and family to take medications prescribed for ADD and ADHD properly. Instructions would include avoiding side effects, timing medication administration to maximize attentiveness, and storing medication properly to avoid the risk of having the medication stolen and abused by others.
3. For the child with anxiety, the nurse can teach the child coping skills and relaxation techniques.
4. The nurse must provide parental support and assist the child in achieving normal development when the child has Giles de la Tourette syndrome.
5. Characteristics of depression can vary from child to child and can be caused by a primary condition or secondary to learned behavior due to dysfunctional family traits.
6. Bipolar disorder is characterized by mood swings that vary between mania and depression. Ten to twenty percent of those with bipolar disorder commit suicide.
7. With anorexia nervosa and bulimia, variations in fluid balance and nutrition can cause serious risks; the LPN/LVN needs to report significant changes immediately.

POWERPOINT LECTURE SLIDES

(NOTE: The number on each PPT Lecture Slide directly corresponds with the Concepts for Lecture.)

1 Autism and Asperger's Syndrome
- Manifestations
  - Infant
    - Lack of response to sound
    - Difficulty sleeping, feeding
    - Avoid eye contact, little response to humans

1a Autism and Asperger's Syndrome
- Manifestations
  - Toddler
    - Unable to communicate verbally, echolalia
    - No fear in unfamiliar environment
    - No fear unfamiliar people
    - Difficult toilet training

1b Autism and Asperger's Syndrome
- Manifestations
  - Child
    - Excessive repetitive behaviors, stereotypy
    - Stiff, unwilling to cuddle, awkward gait
    - Unable to interact socially, significant toy
    - Exaggerated response to pain or minimal response

1c Autism and Asperger's Syndrome
- Diagnosis
  - Symptoms, hearing tests
  - CT scan, MRI, test for lead poisoning
  - Metabolic studies, electroencephalogram

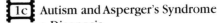

8. The nurse is legally obligated to report to local or state child protective services or law enforcement authorities any suspicion of child abuse. It can occur as physical abuse, emotional abuse, or sexual abuse.

Many parents who abuse their children were abused as children, which indicates a learned pattern of discipline and child rearing.

Shaken baby syndrome is a serious form of physical abuse that may cause permanent brain injury or death.

Bullying is a form of physical and emotional abuse that occurs outside the home.

The primary goal of treatment for nonorganic failure to thrive is adequate nutritional support.

Many children develop dissociation to cope with sexual abuse. The frequently turn to drugs, alcohol, running away, or inflicting pain on themselves or others.

The nurse must be able to recognize physical and psychological or cognitive symptoms of substance abuse.

9. The nurse caring for children and adolescents must give priority to assessing risk factors related to substance abuse.

Risks of fetal alcohol syndrome have three characteristics: growth retardation, CNS abnormalities, and craniofacial abnormalities.

1d Autism and Asperger's Syndrome
- Treatment
  - Provide highly structured environment
  - Provide one-on-one interaction
  - Mainstream into school
  - Give close supervision and consistency, restraint
  - Administer stimulants, SSRIs, mood stabilizers

1e Autism and Asperger's Syndrome
- Nursing Interventions
  - Determine rituals and communication patterns
  - Encourage parents to stay with child
  - Provide safety devices to protect from injury
  - Referrals to support groups

2 ADD and ADHD
- Manifestations
  - ADD
    - Difficulty finishing tasks, easily distracted
    - Move topic to topic in speech
    - Move topic to topic in activities
    - Distractible, difficulty working with others

2a ADD and ADHD
- Manifestations
  - ADHD
    - Difficulty finishing tasks, fidget
    - Loud and disrupt others
    - Difficulty maintaining relationships

2b ADD and ADHD
- Diagnosis
  - Evaluation by health care professional
  - Diagnosis scale
    - 6 of 9 inattentive or hyperactive symptoms
    - Duration longer than 6 months
    - Symptoms in more than one setting

2c ADD and ADHD
- Treatment
  - Change environment, decrease stimuli, provide structure
  - Use behavior modification, reward system
  - Administer stimulants, antidepressants
  - Administer antihypertensives, arousal agents

2d ADD and ADHD
- Nursing Interventions
  - Teach parents medication administration
  - Secure medications from abuse
  - Remove stimulating products from bedroom
  - Offer support for stable, routine environment
  - Refer parents to support groups

3 Anxiety
- Manifestations
  - Feelings of worry, helplessness, insecurity, apprehension
  - Tachycardia, restlessness, diaphoresis, trembling, regression
  - Enuresis, encopresis, withdrawal, overly dependent

3a Anxiety
- Diagnosis
  - Symptoms exhibited
- Treatment
  - Teach coping skills and relaxation techniques
  - Administer antidepressants and antianxiety medications

3b Anxiety
- Nursing Interventions
  - Help to develop coping skills
  - Replace negative thoughts with positive thoughts
  - Use physical activity to decrease stress
  - Avoid caffeine, tobacco, stimulants
  - Replace habits with healthy behaviors

4 Giles de la Tourette Syndrome
- Manifestations
  - Tics, coprolalia, copropraxia
- Treatment
  - Administer pimozide—dopamine receptor antagonist

4a Giles de la Tourette Syndrome
- Nursing Interventions
  - Provide parental support
  - Assist child to achieve normal development
  - Teach stress reduction techniques
  - Assist with home tutoring if needed

5 Depression
- Manifestations
  - Declining school performance, irritability, withdrawal
  - Sleep disorders, appetite disturbance, headache, stomachache
  - Difficulty concentrating, difficulty making decisions

5a Depression
- Treatment
  - Administer antidepressant medications
  - Monitor carefully for behavior changes

6 Bipolar Disorder
- Manifestations with mania
  - Hyperactivity, irritability, aggression, hallucinations

- Manifestations with depression
  - Sadness, sleep and eating disturbances
  - Social withdrawal
  - Suicide

6a Bipolar Disorder
- Treatment
  - Administer lithium, valproate, carbamazepine
  - Administer lamotrigine as a mood stabilizer

7 Anorexia Nervosa and Bulimia
- Manifestations Anorexia Nervosa
  - Cold intolerance, dizziness, constipation, bloating
  - Amenorrhea, lanugo, bradycardia
  - Osteoporosis, fractures, death

7a Anorexia Nervosa and Bulimia
- Manifestations Bulimia
  - Tooth and gum decay
  - Abrasions on back of hand
  - Abdominal distention

7b Anorexia Nervosa and Bulimia
- Treatment
  - Correct malnutrition
  - Provide psychological counseling for client and family
  - Administer total parenteral nutrition, intravenous fluids
  - Administer electrolytes, cardiac medications
  - Contract regarding eating habits

7c Anorexia Nervosa and Bulimia
- Nursing Interventions
  - Firmly enforce prescribed treatments
  - Identify manipulative behaviors
  - Obtain accurate weight, determine exercise habits
  - Measure intake and output
  - Monitor lab values for complications

8 Physical Abuse
- Manifestations
  - Bruises, burns, rope or cord marks
  - Multiple fractures, shortness of breath
  - Sedation from medication, withholding medications

8a Physical Abuse
- Shaken Baby Syndrome
  - Manifestations
    - Seizures, vomiting, lethargy, respiratory difficulties
    - Failure to thrive, mental retardation, paralysis
    - Vision or hearing impairment, developmental delays

8b Physical Abuse
- Bullying
  - Manifestations
    - Anxious, isolated, depressed, suicidal
    - Headaches, stomachaches, anger, aggression
    - Grades suffer, do not feel safe at school

8c Physical Abuse
- Treatment
  - Care by team of professionals
  - Ensure physical safety and recovery from injuries
  - Remove child from situation
  - Assist with emotional recovery
  - Develop plan for abuse-free environment

8d Physical Abuse
- Nursing Interventions
  - Chart bruises objectively
  - Chart subjective statements by parents

8e Emotional Abuse and Neglect
- Manifestations
  - Poor self-esteem, lack of friends
  - Lack of trust in adults, impaired communication
  - Frequent illness, failure to thrive
  - Behavior problems at school, depressed, suicidal

8f Nonorganic Failure to Thrive
- Manifestations
  - <3rd to 5th percentile on growth charts
  - Little subcutaneous fat, reduced muscle mass
  - Lifeless, apathetic, avoid eye contact
  - Flat affect, irritable, difficult to soothe
  - Signs of neglect, foul odor, developmental delays

8g Nonorganic Failure to Thrive
- Treatment
  - Provide adequate nutrition support
  - Promote bonding behaviors
  - Evaluate home environment
  - Ongoing environmental monitoring

8h Sexual Abuse
- Manifestations
  - Physical symptoms
  - Mood changes
  - Cognitive impairment
  - Sexual symptoms
  - Lack of coping skills, drug abuse

8i Sexual Abuse
- Diagnosis
  - History, physical evidence, forensic evidence
- Treatment
  - Refer to mental health professional
  - Ensure physical safety

Sexual Abuse
- Nursing Interventions
  - Explore possibility of sexual abuse in all children
  - Screen for sexual abuse

 Child Abuse
- Reporting
  - Must report to child protective services
  - Report immediately when symptoms recognized
  - Document clearly physical and subjective data
  - Obtain color pictures, notify parents of report
  - Fine or license revoked for not reporting

 Substance Abuse
- Manifestations
  - Physical symptoms
  - Psychological or cognitive symptoms
- Diagnosis
  - Toxicology studies in urine

 Substance Abuse
- Treatment
  - Removal of abused substance
  - Administer sedative-hypnotics, tranquilizers
  - Hospitalize and monitor for withdrawal
  - Psychological therapy

 Substance Abuse
- Nursing Interventions
  - Assess risk factors related to substance abuse
  - Determine child's knowledge of substances
  - Encourage activities to increase self-esteem
  - Ask direct, nonjudgmental questions about abuse
  - Refer for family counseling, support groups

Fetal Alcohol Syndrome
- Manifestations
  - Growth retardation, behavior problems
  - Developmental and cognitive delays
  - Craniofacial abnormalities

Fetal Alcohol Syndrome
- Nursing Interventions
  - Give nutrition support
  - Monitor intake and output
  - Refer mother to alcohol rehabilitation program
  - Monitor mother's care of baby

- Assign students to view the animation on the textbook CD-ROM: Sexual & Physical Abuse.
- Assign students to view the video on the textbook CD-ROM: Identifying Child Abuse (Sexual).
- Show a video on physical and emotional abuse in class. Discuss the long-term impact of abuse on children. Discuss the nursing responsibilities in suspected abuse. Refer to Box 27-4 for manifestations of abuse.
- Have students develop drug cards for the medications used for ADD and ADHD. Identify dosages, side effects, and nursing considerations for administration of the medications.
- Develop case studies of children with various psychosocial disorders. Assign groups of students to complete the case study questions for a case study, and then present the case study to the rest of the class.

SUGGESTIONS FOR CLINICAL ACTIVITIES

- Arrange for students to observe at a child abuse center. Have them write a paper on their observations.
- Assign students to provide nursing care to children with psychosocial disorders. Have them develop a nursing care plan or concept map including the interventions they performed.
- Arrange for students to interview a school nurse to understand the nursing care required for the student with psychosocial disorder. Discuss how the school nurse administers medications to students and what safety measures the nurse must use in regard to the medications.

LEARNING OUTCOME 5

Explain appropriate nursing interventions for children with psychosocial disorders.

CONCEPTS FOR LECTURE

1. Therapies used to assist the child with psychosocial disorders are play therapy, group therapy, family therapy, art therapy, behavior therapy, and cognitive therapy.

    The nurse can assist physicians and mental health professionals to administer therapies to assist the child with psychosocial disorders.

POWERPOINT LECTURE SLIDES

1 Therapies for Psychosocial Disorders
- Play Therapy
  - Allows expression of emotions
  - Play with dolls, toys, clay
  - Used to express anxiety, stress, fears
  - Used to determine child's feelings
  - Teach methods of dealing with negative emotions

1a Play Therapy
- Figure 27-6

1b Therapies for Psychosocial Disorders
- Group Therapy
  - More responsive to peers
  - Assist with verbalizing feelings
  - Accept suggestions from peers
  - Hazard is lack of control by therapist

1c Therapies for Psychosocial Disorders
- Family Therapy
  - Seeks to build strong relationships
  - Promote healing of child
  - Promote future healthy relationships

1d Therapies for Psychosocial Disorders
- Art Therapy
  - Create something that depicts feelings
  - Use to discuss child's feelings
  - Develop methods of managing negative emotions
  - Discover hidden events of abuse or violence

1e Therapies for Psychosocial Disorders
- Behavior Therapy
  ○ To replace negative, unwanted behaviors
  ○ Encourage positive, desirable behaviors
  ○ Use of rewards to reinforce behaviors
  ○ Consistent use of therapy

1f Therapies for Psychosocial Disorders
- Cognitive Therapy
  ○ To recognize negative emotions quickly
  ○ Teach benefits of avoiding emotions
  ○ Teach why negative emotions detrimental
  ○ Teach mental activities to counteract negative emotions

SUGGESTIONS FOR CLASSROOM ACTIVITIES

- Do a relaxation therapy exercise with the students. Dim the lights, play a relaxation music tape, and guide them through a tightening and relaxing muscle exercise.

SUGGESTIONS FOR CLINICAL ACTIVITIES

- Arrange for students to attend an Alcoholics Anonymous meeting or Narcotic Anonymous meeting. Have them compare their observations.
- When caring for children in the acute care setting, have a child draw a picture of what they think about being in the hospital. Have the child explain the picture to the student and then have the student discuss the picture in postconference.

LEARNING OUTCOME 6

Discuss the impact to children of traumatic events and natural disasters.

CONCEPTS FOR LECTURE

1. Children can have negative effects from a traumatic event whether they experience it personally or witness it.

   Children may be affected mentally, emotionally, physically, or morally.

POWERPOINT LECTURE SLIDES

1 Impact of Traumatic Events and Natural Disasters
- Violent crimes, natural disasters, MVAs, abuse
- Negative effects whether experienced or witnessed
- Manifestations
  ○ Feel frightened, confused, insecure
  ○ Feel anger, isolated, anxiety

1a Impact of Traumatic Events and Natural Disasters
- Nursing Interventions
  ○ Discuss event openly and honestly
  ○ Help parents understand child's needs
  ○ Provide reassurance, love, physical contact
  ○ Encourage expression of emotions through drawing
  ○ Maintain normal routine, professional counseling

SUGGESTIONS FOR CLASSROOM ACTIVITIES

- Have students brainstorm traumatic events that can affect children. Discuss the effects of traumatic events at different developmental levels of children. Refer to Box 27-6.

SUGGESTIONS FOR CLINICAL ACTIVITIES

- Have students research the disaster plan for an acute care setting. What is the role of the nurse in a disaster? What is done to make the experience less traumatic for the children on a pediatric unit?

CHAPTER 28
CARE OF THE FAMILY WITH A DYING CHILD

RESOURCE LIBRARY

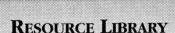 **COMPANION WEBSITE**

Organ donation

 IMAGE LIBRARY

Figure 28-1 Five stages of grief have been identified, but clients do not always experience all five stages.

Figure 28-2 This 3 1/2-year-old's condition has deteriorated rapidly, and death is expected within 2 to 3 days.

Figure 28-3 This teenager and his mother are exploring computer chat rooms of terminally ill children receiving palliative care.

Figure 28-4 When siblings visit the dying child, be prepared to answer questions honestly and in a manner that they can understand.

Figure 28-5 Nurses who work with the dying need to express their own grief in a supportive environment after a child's death.

Figure 28-6 Hospices like Pathways KIDS work with the client and family to provide quality of life for the dying child.

LEARNING OUTCOME 1

Define key terms.

CONCEPTS FOR LECTURE

1. Loss, either real or perceived, is experienced when something is removed from the body or the environment. It may be tangible, such as a missing toy, or intangible, such as loss of health.
2. Grief is a feeling of extreme sadness resulting from a loss.
3. Anticipated loss begins when first hearing of a life-threatening diagnosis or injury.
4. Dysfunctional grief occurs when an individual is unable to accept what has happened and move on with life. Signs should be reported to the registered nurse or physician.
5. Palliative care or palliative management involves a shift in treatment goals to providing relief from suffering.
6. Hospice care is based on the holistic concept of palliative care that emphasizes care to improve the quality of life rather than to cure.

POWERPOINT LECTURE SLIDES

(NOTE: The number on each PPT Lecture Slide directly corresponds with the Concepts for Lecture.)

1 Loss
- Real or perceived
- Something removed from body or environment
- Tangible or intangible

2 Grief
- Feeling of extreme sadness
- Results from a loss

3 Anticipated Loss
- Occurs during life-threatening illness or injury
- Begins the moment of notification
- Anticipate death, permanent damage, disfigurement
- Periods of calm acceptance or emotional stress

3a Anticipated Loss
- Figure 28-2

4 Dysfunctional Grief
- Unable to accept death
- Unable to move on with life
- Manifestations
  ○ Continuous crying, sleep disturbances, eating disturbances

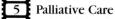
     ○ Difficulty with household activities, unable to work
     ○ Unable to dispose of belongings

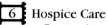 **5** Palliative Care
- Fulfill desires as much as possible
- Death regarded as natural process
- Diagnostic and invasive procedures minimized
- Discourage "heroic" treatment, provide pain relief
- Do not force feedings, individualize care

6 Hospice Care
- Care to improve quality of life
- Carried out in variety of settings
- Comprehensive to focused specialized care
- Delivered by team of health care professionals
- Prognosis of six months or less life expectancy
- Requires physician referral

SUGGESTIONS FOR CLASSROOM ACTIVITIES

- Review key terms in class.
- Compare the terms *palliative care* with *hospice care*. Discuss nursing responsibilities in each type of care. Ask students to discuss their feelings about palliative care and hospice care.

SUGGESTIONS FOR CLINICAL ACTIVITIES

- Arrange for students to visit a hospice unit. Have them interview a hospice nurse to discover the differences in responsibilities from an acute-care nurse.

LEARNING OUTCOME 2

Describe the stages of grief.

CONCEPTS FOR LECTURE

1. According to Kübler-Ross, there are five stages of grief with any major loss.

    Stages of grief are experienced twice: once when loss is anticipated and once when loss actually happens.

    Individuals move through the stages of grief at different rates, and some people experience a stage more than once.

    It is helpful for the nurse to know the stages of grief in order to communicate well with the client.

2. The nurse must promote growth and development and support the family and peers while providing care to the terminally ill child.

    The death of a child is the most painful experience a parent will have to endure.

    Siblings need support and compassion. The nurse needs to explain what is happening in age-appropriate language.

    By acknowledging the grandparents' loss and feelings of helplessness, the nurse communicates empathy for them.

    Nurses who work frequently with the dying child and their family must learn to cope with grief while maintaining their objectivity, empathy, and compassion.

POWERPOINT LECTURE SLIDES

(NOTE: The number on each PPT Lecture Slide directly corresponds with the Concepts for Lecture.)

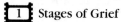 **1** Stages of Grief
- Stage 1—Shock and Disbelief
   ○ Conscious mind trying to process what happened
   ○ Sensory perceptions altered
   ○ Grope for answers and explanations
   ○ May need information repeated several times
   ○ Display wide range of behaviors

1a Stages of Grief
- Stage 2—Anger
   ○ Direct anger at self or others
   ○ Make accusations or threatening comments
   ○ Assault person they believe is responsible
   ○ Nurse needs to maintain objectivity
   ○ Nurse helps to defuse situation

1b Stages of Grief
- Stage 3—Bargaining
   ○ Make deal with others to prevent loss
   ○ Nurse must understand comments
   ○ Nurse must provide support

Family religious and cultural practices related to death should be asked about and honored.

1c Stages of Grief
- Stage 4—Depression
  - State of persistent sadness
  - Lacks energy or enthusiasm to perform ADLs
  - Experience persistent hopelessness, tearfulness, worthlessness
  - Experience times of calm in remembering
  - Nurse helps to explore and understand feelings

1d Stages of Grief
- Stage 5—Acceptance
  - Acceptance of loss of child and dreams
  - Able to make new dreams and plans
  - Encourage to reminisce happy times
  - Help other grieving families

1e Stages of Grief
- Figure 28-1

2 Dying Child
- Infant
  - No concept of illness or death
- Toddler
  - Responds to parent's anxiety
  - Fear body mutilation and pain

2a Dying Child
- Preschooler, beginning school-age
  - Aware of death but not permanence
  - Fear of mutilation
  - Know when condition worsens

2b Dying Child
- Child
  - Keep fears to self

2c Dying Child
- Adolescence
  - Understand death
  - Preoccupied with body image
  - Feel isolated from friends
  - Allow control over events
  - Nurse provides for emotional needs

2d Dying Child
- Figure 28-3

2e Parents of Dying Child
- Provide private room
- Use one spokesperson to inform family
- Assurance everything is being done
- Prepare body before allowing to view
- Encourage talk about feelings

2f Siblings of Child
- Reaction depends on age, development
- May feel punishment for something they did
- Jealous of attention to ill sibling
- Need support and compassion
- Allow to participate in care
- Help to understand finality of death

2g Siblings of Dying Child
- Figure 28-4

2h Grandparents of Dying Child
- Feel intense pain for own child's loss
- Experience helplessness and guilt
- Needs go unrecognized and unmet
- Encourage to express feelings
- Communicate empathy for grandparents

2i Nurses' Grief
- Grieve loss of client
- Feel as if failed client, parents, family
- Begin withdrawal from relationship prior to death
- Feelings of anger, frustration, sadness, powerlessness
- Need to share grief with others

2j Nurses' Grief
- Figure 28-5

2k Culture and Grief
- Understand cultural rites and rituals
- Ask questions about cultural needs
- Provide care with compassion and understanding

SUGGESTIONS FOR CLASSROOM ACTIVITIES

- Compare stages of grief and give examples of client behavior in each stage. Discuss nursing interventions during each stage.
- Compare an infant's, child's, and adolescent's understanding of death. Refer to Table 28-1.
- Arrange for a grief counselor to talk to the students about loss and grief, especially after a child's death.

SUGGESTIONS FOR CLINICAL ACTIVITIES

- Discuss how to communicate with the dying child and family.

LEARNING OUTCOME 3

Describe the signs of impending death.

CONCEPTS FOR LECTURE

1. Although the exact time of death cannot be predicted, physical changes in the child can indicate that death is approaching.

POWERPOINT LECTURE SLIDES

(NOTE: The number on each PPT Lecture Slide directly corresponds with the Concepts for Lecture.)

1 Signs of Impending Death
- Pulse increases, heart rhythm becomes irregular
- Heart slows, blood pressure drops, skin mottled
- Less responsive, coma, reflexes become absent
- Kidneys stop producing urine, peristalsis slows
- Pulmonary edema develops, Cheyne-Stokes breathing
- Apnea, heart stops

SUGGESTIONS FOR CLASSROOM ACTIVITIES

- Present a video on the dying child and care before and after death.

SUGGESTIONS FOR CLINICAL ACTIVITIES

- Discuss how to explain to the family what they will see as death nears.

LEARNING OUTCOME 4

Describe the role of the LPN/LVN in caring for dying children and their families.

CONCEPTS FOR LECTURE

1. As the child deteriorates, the plan should change from curative care to palliative care.

   The nurse must provide emotional support or resources for emotional support to the dying child as well as every member of the family.

2. Nurses' roles in legal issues related to death are determined by the laws of the region and the policies of the health care institution.

   The older child and parents should be encouraged to communicate their wishes about advanced directives and do-not-resuscitate orders.

3. Facility policy must be followed in providing postmortem care, including providing the death certificate, notifying family, and notifying the mortuary.

   Knowledge of client's religious and cultural beliefs helps nurse provide individualized care to clients and their families.

POWERPOINT LECTURE SLIDES

(NOTE: The number on each PPT Lecture Slide directly corresponds with the Concepts for Lecture.)

1 Care for Dying Child
- Change from curative care to palliative care
- Provide comfort measures
  - Change position frequently, frequent oral care
  - Provide liquid tears, administer pain medication
  - Provide alternative pain relieving methods
- Provide emotional support

2 Legalities Related to Death
- Advanced Directives
  - Living will
    - Medical treatment to choose or omit
  - Health care proxy or surrogate
    - Durable power of attorney for health care
  - Witnessed by two people

2a Legalities Related to Death
- Do-Not-Resuscitate Orders
  - No resuscitation for respiratory or cardiac arrest
  - "Comfort measures only"
  - Comfortable, dignified death

2b Legalities Related to Death
- Euthanasia
  - Compassionate putting to death
  - Suffering from incurable or distressing death
- Voluntary euthanasia or assisted suicide
  - Control over time and manner of death
  - Prescribe lethal doses of medication

3 Care After Death
- Provide postmortem care
  - Rigor mortis 2 to 4 hours after death
  - Algor mortis decreasing body temperature
  - Livor mortis skin discoloration
  - Embalming prevents body destruction by bacteria

3a Care After Death
- Certification of Death
  - Pronouncement by physician, coroner, nurse
  - Certificate done when person dies
  - Signed by attending physician
  - Filed with local health or government office
  - Family given copy

3b Care After Death
- Care of Body
  - Check client's religion, comply with wishes
  - Prepare body for viewing, remove equipment
  - Supine position, arms down, head elevated
  - Eyelids and mouth closed
  - Wash soiled body, absorbent pads under body

3c Care After Death
- Labeling of deceased
  - Wrist identification left on
  - Tag ankle or toe and shroud
  - Include name, hospital number, physician's name
- Viewing by parents
  - Stay with parents for support

3d Care After Death
- Calling the mortuary
  - Nurse's responsibility
- Autopsy
  - Physician responsibility, only in certain cases
- Inquest
  - Legal inquiry into cause or manner of death

3e Death-Related Religious and Cultural Practices
- Provide individualized care to client and family
- Be knowledgeable about death-related rituals
- Ask family member's preference
- Verify who will carry out preferences
- Return ritual items to family

SUGGESTIONS FOR CLASSROOM ACTIVITIES

- Discuss cultural and religious beliefs regarding death. Discuss how the nurse can intervene to meet the needs of the family. Refer to Table 28-3.
- Develop case studies of terminally ill or injured children. Assign groups of students to complete the case study questions for a case study, and then present the case study to the rest of the class.
- Have students research the state and local laws regarding autopsy, euthanasia, assisted suicide, and do-not-resuscitate orders. Have them write their own do-not-resuscitate orders.

SUGGESTIONS FOR CLINICAL ACTIVITIES

- Assign students to provide nursing care to children with terminal disorders. Have them develop a nursing care plan or concept map, including the interventions they performed.
- If possible, have students assist with postmortem care. Discuss their feelings about the experience in postconference.

LEARNING OUTCOME 5

Discuss the process of organ donation.

CONCEPTS FOR LECTURE

1. Federal regulations require the family to be given the option of donating the child's organs for research or transplant.
2. Nurses with special education in organ procurement should be called to talk with the family and obtain informed consent.

POWERPOINT LECTURE SLIDES

(NOTE: The number on each PPT Lecture Slide directly corresponds with the Concepts for Lecture.)

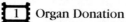 **1** Organ Donation
- Federal regulations require option of donation
- Trained nurse speaks with family
- Informed consent obtained
- Notify physician immediately
- May alter use of life-support medications

SUGGESTIONS FOR CLASSROOM ACTIVITIES

- Arrange for a nurse trained in organ procurement to speak to the students about how to approach parents, obtain an informed consent, and prepare the body for organ donation.

SUGGESTIONS FOR CLINICAL ACTIVITIES

- Have students research the local hospital's policies regarding organ donations.

CHAPTER 1

1. The historic use of medications that produced "twilight sleep" during labor was discontinued because the use of this type of medication caused an increase in the:
1. Cesarean birth rate.
2. Maternal mortality rate.
3. Infant mortality rate.
4. Preterm birth rate.

Answer: 1
Rationale: The cesarean birth rate rose because the anesthesia reduced the ability of the laboring woman to push effectively. The maternal and infant mortality rates were reduced and the preterm birth rate was not affected by the change in anesthesia methods.
Nursing process step: Evaluation
Category of client need: Safe, effective care environment
Cognitive level: Application
Learning outcome 1-1: Describe the historical changes in maternity care and pediatrics
Test-taking tip: When a question is looking at the cause and effect of a situation, consider the most direct relationship between the question and the answer as the correct choice.

2. Changes in the health care delivery system have brought about changes in the way care providers view those that they treat. Which of the following terms implies that the recipient of health care services is an active participant in the health care process with both rights and responsibilities?
1. Client
2. Consumer
3. Advocate
4. Client

Answer: 4
Rationale: *Client* is the term that describes the individual actively participating in his or her own care. The term *client* is associated with an individual who receives care; a *consumer* is an individual who purchases a commodity. An *advocate* is one who promotes productive changes in health care practices.
Nursing process step: Assessment
Category of client need: Health promotion and maintenance
Cognitive level: Application
Learning outcome 1-1: Describe the historical changes in maternity care and pediatrics
Test-taking tip: By knowing the definitions of key terms, the student can choose the correct answer.

3. Which of the following represents the implementation phase of the nursing process?
1. The nurse obtaining vital signs.
2. The nurse reviewing new physician orders.
3. The nurse repositioning a client who reports pain.
4. The nurse discussing medications with a pharmacist.

Answer: 3
Rationale: Repositioning a client represents implementation of a nursing intervention. Obtaining vital signs is nursing assessment. Reviewing new physician orders and discussing medication side effects would be part of the planning phase of the nursing process.
Nursing process step: Implementation
Category of client need: Safe, effective care environment
Cognitive level: Application
Learning outcome 1-2: Describe the steps of the nursing process.
Test-taking tip: By knowing the definitions of key terms and how they relate to the nursing process, the student can choose the correct answer.

4. List the following nursing actions in the order they should occur when the LPN/LVN is using the nursing process.
1. Determines that a client has severe pain in the abdomen following a cesarean section
2. Flushes the IV line and gives 25 mg of Demerol over 2 minutes
3. Documents that the client is able to turn from side to side without grimacing
4. Reviews the physician order sheet and the medication administration record for available drug therapies

Answer: 1, 4, 2, 3
Rationale: The nursing process begins with assessment and determining that the client has pain. The second step is planning, which includes verifying the physician order and checking the medication administration record to determine what drugs and doses can be given to relieve the pain. The next step is implementation and the actual administration of the Demerol, and the final step is evaluation when the client is demonstrating improvement in comfort because the client can move easily from side to side.
Nursing process step: Implementation
Category of client need: Safe, effective care environment
Cognitive level: Application
Learning outcome 1-2: Describe the steps of the nursing process.
Test-taking tip: The student should be able to define and describe the stops of the nursing process.

5. Which of the following situations best represents the infant mortality rates for a population?
1. A hospital has 5 stillbirths and 400 live births annually.
2. A state health department reports 12 deaths in children under age 1 for every 1,000 births each year.
3. There are 10,000 children that die annually in a given country.
4. A county reports 7 SIDS related deaths, 4 AIDS related deaths and 5 accidental deaths in a single year.

Answer: 2
Rationale: The infant mortality rate is the number of deaths during the first year of life out of 1,000 live births. The other statements do not correctly describe infant mortality.
Nursing process step: Assessment
Category of client need: Safe, effective care environment
Cognitive level: Application
Learning outcome 1-3: Describe the benefit of research for nursing practice.
Test-taking tip: By knowing the definitions of key terms, the student can choose the correct answer.

---

6. Which of the following represents a primary care activity?
1. Outclient chemotherapy infusion for a child with leukemia
2. Hospice care for a child with muscular dystrophy
3. Postoperative care following a tonsillectomy
4. Immunization updates as part of a preschool physical examination

Answer: 4
Rationale: Primary care activities are those that represent health promotion or disease prevention activities. Immunizations are a disease prevention activity. Outclient chemotherapy and postoperative care after a tonsillectomy would both be secondary health care activities since they involve an acute disease or situation. Hospice care would be tertiary care.
Nursing process step: Planning
Category of client need: Health promotion and maintenance
Cognitive level: Analysis
Learning outcome 1-4: Describe community-based nursing practice.
Test-taking tip: Look for the answer that is most different from the others.

---

7. The goal of tertiary health care is:
1. Illness prevention.
2. Resolution of acute conditions.
3. Restoration of maximum function.
4. Health maintenance.

Answer: 3
Rationale: Tertiary care includes rehabilitation, chronic, and terminal conditions. The goal is to restore maximum function. Illness prevention and health maintenance are primary care activities and treating acute conditions is secondary health care.
Nursing process step: Diagnosis
Category of client need: Safe, effective care environment
Cognitive level: Application
Learning outcome 1-4: Describe community-based nursing practice
Test-taking tip: By knowing the definitions of key terms, the student can choose the correct answer.

---

8. The community-based LPN/LVN must demonstrate successful integration of a variety of practice roles. Nurses may demonstrate this role diversity when working without compensation at the local free clinic, translating a handout from English to Spanish for parents when their children are admitted to the hospital, and meeting with a registered nurse, respiratory therapist, physical therapist, and chaplain to discuss the care of a homebound client. These nurses are demonstrating which of the following roles? *Select all that apply.*
1. Community volunteer
2. Community educator
3. Cultural competence
4. Consultant
5. Collaborator

Answer: 1, 3, and 5
Rationale: A nurse who works without pay is a community volunteer, a nurse who provides a translated handout for non-English-speaking clients is demonstrating cultural competence, and a nurse who meets with other professionals to plan care is in the role of collaborator. These examples are not of a community educator or consultant.
Nursing process step: Planning
Category of client need: Safe, effective care environment
Cognitive level: Application
Learning outcome 1-5: Describe LPN/LVN roles in maternal-child nursing.
Test-taking tip: Look for specific answers that best fit the roles described.

9. Which of the following is objective data? *Select all that apply.* 1. Temperature 98.7°F 2. Pain 5/10 3. Incision is reddened 4. Hemoglobin 12.6 5. Nausea	Answer: 1, 3, and 4 Rationale: Objective data is data that are observed or measured, including vital signs, assessments, and lab tests. Information that the client reports, such as pain or nausea, is subjective data. Nursing process step: Assessment Category of client need: Safe, effective care environment Cognitive level: Analysis Learning outcome 1-5: Describe LPN/LVN roles in maternal-child nursing. Test-taking tip: By knowing the definitions of key terms, the student can choose the correct answer.
10. Which statement is true regarding homeopathy? 1. It is a Japanese technique of energy healing. 2. Pressure applied to trigger points helps to balance energy. 3. It utilizes natural techniques, such as vitamins and diet, to restore health. 4. A small amount of a substance will stimulate the immune response.	Answer: 4 Rationale: Homeopathy is a health belief system that encourages the stimulation of the immune system by a small amount of a disease trigger. Reiki is a Japanese system of energy healing and acupuncture that uses trigger points that promote healing and energy balance. Naturopathy uses vitamins and diet as part of the health restoration process. Nursing process step: Implementation Category of client need: Health promotion and maintenance Cognitive level: Application Learning outcome 1-4: Describe community-based nursing practice. Test-taking tip: By knowing the definitions of key terms, the student can choose the correct answer.
11. Which of the following clients should the LPN/LVN check on first at the start of a morning shift? 1. The postpartum client and her newborn who are planning to be discharged later in the morning 2. The newborn who is being treated with phototherapy using a BiliBlanket 3. The first day postoperative cesarean client who has an IV antibiotic due in 1 hour 4. The woman at 8 weeks gestation admitted from the emergency room for heavy vaginal bleeding 2 hours ago	Answer: 4 Rationale: The client who is bleeding heavily at 8 weeks gestation is at the greatest risk when the nurse prioritizes care by airway, breathing, and circulation; the bleeding would be the key factor in the prioritization. The client about to be discharged would be stable and not likely to need immediate assessment. The newborn being treated with phototherapy should be seen as a second priority but would not be as acute as the bleeding client. The antibiotic should be administered within 1 hour of the designated time. Nursing process step: Planning Category of client need: Safe, effective care environment Cognitive level: Analysis Learning outcome 1-6: Prioritize nursing care to assess the most unstable or critical clients first. Test-taking tip: Look for answer choices that provide the safest possible environment for the client.
12. The LPN/LVN can evaluate whether or not it would be appropriate to perform a given task if the task meets which of the following criteria? *Select all that apply.* 1. Permitted by the State Board of Nursing 2. Part of the nurse's basic education program 3. No other personnel are available to perform the task 4. The client's life is in jeopardy if the task is not performed 5. The employer has policies and procedures on file for the task	Answer: 1, 2, and 5 Rationale: When an LPN/LVN is deciding whether performance of a task is appropriate, it must be determined if the task is within the scope of nursing practice as described by the State Board of Nursing and if the employer has documented within the facility how and when the task should be performed. The nurse should also know how to perform the task, and that would be documented if the task were part of the basic education program or the nurse has received appropriate supervision/training to perform the task. The nurse should not perform the task even if there is no one else available to perform the task or the client is in jeopardy. Nursing process step: Implementation Category of client need: Safe, effective care environment Cognitive level: Application Learning outcome 1-6: Describe decision making and prioritizing as they relate to nursing scope of practice Test-taking tip: Look for answer choices that provide the safest possible environment for the client.

13. Which of the following situations describes the evaluation step of the nursing process?
1. The nurse who repeats a temperature after giving Tylenol to a febrile client.
2. The nurse who documents intake and output in the client's chart.
3. The nurse who wraps a baby in a warm blanket after a bath.
4. The nurse who notifies a physician when a child has a pulse rate of 180.

Answer: 1
Rationale: Evaluation is the part of the nursing process that includes reassessment of the client after the nurse has provided an intervention for a problem. Retaking a temperature allows the nurse to determine the effectiveness of the Tylenol administration. Documentation and client care are part of the implementation phase of the nursing process. Contacting a physician is part of the diagnosis phase of the nursing process.
Nursing process step: Evaluation
Category of client need: Health promotion and maintenance
Cognitive level: Application
Learning outcome 1-2: Describe the steps of the nursing process.
Test-taking tip: By knowing the definitions of key terms and the steps of the nursing process, the student can choose the correct answer.

14. An LPN/LVN should determine the competence of an individual to perform a given task. If the individual has been certified as a Nursing Assistant, the nurse should:
1. See a copy of the certification.
2. Teach a class for CNAs before delegation.
3. Observe the CNA as the task is performed.
4. Discuss the procedure with the CNA.

Answer: 3
Rationale: Before delegating a task, the licensed nurse should determine the competency of the CNA and that can best be accomplished by observation. The other choices would not give the nurse the proof that the CNA could safely complete the task.
Nursing process step: Implementation
Category of client need: Safe, effective care environment
Cognitive level: Application
Learning outcome 1-7: Describe the delegation process related to nursing scope of practice.
Test-taking tip: By knowing the definitions of key terms, the student can choose the correct answer.

15. Which of the following represents appropriate delegation?
1. The CNA asks another CNA to remove the Foley catheter of a postoperative client
2. The registered nurse asks the LPN/LVN to obtain vital signs and an assessment of the client immediately following a seizure
3. The LPN/LVN delegates vital signs for a client receiving a blood transfusion to the CNA
4. The LPN/LVN delegates to the unlicensed assistive personnel to record the intake and output for a client following surgery

Answer: 4
Rationale: Recording intake and output for a client following surgery is a task that would be appropriate for delegation, and the LPN/LVN can delegate to the CNA. One CNA cannot delegate to another CNA. A client who just had a seizure would not be an appropriate client for the RN to delegate any tasks for care by other personnel. A client who is receiving a blood transfusion should only be assessed by licensed personnel.
Nursing process step: Planning
Category of client need: Safe, effective care environment
Cognitive level: Analysis
Learning outcome 1-7: Describe the delegation process related to nursing scope of practice.
Test-taking tip: Look for an answer that describes appropriate nursing actions.

CHAPTER 2

1. A parent may lose the right to make health care decisions for their child if (*select all that apply*):
1. The parent is mentally incapacitated.
2. The child has been living separately from the parent for 6 months or more.
3. The child professes to follow a religion that prohibits certain medical treatments.
4. The child is a suspected victim of abuse or neglect.
5. The parent has refused life-saving treatments for a child.

Answer: 1, 4, and 5
Rationale: When a parent cannot demonstrate mental competence, a child is abused while in the care of the parents, or the parents refuse life-saving medical care for a child, parental rights may be terminated. A child may live separately from the parents and the parent may still have the right to make decisions for a child. The child's religious beliefs do not affect parental rights.
Nursing process step: Diagnosis
Category of client need: Safe, effective care environment
Cognitive level: Application
Learning outcome 2-1: Describe federal initiatives to protect children.
Test-taking tip: Look for the answer that allows for the safest child care situations.

2. Which of the following adolescents could be considered emancipated?
1. The 14-year-old who resides 9 months a year at a boarding school
2. The 15-year-old living with grandparents in a different state
3. The 17-year-old sent to a juvenile detention center by the courts
4. The 16-year-old living with her husband and newborn baby

Answer: 4
Rationale: Emancipated adolescents will make their own health care decisions. The married teen who has a baby would be responsible for her own health and that of her child. The others would all have individuals who would make health care decisions for them, including parents, school officials, grandparents, or court appointees, so would not be considered emancipated.
Nursing process step: Planning
Category of client need: Safe, effective care environment
Cognitive level: Analysis
Learning outcome 2-2: Describe parents' rights as they relate to the care of children.
Test-taking tip: The nurse should know the legal rights of the client and protect those rights while providing client care.

---

3. Which of the following situations represents a violation of a Patient's Bill of Rights?
1. The 3-year-old child cries and screams, "No, No," and the nurse continues to restrain the child for placement of an intravenous catheter
2. The nurse discusses the client's treatment with the social worker, therapist, and chaplain as part of the management team
3. The client is placed in a ward-style room with three other children. The only privacy is provided by curtains that can enclose three sides of the bed
4. The nurse leaves the client's chart open on the bedside table in the room of an infant when the nurse is called to another client's room

Answer: 4
Rationale: The nurse is legally responsible to protect client information, such as the chart, from public view. A 3-year-old child cannot refuse treatment in this way, and the nurse is protecting the child from injury by continuing to restrain the child. It is appropriate to discuss the client with the case management team to provide client care. A ward situation does not violate client privacy unless the nurse fails to draw the curtain during procedures.
Nursing process step: Implementation
Category of client need: Safe, effective care environment
Cognitive level: Analysis
Learning outcome 2-3: Describe client rights as they relate to children.
Test-taking tip: The nurse should be aware of how to protect client information.

---

4. The nurse is breaking client confidentiality when:
1. The nurse calls the parents of a 14-year-old who has requested birth control.
2. The nurse reports to a nurse supervisor that a 12-year-old has threatened suicide.
3. The nurse reports that a 4-year-old has a large bruise on the buttocks.
4. The nurse reports to the local health department that a client has tested positive for rubella.

Answer: 1
Rationale: The adolescent may request birth control without parental notification; if the nurse notifies the parents, the client may no longer trust the nurse. Certain diseases and risks (including suicide threats and abuse) must be reported to the appropriate authorities.
Nursing process step: Implementation
Category of client need: Safe, effective care environment
Cognitive level: Application
Learning outcome 2-3: Describe client rights as they relate to children.
Test-taking tip: By knowing what to do with client information and guarding that information, the question can be answered.

---

5. A nurse does not want to discuss end-of-life issues such as living wills and advance directives with the family of a terminally ill child. This represents a violation of:
1. Patient's Bill of Rights
2. HIPAA regulations
3. Patient Self-Determination Act
4. Nurses Code of Ethics

Answer: 3
Rationale: Living wills and advance directives are part of the treatment issues covered by the Patient Self-Determination Act. HIPPA regulations are in place to protect client identity and the inappropriate release of health care information. The Patient's Bill of Rights defines how clients can participate in their health care. The Code of Ethics for nurses is created by professional nursing organizations to establish professional practice guidelines.
Nursing process step: Implementation
Category of client need: Safe, effective care environment
Cognitive level: Analysis
Learning outcome 2-1: Describe Federal initiatives to protect children.
Test-taking tip: The nurse should know the legal rights of the client and participate in care so that the client's rights are protected.

6. *Healthy People 2010* is a program that includes:
1. A health care funding system for high-risk, low-income women of reproductive age.
2. National Health Care goals and objectives to promote a healthier population.
3. Federal funding to supplement school lunches for children living in poverty.
4. State-mandated programs to provide health care for children without private insurance.

Answer: 2
Rationale: *Healthy People 2010* is the follow-up program to *Healthy People 2000*, which set goals and interdisciplinary outcomes for encouraging *all* Americans to develop healthier lifestyles. The other programs each address specific segments of the population only.
Nursing process step: Evaluation
Category of client need: Health promotion and maintenance
Cognitive level: Application
Learning outcome 2-1: Describe federal initiatives to protect children
Test-taking tip: Nurses should be aware of programs that offer clients opportunities and provide services.

7. The nurse sees that a 3-year-old has had multiple injuries in the past year, including a broken arm, large scalp laceration, and several broken ribs. The most appropriate nursing action is to:
1. Report to local authorities according to facility policy the suspicious assessment findings.
2. Remind the parents that children are prone to injuries and provide a handout on home safety.
3. Document in the client's chart in brief general terms to avoid liability.
4. Notify both parents of any suspicions and record exactly what each parent says.

Answer: 1
Rationale: The nurse is legally obligated to report suspected abuse and the facility policy is the correct document to consult and follow. The nurse who concludes that the injuries are accidental may place the client at risk for further injuries. All documentation should be detailed and very specific, and the parents should be separated from the child until the authorities decide a proper course of action.
Nursing process step: Assessment
Category of client need: Safe, effective care environment
Cognitive level: Application
Learning outcome 2-4: Name situations in which the nurse must legally report to public agencies.
Test-taking tip: Look for answer choices that provide the safest possible environment for the client.

8. Ethical issues affecting mothers and children:
1. May require resolution through the legal system and the courts.
2. Should always be explained to the client and family by the physician.
3. Are complicated issues because there are rarely laws that define the solutions.
4. Often require that the nurse make decisions for the client based on the profession's Code of Ethics.

Answer: 1
Rationale: Ethical issues are often without a right or wrong answer and may only be resolved in the courts. The nurse is responsible for providing information to the client; the nurse will never make decisions for the client. The nurse should provide information so that the client and family can make informed decisions about their care. Laws often offer solutions to ethical dilemmas, but sometimes laws can complicate ethical discussions.
Nursing process step: Evaluation
Category of client need: Safe, effective care environment
Cognitive level: Application
Learning outcome 2-5: Describe the difference between legal and ethical issues.
Test-taking tip: Choose answers that offer the broadest explanation to the problem as stated. Terms such as *always* and *never* and choices that seem out of the ordinary often are used to distract or confuse the student.

9. In describing the scope of nursing practice, the practical/vocational nurse is correct when stating:
1. "If I have studied a procedure and my supervisor has documented my competency, then that procedure becomes part of my scope of practice."
2. "The state board of nursing establishes general guidelines for my scope of practice, but my employer is able to authorize more advanced skills if those skills are part of my job."
3. "The scope of nursing practice changes from one practice setting to another. Inpatient nursing has a much narrower scope of practice than community-based nursing practice."

Answer: 4
Rationale: The state board of nursing determines the scope of nursing practice, and there may be differences from one state to another. Within the confines of state regulations, nurses' roles within a practice facility may be modified. For example, a facility may provide a more limited scope of nursing practice, though it is not able to broaden the scope of a nurse's practice. Scope of nursing practice is not site dependent but applies to all nurses in any setting.
Nursing process step: Planning
Category of client need: Safe, effective care environment
Cognitive level: Application
Learning outcome 2-5: Describe the difference between legal and ethical issues.
Test-taking tip: By knowing key definitions, such as scope of practice, the student can select the answer that fits the definition.

4. "My scope of practice will change if I move to another state. I may gain or lose the ability to perform certain procedures or tasks."

---

10. Choose all of the following that represent appropriate documentation as part of a nursing note.
   1. "Client's mother was rude to the respiratory therapist."
   2. "I gave the client morphine for her pain."
   3. "The leg wound measured 2 × 4 cm."
   4. "The doctor circumcised the client."
   5. "18-gauge Foley catheter inserted using sterile technique."

Answer: 3 and 5
Rationale: The description of a wound should be detailed, and including specific measurements is appropriate. It is important to document completely, including the size of the catheter and how it was inserted (with sterile technique). The other choices offer information that is not appropriate or complete. Documentation should be objective and not appear to judge an individual. Describing the mother as rude should not be part of the client chart. The morphine should be documented as to dosage, route, and pain level. The circumcision note is not complete, as it does not include the type of circumcision, anesthesia, and how the procedure was tolerated by the client.
Nursing process step: Implementation
Category of client need: Safe, effective care environment
Cognitive level: Application
Learning outcome 2-7: Describe the practical and vocational nurse's role in legal/ethical issues.
Test-taking tip: Following the rules of documentation will help to evaluate the choices.

---

11. The nurse has documented the following in the client's chart: "05/01/07, 0800, 100 mg ampicillin given." What else should be documented in the client's record?
   1. Drug strength
   2. Expiration date
   3. Route of administration
   4. Physician's name

Answer: 3
Rationale: Always document the dose, route, and time of medication administration. The other choices are not part of the documentation process.
Nursing process step: Implementation
Category of client need: Safe, effective care environment
Cognitive level: Analysis
Learning outcome 2-7: Describe the practical and vocational nurse's role in legal/ethical issues.
Test-taking tip: Know the steps involved in safe administration of medications.

---

12. The underlying principle for ethical decision making by the vocational/practical nurse is:
   1. Protect the client from injury.
   2. Use technology only to save time.
   3. Prevent malpractice lawsuits.
   4. Develop high moral standards for all nurses.

Answer: 1
Rationale: The goal of client care decision making is "do no harm." The other choices are part of nursing practice, but not the basic principle for ethical decision making.
Nursing process step: Planning
Category of client need: Safe, effective care environment
Cognitive level: Application
Learning outcome 2-6: Describe common legal and ethical issues that can affect the mother, child, and family.
Test-taking tip: Choose answers that offer the broadest explanation to the problem as stated.

---

13. The parents of a child newly identified with a terminal diagnosis ask to talk about the diagnosis with the nurse. The nurse should:
   1. Refuse to discuss any issues with the parents until they sign the "do not resuscitate" order.
   2. Tell the parents that it is best that the child not know about the diagnosis.
   3. Recommend that the family meet with the social worker, nursing staff, and chaplain.
   4. Tell the parents that it is always best to take the child home and contact hospice for care.

Answer: 3
Rationale: A care team should be made available to discuss all treatment options from a holistic point of view. The other choices—the "do not resuscitate" order, keeping the diagnosis from the client, and the recommendation of hospice home care—all involve the nurse determining what is best. The nurse should remain objective and supportive of the client and family wishes.
Nursing process step: Implementation
Category of client need: Safe, effective care environment
Cognitive level: Analysis
Learning outcome 2-6: Describe common legal and ethical issues that can affect the mother, child, and family.
Test-taking tip: Know the role of the nurse in supporting clients as they make an ethical decision. Look for choices that are very different from each other. Three of these choices involve the nurse providing a solution for the client; only one choice offers the client a role in the decision making.

---

14. A couple decides that they no longer want any of the embryos from their in vitro fertilization attempts. The nurse should inform the couple that:
1. If their embryos die, they will be financially responsible for funeral expenses.
2. The embryos should be donated to a laboratory for research.
3. They can terminate parental rights and give the embryos to another couple.
4. They will need to follow state and federal laws and examine their own philosophical beliefs.

Answer: 4
Rationale: The role of the nurse in legal/ethical issues is to listen, support, and inform clients about any laws affecting their decision. The nurse should help the clients determine what is best for them within their own belief system. The other choices are not reasonable and involve the nurse limiting the choice given to the clients.
Nursing process step: Planning
Category of client need: Safe, effective care environment
Cognitive level: Application
Learning outcome 2-6: Describe common legal and ethical issues that can affect the mother, child, and family.
Test-taking tip: Look for the broadest answer. Very specific answers are often given to distract from the general answer.

15. The parents of a child born with a minor cardiac defect have refused any treatment for the problem. With medication and a minor procedure, the child has an excellent prognosis. Which of the following groups would address this situation?
1. The hospital ethics committee
2. The Joint Commission of Hospital Accreditation (JCAHO)
3. The state board of nursing
4. The local police or sheriff's department

Answer: 1
Rationale: This case should be evaluated by the hospital ethics committee. The other organizations, the Joint Commission and state board of nursing do not have any responsibility in specific cases involving ethics. The police or sheriff's department would not be involved in this situation.
Nursing process step: Evaluation
Category of client need: Safe, effective care environment
Cognitive level: Application
Learning outcome 2-7: Describe the practical and vocational nurse's role in legal/ethical issues.
Test-taking tip: Know the role of the nurse in supporting clients as they make an ethical decision.

CHAPTER 3

1. The following groups are living together and working together to raise children. Which one represents a nuclear family?
1. A single mother living with her parents and 2 children
2. A homosexual couple with 1 biological child and 1 adopted child
3. An unmarried couple and their 3 children
4. A married couple and her 2 children from a previous relationship

Answer: 3
Rationale: A nuclear family is a couple and their biological children. A single mother living with her parents and children represents an extended family. Adopted children are not part of nuclear families, and children who were born during previous relationships represent blended families.
Nursing process step: Assessment
Category of client need: Health promotion and maintenance
Cognitive level: Analysis
Learning outcome 3-1: Describe family assessment techniques, such as genogram and ecomap.
Test-taking tip: Look for answers that meet the definitions of the key terms in the chapter.

2. The following genogram represents what relationship between JW and BW?

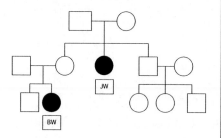

1. Sisters
2. Cousins
3. Mother, daughter
4. Aunt, niece

Answer: 4
Rationale: The relationship between JW and BW show different generations and are not a direct link. The genogram shows that JW is sister to the mother of BW, or aunt and niece. The other relationships are shown on the genogram but not represented by the two designated individuals.
Nursing process step: Assessment
Category of client need: Health promotion and maintenance
Cognitive level: Analysis
Learning outcome 3-1: Describe family assessment techniques, such as genogram and ecomap.
Test-taking tip: Know the key terms in the chapter and look for simple uses of the definitions.

3. Which of the following is a true statement regarding families? 1. A healthy family system will have closed boundaries to protect its members 2. Blended families are defined as families that include at least three generations 3. Adaptable families will change as needed to solve problems 4. Modern families are characterized only by the relationship between parent and child	Answer: 3 Rationale: A family that is flexible will manage changes and solve problems, as they have the ability to adapt roles, boundaries, and system functioning. Closed boundaries will not allow the family to accept new ideas, and they will not be able to manage stress or crisis. A blended family is one in which one or more children are from previous relationships and not the biological children of both parents. Modern families are defined by culture, new role performance, and how these new roles have developed in defining families. Nursing process step: Diagnosis Category of client need: Health promotion and maintenance Cognitive level: Analysis Learning outcome 3-3: Describe the characteristics of family systems. Test-taking tip: Know the key terms in the chapter and look for simple use of the definitions.
4. The nurse may be invading a client's personal space when (*select all that apply*): 1. Placing personal belongings in a drawer or closet. 2. Leaving the door to the room open while the client is sleeping. 3. Stooping to face the client eye to eye when explaining a procedure. 4. Sitting on the side of the bed to assist the client with eating a meal. 5. Placing newborn twins in the same baby bed.	Answer: 1, 3, 4 Rationale: While the amount of space an individual requires can vary from one culture to another, moving personal belongings and being too close to an individual represent invasions of personal space. Leaving a door open would not violate personal space. Newborn twins have integrated each other into their personal space and would most likely be comforted by the presence of their sibling. Nursing process step: Implementation Category of client need: Health promotion and maintenance Cognitive level: Application Learning outcome 3-2: Describe the effect of cultural and religious beliefs on family functioning. Test-taking tip: When answering a question with multiple answers, look for answers that are the most similar. The correct answers here all include the nurse and the client interacting.
5. The client and nurse may use nonverbal communication. The nurse is correctly interpreting nonverbal communication when: 1. The nurse obtains a rectal temperature for an infant with flushed, moist skin. 2. The nurse provides a snack to the child when the mother reports that the child is hungry. 3. The nurse questions the child about pain after the child pulls back when the IV site is touched. 4. The nurse picks up to cuddle a toddler who is laughing and smiling while sitting on a parent's lap.	Answer: 3 Rationale: Guarding behaviors, grimacing, and facial expressions are nonverbal cues for pain management and the nurse who recognizes these cues will ask about pain. An infant with flushed, moist skin is exhibiting physiologic symptoms, not nonverbal communication. The mother who requests a snack is interpreting cues from the child and no nonverbal assessments are described in this answer. A child who is laughing and smiling in the parent's lap may not want to be held by the nurse since toddlers are often shy of strangers. The nurse should recognize that the nonverbal cues in this example are a response to the presence of the parent and do not indicate a desire to be held by the nurse. Nursing process step: Assessment Category of client need: Psychosocial integrity Cognitive level: Analysis Learning outcome 3-2: Describe the effect of cultural and religious beliefs on family functioning. Test-taking tip: Look for an answer that describes appropriate nursing actions.
6. A future-oriented family may include a family that: 1. Makes decisions based on ancestral patterns and beliefs. 2. May sacrifice family vacations to save for college expenses. 3. Provides all the latest electronics for family entertainment. 4. Defers major decision making to a family elder such as a grandparent.	Answer: 2 Rationale: A future-oriented family will sacrifice immediate pleasures in order to meet future goals, so delaying a vacation now would help meet the future goal of attending college. A family that looks to the past would place a high value on ancestral beliefs and defer to elders in the family. A present-oriented family would provide for immediate needs and desires and might not think about the implications of this on the future. Nursing process step: Planning Category of client need: Health promotion and maintenance Cognitive level: Analysis Learning outcome 3-3: Describe the characteristics of family systems. Test-taking tip: The correct answer will be the answer that fits with the question. In this case, look for the answer that discusses the future.

7. A healthy family will have family roles that are: 1. Associated with family structure, culture, and gender. 2. Always the same as long as family members remain in the same household. 3. Able to change from day to day to help the family cope with emergencies. 4. Dependent on economics, with the person with the greatest wealth having the most powerful roles.	Answer: 1 Rationale: Family roles are not the same for all families. The family that allows for role development based on structure, culture, and gender will be healthier than the family that sets narrow guidelines for role performance. Roles must be flexible and change as the family develops, but day-to-day role changes could create stress and would not allow the family to cope with an emergency since clear roles are needed to cope effectively with stress and crisis. Roles may often be based on age or other factors not associated with wealth. Nursing process step: Diagnosis Category of client need: Health promotion and maintenance Cognitive level: Analysis Learning outcome 3-3: Describe the characteristics of family systems. Test-taking tip: Look for an answer that may be more general. Sometimes very specific answers have too much information to distract from the correct answer.
8. The purpose of an ecomap as part of a family assessment is to: 1. Demonstrate family values and ethics. 2. Diagnose family risk factors. 3. Diagram family relationships and health patterns. 4. Show how the family interacts with outside agencies and groups.	Answer: 4 Rationale: An ecomap is a visual representation of the relationships of a family and the environment, including outside social influences. An ecomap does not include values and ethics or risk factors. A genogram will diagram relationships and disease patterns. Nursing process step: Assessment Category of client need: Health promotion and maintenance Cognitive level: Application Learning outcome 3-1: Describe family assessment techniques, such as a genogram and ecomap. Test-taking tip: By knowing the definitions of key terms in the chapter, the student should be able to choose which answer best fits the question.
9. Which of the following represents a parenting style that allows children maximum control over their environment? 1. The authoritative parent who sets a curfew for teens 2. The parent who coaches their child in sports for many years 3. The permissive parent who allows a child to choose what to eat 4. The authoritarian parent who establishes many rules for the child	Answer: 3 Rationale: Parenting styles can differ from one family to another, and permissive parents allow children to have the most control in what they do, eat, etc. An authoritative parent sets guidelines for the child. Coaching a child in sports does not indicate what type of parenting style is being followed. An authoritarian style of parenting allows the child little input and values obedience. Nursing process step: Planning Category of client need: Health promotion and maintenance Cognitive level: Application Learning outcome 3-3: Describe the characteristics of family systems. Test-taking tip: By knowing the definitions of key terms in the chapter, the student should be able to choose which answer best fits the question.
10. Which of the following families are developing appropriately? *Select all that apply.* 1. The family with a newborn that has prepared a nursery and bought clothing and baby care supplies 2. The newlyweds who have decided together to not have children for several years 3. The family that teaches their school-age children at home and does not participate in social groups 4. The family with teenagers in which the teenagers are expected to work in the family business after school and on weekends 5. The "empty nest" family that has opened a new business and spends long hours each day working together	Answer: 1, 2, 5 Rationale: The developmental goal of the early childbearing family is to nurture and bond with the child. When the parents prepare the home environment for the child, they are demonstrating acceptance of their new roles as parents. The couple beginning their family who decide to wait to have children are showing that they are communicating and resolving important issues together. The empty-nest couple are adapting well when they pursue career goals and establish new roles after the children are out of the household. A family with school-age children that does not foster socialization of the children may be creating a situation in which the children fall behind in their social development. Teenagers should be encouraged to begin making decisions and can do so when they spend more time with their peers than with their family. Teenagers who spend most of their free time working may miss the opportunity to develop independence while still under the protection of the family. Nursing process step: Assessment Category of client need: Health promotion and maintenance Cognitive level: Analysis Learning outcome 3-4: Describe the normal changes a family undergoes over time. Test-taking tip: When answering a question with multiple answers, look for answers that are the most similar.

11. The nurse suspects child abuse in which of the following situations?
1. The 14-year-old who attempts suicide
2. The 4-year-old who still needs a diaper at night
3. The 6-year-old with a broken arm from a trampoline injury
4. The 15-year-old who is pregnant; the father is a 17-year-old school friend

Answer: 1
Rationale: One of the indicators of abuse is attempted suicide. A 4-year-old who still needs a diaper can be normal development. A broken arm is a normal consequence of a trampoline injury. If injuries were inconsistent with the explanation offered, then the nurse could consider abuse. Pregnancy with a peer would not be considered abuse unless more information were provided in the answer.
Nursing process step: Diagnosis
Category of client need: Safe, effective care environment
Cognitive level: Analysis
Learning outcome 3-5: Describe the characteristics of a family under stress.
Test-taking tip: By knowing the definitions of key terms in the chapter, the student should be able to choose which answer best fits the question.

---

12. A family comes to the community-based clinic seeking care for a sick child. During this visit, the mother states, "He brings every illness home from school. That's why I can't keep any of the other children healthy. He doesn't do anything right. I spend more time cleaning up after him than all the other children combined." The nurse should:
1. Ask the mother whether the child has been tested for learning disabilities.
2. Notify the authorities that the child is probably the victim of child abuse.
3. Provide the mother with the name of a good day care center.
4. Tell the nurse supervisor and make a referral to a family counselor.

Answer: 4
Rationale: The nurse should recognize that this child is a scapegoat and this is a sign of an unhealthy family. Appropriate action would be to report the situation to the nurse supervisor and then seek help for the family. There is not enough information to determine whether the child is being abused or has any learning disabilities, so it would not be appropriate for the nurse to act based on these principles. Referring the mother to a day care center would not be appropriate with the information provided.
Nursing process step: Implementation
Category of client need: Safe, effective care environment
Cognitive level: Analysis
Learning outcome 3-5: Describe the characteristics of a family under stress.
Test-taking tip: Recognizing healthy and unhealthy behaviors is a nursing responsibility and the correct answer will include nursing actions.

---

13. A family is preparing for discharge from the hospital following a child's surgery. A handout is reviewed with the parents. It includes the date and time of the follow-up appointment with the surgeon, medication prescriptions, home care referral and phone number, wound care instructions, and signs and symptoms of complications. What additional information should be included before the family leaves the facility?
1. A copy of the operative report
2. Medication classifications and side effects
3. A follow-up appointment with the anesthesiologist
4. Normal weight and height guidelines and a copy of a growth chart

Answer: 2
Rationale: It is the nurse's responsibility to provide information about the prescriptions at the time of discharge and to make sure that parents know when to seek care should harmful side effects occur. The operative report would not be a normal discussion during the discharge process. The anesthesiologist usually will follow up with the client during the hospitalization and not as a return visit since most anesthesia-related issues are immediate and resolved prior to discharge. Height and weight guidelines are generally part of well-child evaluations and not likely to be addressed as part of the hospital discharge following surgery.
Nursing process step: Evaluation
Category of client need: Safe, effective care environment
Cognitive level: Application
Learning outcome 3-6: Identify the role of the Practical/Vocational Nurse in family assessment and care.
Test-taking tip: The student should recognize that safe nursing care will include complete and thorough discharge planning and evaluation.

---

14. The vocational/practical nurse is obtaining a health history for a pregnant client at the beginning of her pregnancy. Which of the following assessments could place this client at risk for preterm labor?
1. The client works part time in a grocery store
2. This is the second pregnancy for the client

Answer: 3
Rationale: Risk factors for the development of preterm labor include poor nutritional status, and this client is underweight for height. A part-time job would not increase the risk of preterm labor. First pregnancies are more at risk for preterm labor; a second pregnancy does not increase this client's risk. The hemoglobin and hematocrit do not indicate anemia and would not increase the risk of preterm labor.
Nursing process step: Diagnosis
Category of client need: Health promotion and maintenance
Cognitive level: Analysis

| 3. The client weighs 110 pounds and is 66 inches tall | Learning outcome 3-7: Apply the nursing process to care of the family. |

3. The client weighs 110 pounds and is 66 inches tall
4. The client has a hemoglobin of 14 and a hematocrit of 41

Learning outcome 3-7: Apply the nursing process to care of the family.
Test-taking tip: When evaluating risks, look for the answer that is most abnormal or most different from the others.

---

15. Cultural variations can lead to conflict between clients and nurses. A cultural variation that encourages individuals to place their personal needs before the needs of the extended family is a characteristic common in the:
1. Rasa Latina culture.
2. Asian Pacific culture.
3. Black American culture.
4. Caucasian American culture.

Answer: 4
Rationale: The Caucasian American culture values the individual, so it is acceptable to place personal needs before the needs of the family. The other cultures listed are very family oriented and will nearly always sacrifice individual needs and comforts for the greater good of the family.
Nursing process step: Diagnosis
Category of client need: Psychosocial integrity
Cognitive level: Application
Learning outcome 3-7: Apply the nursing process to care of the family.
Test-taking tip: When comparing cultures, avoid stereotypes and look for generalities that are common within a culture.

CHAPTER 4

1. A genetic condition such as sickle cell disease requires a gene from the mother and the father for the disease to be expressed in the offspring. This is referred to as:
1. Autosomal recessive.
2. Mixed dominance.
3. Transposition.
4. A trisomy.

Answer: 1
Rationale: A recessive characteristic will only be expressed in the offspring if the gene is inherited from both parents. Mixed dominance can be expressed if inherited from one parent. Transposition and trisomy formation occur within the individual and are not inherited.
Nursing process step: Assessment
Category of client need: Physiological integrity
Cognitive level: Application
Learning outcome 4-2: Describe basic information about genes in relation to reproduction.
Test-taking tip: Learning the definitions of key terms will help the student pick the right answer.

---

2. Spermatogenesis:
1. Begins at puberty under the influence of follicle-stimulating hormone (FSH).
2. Produces sperm that contain 46 chromosomes in 23 pairs.
3. Can only occur if the temperature in the testes is 3°F higher than body temperature.
4. Occurs when spermatids stored in the prostate gland are transformed into sperm.

Answer: 1
Rationale: Puberty is marked by an increase in pituitary hormones, with one result being the beginning of sperm production. Sperm contain 23 unpaired chromosomes. The temperature of the testes must be lower than body temperature for sperm to survive. Spermatids mature into sperm in the epididymis and not in the prostate.
Nursing process step: Assessment
Category of client need: Physiological integrity
Cognitive level: Application
Learning outcome 4-1: Explain the developmental steps of spermatogenesis and oogenesis.
Test-taking tip: Learning the definitions of key terms will help the student pick the right answer.

---

3. You are the nurse evaluating the effectiveness of teaching for an adolescent boy following instruction for testicular self-examination (TSE). Which of the following statements indicates that further instruction is needed? *Select all that apply.*
1. "I should first look at my scrotum and penis in good light."
2. "I can check my testicles for lumps in the shower."
3. "I should check for cancer in my testicles at least twice a year."
4. "Normal discharge from my penis is clear or white and does not need to be reported."
5. "Testes usually feel hard and firm with two distinct lobes."

Answer: 3, 4, 5
Rationale: Testicular self-examination (TSE) should be performed monthly, beginning in adolescence. Any penile discharge should be reported to the care provider when first discovered. Testes should be smooth and soft. Hard and firm lobes should be reported as an abnormal finding during testicular self-examination.
Nursing process step: Evaluation
Category of client need: Health promotion and maintenance
Cognitive level: Analysis
Learning outcome 4-3: List the essential and accessory organs of the male and female reproductive system.
Test-taking tip: The correct answers will describe the steps of testicular self-examination.

4. Choose all of the following that relate to testicular self-examination (TSE).
1. Inspection of the penis and scrotum for lesions or discharge
2. Measurement of the scrotum for edema and symmetry
3. Palpation of the prostate for lumps, tenderness, or discharge
4. Checking each testicle for thickening or hardening
5. Recording the date of the examination and examining again in one month

Answer: 1, 4, and 5
Rationale: The process of testicular self-examination includes monthly inspection and palpation of the penis, scrotum, and testicles. Abnormalities such as thickening, a lump, or discharge might be found. Measurement is not part of the self-examination process, and the prostate cannot be examined as part of a self-examination process.
Nursing process step: Implementation
Category of client need: Health promotion and maintenance
Cognitive level: Analysis
Learning outcome 4-3: List the essential and accessory organs of the male and female reproductive system.
Test-taking tip: Look for the logical progression of procedures from start to finish. Avoid answers that sound too complicated or unusual.

5. You are the nurse discussing lab results with the parents of a 15-year-old client diagnosed with low testosterone levels. Your assessment is most likely to also reveal the following:
1. A deepening voice.
2. Abundant chest hair.
3. Narrow hips and shoulders.
4. Adequate sperm production.

Answer: 3
Rationale: If a client has low testosterone, he will not develop secondary sex characteristics and the shoulders will be narrow. As testosterone levels increase, it is expected that the voice will become deeper, the chest will develop hair, and sperm production will begin.
Nursing process step: Evaluation
Category of client need: Physiological integrity
Cognitive level: Analysis
Learning outcome 4-4: Describe the general function of each organ of the male and female reproductive systems.
Test-taking tip: Look for the answer that is most different from the others. Three choices represent sexual physical maturation.

6. A male client could not have a penile erection if:
1. The nerves that control contraction of the muscles of the penile shaft were injured.
2. There was diminished blood flow through the corporal cavernosa.
3. The flow of seminal fluid through the ejaculatory duct was blocked.
4. The prostate gland was enlarged and partially blocking urethral outflow.

Answer: 2
Rationale: Sexual arousal stimulates increased blood flow to the penis and causes an erection to occur. The other choices do not contribute to development of an erection.
Nursing process step: Diagnosis
Category of client need: Physiological integrity
Cognitive level: Application
Learning outcome 4-4: Describe the general function of each organ of the male and female reproductive systems.
Test-taking tip: The correct answer is one that is physiologically possible based on knowledge of anatomy and physiology.

7. As a young woman reaches puberty, she will experience an increase in ovarian hormone production. An increase in estrogen will produce:
1. Increased vascularization of the endometrium.
2. Increased number of eggs that are available for development.
3. Increased development of breast tissue and growth of pubic hair.
4. The onset of menses and beginning of monthly menstrual flow.

Answer: 3
Rationale: Estrogen is an ovarian hormone that increases at puberty and stimulates the development of secondary sex characteristics. Progesterone stimulates vascularization of the endometrium. The number of eggs in the ovary declines throughout a female's lifetime; they are present from birth and at no time is there an increase in the number of eggs in the ovary. Menses begins following a decline in progesterone if the egg is not fertilized after ovulation.
Nursing process step: Diagnosis
Category of client need: Physiological integrity
Cognitive level: Application
Learning outcome 4-5: Discuss the primary functions of the sex hormones.
Test-taking tip: The correct answer is one that is physiologically possible based on knowledge of anatomy and physiology.

8. You are the nurse teaching a young woman about her menstrual cycle. You are sure that she understands how to measure her cycle when she says:
1. "The first day of my cycle will be the day that I ovulate."
2. "The day my period stops is the first day of my cycle."
3. "My cycle starts the day after I ovulate and ends when my period starts."

Answer: 4
Rationale: The onset of menses is considered the first day of the menstrual cycle, so cycles can be compared from one woman to another. Many women do not know when ovulation occurs and so may not be able to recognize the start of a cycle if that were the basis for counting the menstrual cycle. Some women do not ovulate with each menstrual cycle. The last day of the menses is not used to evaluate any part of the menstrual cycle.
Nursing process step: Evaluation
Category of client need: Health promotion and maintenance
Cognitive level: Analysis

4. "Each time I start my period, I start a new menstrual cycle."	Learning outcome 4-6: Discuss the phases of the menstrual cycle and correlate each with physical changes during a 28-day cycle. Test-taking tip: The correct answer is one that is physiologically possible based on knowledge of anatomy and physiology.
9. In teaching a client about ovulation, the nurse should include the following statement: 1. Follicles within the ovary contain the ovum or egg and mature under the influence of estrogen and follicle-stimulating hormone (FSH). 2. The ovum will pass directly from the ovary into the uterus where fertilization most often occurs. 3. Increases in progesterone will stimulate the cell division called meiosis that creates a mature ovum. 4. Every ovum that develops has the genetic potential to develop into either a male or female, usually one-half become boys and one-half become girls.	Answer: 1 Rationale: A follicle is a cyst-like structure that will mature as follicle-stimulating hormone levels and estrogen levels increase. Fertilization most often occurs in the fallopian tube, not the uterus. Progesterone levels are low during the time when the ovum matures. All ovum contain only female genetic potential. It is the sperm that determines the sex of the developing embryo. Nursing process step: Evaluation Category of client need: Health promotion and maintenance Cognitive level: Analysis Learning outcome 4-6: Discuss the phases of the menstrual cycle and correlate each with physical changes during a 28-day cycle. Test-taking tip: The correct answer is one that is physiologically possible based on knowledge of anatomy and physiology.
10. In a lactating woman, colostrum passes from the lactiferous sinus through the nipple pores under the influence of: 1. Estrogen. 2. Progesterone. 3. Follicle-stimulating hormone. 4. Oxytocin.	Answer: 4 Rationale: The "let-down reflex," which allows colostrum and later milk to pass from the nipple, is under the hormonal control of oxytocin. The other hormones listed do not contribute to milk let-down. Nursing process step: Assessment Category of client need: Physiological integrity Cognitive level: Application Learning outcome 4-7: Explain the process of lactation Test-taking tip: By learning the definitions of key terms, many questions that use the term can be answered correctly.
11. A breastfeeding mother should be taught that milk production can be increased during lactation by: 1. Waiting longer between feedings, at least 4–6 hours. 2. Taking one estrogen tablet daily to boost levels and increase milk production. 3. Feeding more often for shorter periods of time, alternating breasts. 4. Making sure the breast is completely empty at each feeding.	Answer: 4 Rationale: Milk production is stimulated when the breast is completely emptied. Decreased feedings and estrogen tablets may decrease milk production instead of increasing production. The amount of milk produced is dependent on the volume of milk used. This follows the principle of supply and demand. Nursing process step: Implementation Category of client need: Physiological integrity Cognitive level: Analysis Learning outcome 4-7: Explain the process of lactation. Test-taking tip: Look for the answer that is most different from the others.
12. Teaching a client about breast self-examination should include the following instructions: 1. Palpate each breast with the opposite hand, after placing a small pillow under the shoulder. 2. It is good practice to perform breast self-examination about the time of ovulation. 3. All women should begin practicing breast self-examination just after having their first baby. 4. The breasts should be palpated one at a time using the thumb and forefinger to apply gentle pressure.	Answer: 1 Rationale: Correct performance of breast self-examination includes elevation of the shoulder to maximize the surface of the breast and to facilitate examination. Ovulation is a poor time for breast self-examination because of the hormonal stimulation of the breast tissue. Breast self-examination should begin with puberty. The pad of the fingers, not the thumb, should be used for palpation. Nursing process step: Evaluation Category of client need: Health promotion and maintenance Cognitive level: Analysis Learning outcome 4-6: Discuss the phases of the menstrual cycle and correlate each with physical changes during a 28-day cycle. Test-taking tip: When evaluating a procedure, review the procedure from start to finish and choose answers that most closely follow the procedure.

13. The role of the prostate gland in the male is to:
1. Produce testosterone to stimulate sperm production.
2. Secrete a fluid into semen that helps the sperm retain motility.
3. Provide a lubricant for the penis to easily enter the vagina during intercourse.
4. Increase blood flow to the erectile tissue of the penis and support the erection.

Answer: 2
Rationale: The prostate gland produces a thin milky fluid that, when added to the seminal vesicles, prolongs sperm motility and survival. Testosterone is produced in the testes, not the prostate gland. The Cowper's glands produce a lubricating fluid to allow for penile lubrication. The prostate does not play a role in penile erection.
Nursing process step: Implementation
Category of client need: Physiological integrity
Cognitive level: Application
Learning outcome 4-4: Describe the general function of each organ of the male and female reproductive systems.
Test-taking tip: Look for answers that are physiologically possible and describe actual physiological changes.

14. A teen is concerned about whether her first sexual experience will be painful when the hymen is torn. What assessment information would be important for the nurse to know?
1. The size of the clitoris and labia majora
2. Whether the client has ever had a vaginal infection
3. Whether the client uses tampons during her menses
4. The size and shape of the pelvic outlet

Answer: 3
Rationale: The hymen may be torn prior to first sexual intercourse. Activities such as tampon use and sports may be contributing factors. The size of the genitalia and pelvic outlet are not factors when considering pain and the tearing of the hymen. A history of vaginal infections does not impact discomfort with the first intercourse experience.
Nursing process step: Assessment
Category of client need: Physiological integrity
Cognitive level: Application
Learning outcome 4-4: Describe the general function of each organ of the male and female reproductive systems.
Test-taking tip: The correct answer is often the answer most unlike the others. The use of tampons represents an activity that could affect tearing the hymen. Infection and size would not have any impact on the hymen.

15. The excitement phase of the sexual response cycle includes:
1. Heart rate of 150, BP rises from 120/80 to 160/124
2. Contractions of the pelvic floor muscles and the anal sphincter
3. Nipple erection and enlargement of the areola
4. Emotional outbursts such as laughing or crying

Answer: 3
Rationale: Nipple erection and darkening and enlargement of the areola all occur early in the sexual response cycle and represent the excitement phase. The other answers reflect physical changes occurring during the orgasmic and resolution phases of the cycle.
Nursing process step: Assessment
Category of client need: Physiological integrity
Cognitive level: Application
Learning outcome 4-4: Describe the general function of each organ of the male and female reproductive systems.
Test-taking tip: The correct answer is the one that occurs first in the cycle and represents the lowest level of physical response.

CHAPTER 5

1. Teaching a client the best ways to manage fibrocystic breast disease should include:
1. Symptoms will resolve if dietary changes include decreasing caffeine and increasing sodium intake.
2. Breastfeeding should be avoided by women whose breasts contain multiple fluid-filled cysts.
3. There may be an increased risk of breast cancer if the disease onset occurred before the age 30.
4. The natural aging process helps to resolve cyst formation as hormone levels fall with the onset of menopause.

Answer: 4
Rationale: Fibrocystic breast disease is caused by hormonal changes of estrogen and progesterone, so that when menopause occurs, the symptoms resolve. Limiting caffeine may help some women, but sodium restriction has not been shown to be effective. Breastfeeding is not affected by fibrocystic disease and age of onset will not increase the risk of cancer.
Nursing process step: Implementation
Category of client need: Physiological integrity
Cognitive level: Application
Learning outcome 5-1: Define key terms.
Test-taking tip: Look for answers that demonstrate plausible choices and relationships, such as the decreasing cyst formation with lower hormone levels.

2. Which of the following clients is describing a breast change most consistent with breast cancer? The client reporting:
1. Breast tenderness and nipple discoloration.
2. Breast asymmetry and a hard painless lump.
3. A round easily movable mass with serous nipple discharge.
4. Rough reddened skin and hardened nipple pores.

Answer: 2
Rationale: Breast cancers are typically unilateral and will cause breast asymmetry. Cancerous lumps are often firm and painless. The other choices (breast tenderness, round movable mass, with discharge) include changes related to fibrocystic disease, infection, or fibroadenoma, a benign breast condition. Nipple discoloration, rough reddened skin and hardened nipple pores would be skin changes related to hormones, infection, or other benign conditions but do not indicate cancer.
Nursing process step: Diagnosis
Category of client need: Health promotion and maintenance
Cognitive level: Analysis
Learning outcome 5-2: Describe possible causes of reproductive issues.
Test-taking tip: Look for answers that describe changes consistent with the described disease.

3. Postoperative care for a woman following a mastectomy will include arm exercises to:
1. Strengthen the affected muscles.
2. Increase firmness in the remaining breast tissue.
3. Decrease pain as the surgical site heals.
4. Promote drainage after lymphatic disruption.

Answer: 4
Rationale: A mastectomy includes the removal of lymph nodes and the recommended exercises will help promote drainage and prevent swelling. The exercises will not help strength muscles, increase breast firmness, or help with pain control.
Nursing process step: Planning
Category of client need: Physiological integrity
Cognitive level: Application
Learning outcome 5-3: Discuss the medical and surgical interventions used to treat the client with reproductive issues.
Test-taking tip: Often the simplest explanation is the correct answer.

4. You are the nurse providing care for a client reporting symptoms of bloating, irritability, and breast tenderness. The symptoms recur monthly about 3 weeks after the onset of the menstrual cycle. Based on your knowledge, you recommend:
1. Vitamin B_6 and calcium.
2. Low carbohydrate diet and ibuprofen.
3. Melatonin and saw palmetto.
4. Acupuncture and fluid restriction.

Answer: 1
Rationale: Treatment for premenstrual syndrome includes increasing vitamin B_6 and calcium. The other choices do not have a role in PMS management.
Nursing process step: Planning
Category of client need: Physiological integrity
Cognitive level: Analysis
Learning outcome 5-5: Provide appropriate care for the couple with reproductive issues.
Test-taking tip: Look for answers that have a direct relationship to the stated problem.

5. A client has just been diagnosed with cervical dysplasia. The client demonstrates understanding of this condition when she states:
1. "Treatment will most likely begin with a hysterectomy, followed by chemotherapy."
2. "I will not be able to have any more children after laser treatments for removal of the cancerous tumor."
3. "My tests show changes in the cells on my cervix that may have been caused by exposure to a virus."
4. "Cervical dysplasia usually resolves without any invasive treatment, if I quit smoking, always use condoms, and avoid douching."

Answer: 3
Rationale: Cervical dysplasia has been linked to human papilloma virus exposure. The dysplastic changes are not cancer but warrant close observation. Treatment options include removal by laser or cryotherapy. A hysterectomy would be overly aggressive and appropriate treatment will not affect fertility. Avoiding treatment might allow progression of the disease to cervical cancer.
Nursing process step: Evaluation
Category of client need: Physiological integrity
Cognitive level: Analysis
Learning outcome 5-1: Define key terms.
Test-taking tip: By learning the key terms in the chapter, the student can apply the definition to the question.

6. A woman has reported frequent pelvic fullness accompanied by pain with intercourse and constipation, and she has felt something protruding from her vagina. Visual assessment reveals the end of the cervix visible at the vaginal opening. Since the woman is postmenopausal but otherwise in good health, the most likely treatment for this condition will be:
1. Kegel exercises daily.
2. Complete hysterectomy.
3. Placement of a vaginal pessary.
4. Laser ablation followed by chemotherapy.

Answer: 2
Rationale: The description provided is of uterine prolapse, which will most often be treated by hysterectomy. Kegel exercises might help pelvic floor relaxation but would not help resolve uterine prolapse. A pessary might be used for someone who was not a good surgical risk, and laser surgery and chemotherapy are not used to treat uterine prolapse.
Nursing process step: Diagnosis
Category of client need: Physiological integrity
Cognitive level: Application
Learning outcome 5-3: Discuss the medical and surgical interventions used to treat the client with reproductive issues.
Test-taking tip: Often the simplest explanation is the correct answer.

7. The nurse is caring for a woman following a rape. The nurse's responsibilities include:
1. Verify the presence of sperm to verify the rape took place.
2. Assisting the woman to shower and douche to prevent infection.
3. Screening the victim for the presence for alcohol and illegal drugs.
4. Offer emotional support since the woman may feel angry and humiliated.

Answer: 4
Rationale: An important nursing role is providing emotional support for the victim. There may not be sperm if the rapist used a condom or did not ejaculate. Showering and douching could destroy evidence. The victim's use of alcohol or drugs would not be part of every evaluation.
Nursing process step: Implementation
Category of client need: Safe, effective care environment
Cognitive level: Application
Learning outcome 5-4: Identify nursing diagnoses and nursing interventions to assist the couple with reproductive issues.
Test-taking tip: When a question asks about nursing roles, consider the role of the nurse in the given situation.

8. Which man should see his physician immediately to be evaluated for testicular cancer?
1. The 60-year-old who reports having to urinate at least twice each night
2. The 19-year-old with an enlarged tender scrotum and a purulent penile discharge
3. The 26-year-old with one normal feeling testicle and one testicle that is hard but not tender
4. The 38-year-old that has found a painless indurated lesion 1 × 2 cm in diameter on the dorsal surface of the penis

Answer: 3
Rationale: Testicular cancer may produce tissue changes that include a hard area on the testicle. This will be painless. Frequent urination is a symptom of prostate, not testicular, enlargement. An enlarged tender scrotum, penile discharge, and lesion would all indicate infection.
Nursing process step: Diagnosis
Category of client need: Health promotion and maintenance
Cognitive level: Analysis
Learning outcome 5-5: Provide appropriate care for the couple with reproductive issues.
Test-taking tip: Look for answers that have a direct relationship to the stated problem.

9. You are providing instructions for a man with a new prescription for Viagra (sildenafil). You should include:
1. Call the physician if erection lasts more than 24 hours.
2. It may take up to 1 hour before the effects of the drug are evident.
3. Respiratory distress is a common but serious side effect of the drug.
4. Additional doses may be taken if the medication effects end too soon.

Answer: 2
Rationale: Dosing with Viagra should take place 1 hour before sexual activity is anticipated. The client should call the physician if the erection lasts more than 4 hours. Cardiovascular collapse, including hypertension or heart failure, is an uncommon side effect, and only one dose a day should be taken.
Nursing process step: Implementation
Category of client need: Physiological integrity
Cognitive level: Application
Learning outcome 5-4: Identify nursing diagnoses and nursing interventions to assist the couple with reproductive issues.
Test-taking tip: Know the side effects of medications.

10. Following a surgical transurethral resection of the prostate (TURP) for benign prostatic hyperplasia (BPH), the client can expect:
1. A urethral catheter with bladder irrigation.
2. Surgical dressing changes twice daily.
3. Infertility due to ligation of the vas deferens.
4. Chemotherapy treatments that will start within 2 weeks.

Answer: 1
Rationale: Bladder irrigation is necessary to prevent clot formation that might obstruct the urethra. Since the surgical access is through the urethra, there is no incision and no dressing changes. Fertility is not affected, and chemotherapy is not indicated because of the benign diagnosis.
Nursing process step: Planning
Category of client need: Physiological integrity
Cognitive level: Application
Learning outcome 5-3: Discuss the medical and surgical interventions used to treat the client with reproductive issues.
Test-taking tip: When evaluating a procedure, the correct intervention will often be the one that is directly related to the procedure.

11. Gonorrhea and chlamydia pose a threat to newborns because:
1. The organisms can cause birth defects if acquired during early pregnancy.
2. The infection may restrict fetal growth and prevent lung development.
3. The baby may encounter the organisms in the birth canal during delivery.
4. The treatment for these diseases may cause irreversible mental retardation.

Answer: 3
Rationale: Untreated gonorrhea and chlamydia may cause eye or respiratory infections if the baby acquires the infection when passing through the birth canal. These organisms do not ascend into the uterus and cause the other problems described.
Nursing process step: Evaluation
Category of client need: Physiological integrity
Cognitive level: Application
Learning outcome 5-2: Describe possible causes of reproductive issues.
Test-taking tip: Look for answers that are physiologically possible for the conditions described.

12. Client teaching regarding use of a vaginal diaphragm should include that:
1. Effectiveness can be increased if spermicide is applied just before insertion of the diaphragm.
2. The open end of the diaphragm should be placed just inside the vagina.
3. The diaphragm should be left in place for 2 hours after intercourse.
4. The diaphragm should be carefully removed immediately following ejaculation.

Answer: 1
Rationale: The use of a spermicide with a diaphragm will place spermicide next to the cervix where it can be effective if any sperm should contact the cervix. The open end of the diaphragm should cover the cervix. The diaphragm should be left in place for at least 6 hours following intercourse and not be removed following ejaculation.
Nursing process step: Planning
Category of client need: Health promotion and maintenance
Cognitive level: Application
Learning outcome 5-4: Identify nursing diagnoses and nursing interventions to assist the couple with reproductive issues.
Test-taking tip: When evaluating patient education, consider a simple explanation instead of an explanation that seems confusing or unclear.

13. A client is considering a vasectomy. When teaching about the procedure, the nurse should include which of the following? *Select all that apply.*
1. The procedure should be considered permanent.
2. The procedure involves ligation of the seminal vesicles.
3. Additional birth control should be used until no sperm are present.
4. The client will be unable to ejaculate for at least 1 week after the procedure.
5. Impotence is a common side effect after a vasectomy.

Answer: 1, 3
Rationale: A vasectomy is a form of permanent sterilization that involves ligation of the vas deferens. There will still be sperm remaining in the seminiferous tubules; it will take up to 6 ejaculations to clear the sperm from the tubules, so the couple will need to use another form of birth control. Ejaculation is possible and there may be some scrotal swelling, but impotence is not a problem following vasectomy.
Nursing process step: Planning
Category of client need: Physiological integrity
Cognitive level: Application
Learning outcome 5-5: Provide appropriate care for the couple with reproductive issues.
Test-taking tip: When evaluating client education, consider a simple explanation instead of an explanation that seems confusing or unclear.

14. You are the nurse providing care for a birth mother who has chosen to have a closed adoption. Which of the following is likely to be part of this type of adoption? *Select all that might apply.*
1. The birth mother will meet the adoptive parents
2. The birth mother is able to hold the baby

Answer: 2, 3, 4
Rationale: In a closed adoption, the biological parents have no information about the adoptive parents and the adoptive parents have information about the health history and limited demographic information about the birth parents. The birth mother is able to hold the baby and may use a lawyer or adoption agency to maintain privacy. The adoptive child could contact and visit the birth mother if the adoption were an open adoption.
Nursing process step: Implementation
Category of client need: Safe, effective care environment

3. The birth mother may use a lawyer to manage the adoption
4. The adoptive family has some information about the birth mother
5. The adoptive child can visit the birth mother

Cognitive level: Analysis
Learning outcome 5-4: Identify nursing diagnoses and nursing interventions to assist the couple with reproductive issues.
Test-taking tip: By recognizing the difference between an open and closed adoption, the student will be able to choose the correct answers.

---

15. You are the nurse caring for a client experiencing an incomplete spontaneous abortion at 8-weeks gestation. You anticipate:
1. Minimal bleeding with no additional medical treatment.
2. Antibiotic therapy following discharge.
3. Surgical curettage to control the bleeding.
4. Teaching the mother that she probably has an incompetent cervix.

Answer: 3
Rationale: An incomplete abortion means that fetal tissue remains in the uterus and bleeding will continue until all fetal tissue is removed. A complete abortion will have minimal bleeding. Antibiotics are not routinely used following a spontaneous abortion, and there is no information given that describes an incompetent cervix.
Nursing process step: Planning
Category of client need: Physiological integrity
Cognitive level: Analysis
Learning outcome 5-5: Provide appropriate care for the couple with reproductive issues.
Test-taking tip: By learning the key terms in the chapter, the student can apply the definition and choose the correct answer.

CHAPTER 6

1. A woman is planning to become pregnant within 3 months. She should modify her diet to include more green leafy vegetables, wheat germ, and broccoli because:
1. These foods are high in fiber and will prevent constipation.
2. These high iron foods will insure healthy fetal development.
3. Increased folic acid will help to prevent birth defects.
4. A low-fat diet will decrease morning sickness.

Answer: 3
Rationale: Increased folic acid is a primary prevention method for prevention of open neural tube defects and should be included in preconception counseling. These foods do contain fiber and iron, but just eating them may not positively prevent constipation or positively insure healthy fetal development. These foods might be part of a low fat diet, but in planning a pregnancy, you would not be concerned with morning sickness before the pregnancy is established.
Nursing process step: Planning
Category of client need: Health promotion and maintenance
Cognitive level: Analysis
Learning outcome 6-5: Discuss nutritional requirements during pregnancy.
Test-taking tip: Answers that use absolute terms such as "will prevent "or "will insure" are unlikely to be the correct answer.

---

2. In order to increase the chances of fertilization of an ovum, the couple attempting to establish a pregnancy should know that:
1. The greatest chance of fertilization occurs 48 hours following ovulation.
2. Sperm placed in the vagina by ejaculation has a greater chance of fertilization than artificial insemination.
3. Sperm motility and viability may be decreased by male cigarette smoking.
4. A woman who uses alcohol, even in small amounts, can decrease the chance of becoming pregnant.

Answer: 3
Rationale: Sperm quality is affected if the male smokes cigarettes. The effects can be reversed if the male quits smoking 3–4 months before conception. The ovum is viable for only 24 hours. There is no real difference in how the sperm reach the cervix, although most pregnancies occur following male ejaculation in the vagina. Alcohol will affect fetal development but does not decrease the chance of becoming pregnant.
Nursing process step: Planning
Category of client need: Physiological integrity
Cognitive level: Application
Learning outcome 6-2: Describe factors that influence prenatal development.
Test-taking tip: The correct answer is often the one that makes the most sense from a physiologic standpoint.

---

3. The role of amniotic fluid during pregnancy is to (*select all that apply*):
1. Regulate temperature.
2. Prevent infection.
3. Provide nutrition.
4. Filter toxins.
5. Allow easy movement.

Answer: 1, 5
Rationale: Amniotic fluid helps to maintain a constant temperature in the uterus. The buoyancy of the amniotic fluid provides support and resistance to aid movement and muscle development. The amniotic fluid has no role in immunity and cannot nourish the fetus or filter toxins. These are all functions of the placenta.
Nursing process step: Diagnosis
Category of client need: Physiological integrity
Cognitive level: Analysis
Learning outcome 6-2: Describe factors that influence prenatal development.
Test-taking tip: Know the function of key components of the system being evaluated.

---

4. The role of the placenta in fetal development includes: 1. Transporting blood from the mother to the fetus. 2. Storing oxytocin to prepare for labor contractions. 3. Producing relaxin to allow for pelvic stretching. 4. Protecting the fetus from maternal drug use.	Answer: 3 Rationale: One of the functions of the placenta is hormone production, and relaxin is a placental hormone. Blood cells do not cross between the mother and fetus. Oxygen, amino acids, and other substances cross the placental barrier from the mother, and fetal waste will cross the placenta to the mother's system. The placenta does not store oxytocin, which is a product of the posterior pituitary gland. Nursing process step: Diagnosis Category of client need: Physiological integrity Cognitive level: Analysis Learning outcome 6-3: Describe fetal development. Test-taking tip: Know the function of the major organs involved in pregnancy.
5. Fetal circulation and the fetal cardiovascular system include the following pregnancy-related adaptation: 1. Oxygenated blood is carried from the placenta to the fetus through the umbilical arteries. 2. The fetal lungs require increased blood flow because the fetal heart rate is nearly double the adult heart rate. 3. Maternal blood passes through the umbilical vein to the fetal liver for filtering of toxins. 4. The foramen ovale allows for some blood from the right atrium to pass directly into the left atrium.	Answer: 4 Rationale: Oxygenated blood enters the right atrium and can pass directly to the left atrium through the foramen ovale and can then enter the fetal systemic circulation. Blood comes from the placenta to the fetus in the umbilical vein. The blood flow is reduced to the fetal lungs because all oxygen enters the fetus via the placenta. Maternal blood does not enter the fetus but remains outside the amniotic sac, providing nutrients and oxygen into the intervillous spaces for transport to the fetus. Nursing process step: Diagnosis Category of client need: Physiological integrity Cognitive level: Analysis Learning outcome 6-3: Describe fetal development. Test-taking tip: Know the developmental process for the major organs involved in fetal development.
6. As the nurse teaching a pregnant woman about fetal lung development, it is important to include that: 1. Survival chances are low before 24 weeks because of inadequate surfactant production. 2. By 20 weeks gestation, the fetal lungs contain the same number of alveoli as an adult. 3. Gas exchange in the lungs begins at about 35 weeks gestation. 4. Fetal lungs are filled with amniotic fluid so that the lungs will inflate after birth.	Answer: 1 Rationale: Surfactant prevents alveoli collapse and allows the lungs to function. Production is not adequate to sustain lung function until 24 weeks, but the lungs are still very immature and the 24-week newborn will need considerable respiratory support. Alveoli are generated throughout an individual's life and the small lungs of the newborn do not contain as many alveoli as an adult. Gas exchange occurs within the placenta until after birth. The amniotic fluid in the fetal lungs must clear before the lungs can inflate. Surfactant is needed to maintain alveoli inflation. Nursing process step: Implementation Category of client need: Physiological integrity Cognitive level: Analysis Learning outcome 6-3: Describe fetal development. Test-taking tip: Know the developmental process for the major organs involved in fetal development.
7. Place in order the following fetal developmental milestones as they would normally occur, starting with the earliest and ending with the last. 1. The eyelids begin to open and close 2. Blood cells are manufactured by the liver 3. Surfactant levels are adequate for respiration 4. The kidneys produce urine	Answer: 2, 4, 1, 3 Rationale: Fetal development proceeds at a predictable rate and sequence. The liver can manufacture red blood cells by 5 weeks, the kidneys produce urine by 12 weeks, the eyelids are fused until 28 weeks, and surfactant production is adequate at 35 weeks gestation. Nursing process step: Assessment Category of client need: Physiological integrity Cognitive level: Analysis Learning outcome 6-3: Describe fetal development. Test-taking tip: Know the developmental process for the major organs involved in fetal development.

8. Which of the following clients is demonstrating a probable sign of pregnancy?
1. The woman who has little appetite and vomits nearly every day
2. The woman who has not had a menstrual period for 3 months
3. The woman who reports fluttering abdominal sensations
4. The woman who had a positive home pregnancy test

Answer: 4
Rationale: Probable signs are objective findings such as a positive pregnancy test. The other signs are all subjective or presumptive signs of pregnancy. Presumptive signs may be attributed to other conditions
Nursing process step: Assessment
Category of client need: Physiological integrity
Cognitive level: Analysis
Learning outcome 6-4: Identify signs of pregnancy and maternal changes throughout pregnancy.
Test-taking tip: The nurse should be able to help clients interpret symptoms and determine the significance of symptoms.

9. Which of the following tests would be best to positively confirm a pregnancy that is estimated to be about 4-weeks gestation?
1. Transvaginal ultrasound
2. Pelvic x-ray
3. Abdominal ultrasound
4. Doppler auscultation of fetal heart tones

Answer: 1
Rationale: At 4 weeks gestation, the uterine contents could only be visualized transvaginally. Pelvic x-rays are rarely used during pregnancy and would not be used at such a sensitive period of fetal development. The pregnancy within the uterus would not easily be visualized by an abdominal ultrasound, and Doppler auscultation of fetal heart tones would be expected by about 10 weeks gestation.
Nursing process step: Implementation
Category of client need: Safe, effective care environment
Cognitive level: Application
Learning outcome 6-4: Identify signs of pregnancy and maternal changes throughout pregnancy.
Test-taking tip: Consider which procedure would be best for a very early pregnancy.

10. You are the nurse positioning a pregnant woman of 24 weeks gestation in a supine position for fundal height measurement. She becomes pale, dizzy, and nauseated. Your first action should be to:
1. Provide oxygen.
2. Go get the crash cart.
3. Assess blood pressure.
4. Prop the hip at an angle.

Answer 4
Rationale: The client described is experiencing supine hypotension because the pregnant uterus has compressed the vena cava and restricted blood flow from the lower extremities. By shifting the weight of the uterus with a hip roll, blood flow will be restored and symptoms should resolve. None of the other actions would relieve the symptoms described but may be appropriate if the hip tilt does not relieve symptoms.
Nursing process step: Implementation
Category of client need: Physiological integrity
Cognitive level: Analysis
Learning outcome 6-6: Discuss common maternal discomforts during pregnancy and their treatment.
Test-taking tip: Prioritization of nursing actions often starts with the simplest action first, such as changing maternal position.

11. Teaching the pregnant woman about changes during pregnancy should include:
1. Muscle cramps may be relieved by increased potassium intake and exercise.
2. Striae gravidarum (stretch marks) are caused by pregnancy hormones and will disappear completely after delivery.
3. Placental hormones affect glucose metabolism by decreasing the effectiveness of insulin and stimulating insulin production.
4. Electrolyte imbalances may be caused by changes in kidney function, such as increased glomerular filtration and decreased tubular reabsorption.

Answer: 3
Rationale: During pregnancy, there is an increased amount of glucose present in the bloodstream. The pregnant woman's cells demonstrate reduced sensitivity to insulin. The pancreas does not produce adequate amounts of insulin to meet the woman's needs. Muscle cramps may be relieved by calcium and phosphorus. Striae gravidarum are permanent changes from disruption of connective tissue, but they often change from red to silver or white over time. Pregnant women have an increased glomerular filtration rate but it is accompanied by an increased tubular reabsorption rate, so balance is maintained.
Nursing process step: Evaluation
Category of client need: Physiological integrity
Cognitive level: Application
Learning outcome 6-6: Discuss common maternal discomforts during pregnancy and their treatment.
Test-taking tip: The correct answer will include those actions that follow principles of physiology, such as glucose metabolism.

12. The nurse's responsibilities during an amniocentesis include:

1. Administering Rh immune globulin if the woman is Rh negative.
2. Using sterile technique to place a Foley catheter in the bladder.
3. Obtaining informed consent and answering any questions posed by the woman.
4. Inserting the needle into the uterus and withdrawing a sample of amniotic fluid.

Answer: 1

Rationale: Since there is a risk of bleeding with the procedure, the Rh status of the mother should be evaluated and RhoGAM administered if appropriate. There is no need for a Foley catheter during this procedure. It is the role of the physician to answer questions associated with obtaining informed consent, and it is the role of the physician to obtain the amniotic fluid by inserting a needle into the uterus.

Nursing process step: Implementation

Category of client need: Physiological integrity

Cognitive level: Analysis

Learning outcome 6-7: Discuss prenatal care and client teaching related to prenatal care.

Test-taking tip: The correct answer will always be a nursing action and not a physician responsibility.

---

13. You are documenting the obstetric history of a pregnant woman during her first prenatal visit using the G P/T PAL notation system. She reports that this will be her third child. She delivered her first child at 32 weeks and her second child at 40 weeks. She had a miscarriage 5 years ago of unknown age and another miscarriage at 7 weeks last year. Which of the following represents the correct documentation of this history?

1. 4 1 2 1 2
2. 5 1 1 2 2
3. 4 2 0 2 3
4. 5 2 1 1 3

Answer: 2

Rationale: The first number represents the total number of pregnancies, which is 5 (the current pregnancy, 2 live children, and 2 spontaneous abortions). The second number is 1 for 1 term delivery at 40 weeks. The third number is 1 for the preterm delivery at 32 weeks. The fourth number is 2 for the 2 spontaneous abortions (miscarriages), and the last number is 2 for her two living children.

Nursing process step: Assessment

Category of client need: Health promotion and maintenance

Cognitive level: Application

Learning outcome 6-7: Discuss prenatal care and client teaching related to prenatal care.

Test-taking tip: Analyze the question carefully and organize the data according to the order requested.

---

14. Nutritional needs change during pregnancy and the pregnant woman should be instructed to:

1. Add about 500 extra calories daily during the pregnancy.
2. Use fruits and vegetables to provide ½ of the total daily calories.
3. Add 2 servings of milk or dairy for extra calcium.
4. Avoid dried peas, beans and other gas-forming foods.

Answer: 3

Rationale: The calcium needs increase as fetal bone development requires extra calcium, and the mother could suffer bone loss if she doesn't increase her dietary intake. Recommendations include 300 additional calories daily during the pregnancy. Also, 4-6 servings of fruits and vegetables are recommended, and dried peas and beans are good sources of protein during pregnancy.

Nursing process step: Planning

Category of client need: Health promotion and maintenance

Cognitive level: Application

Learning outcome 6-5: Discuss nutritional requirements during pregnancy.

Test-taking tip: Follow healthy food guidelines and include minor changes for pregnancy.

---

15. Hot tubs should be avoided during pregnancy since:

1. They may expose the fetus to infection.
2. The shifting weight of the uterus may make the woman at risk for falling.
3. Chemicals in the water can harm the fetus.
4. The temperature of the water may overheat both mother and fetus.

Answer: 4

Rationale: The pregnant woman should avoid overheating and hot tubs can contribute to overheating. The uterus protects the fetus from infection and chemical exposure. The woman is at risk for falls at any time during late pregnancy not just around hot tubs.

Nursing process step: Evaluation

Category of client need: Safe, effective care environment

Cognitive level: Application

Learning outcome 6-7: Discuss prenatal care and client teaching related to prenatal care.

Test-taking tip: Look for the greatest risk among the choices; overheating could cause the greatest adverse effect for the fetus.

---

1. The hormonal theory regarding the onset of labor is based on maternal hormone level changes. Which hormone will decrease as labor approaches?
1. Estrogen
2. Progesterone
3. Oxytocin
4. Fetal cortisol

Answer: 2

Rationale: Progesterone causes smooth muscles to relax; thus as the progesterone declines, the uterus is more sensitive to contractions. Estrogen, oxytocin, and fetal cortisol levels will all increase as labor approaches.

Nursing process step: Diagnosis

Category of client need: Physiological integrity

Cognitive level: Application

Learning outcome 7-3: Describe variables affecting labor and delivery.

Test-taking tip: Know the definitions of key terms so that when those terms are used in questions, the question will be easier to answer.

---

2. In order to determine if a primigravida at term is in labor, the LVN/LPN is questioning the client about her contractions. Which of the following statements by the client would be the most probable indication that this is true labor?
1. "Some contraction pains last one minute and some are much shorter."
2. "When my labor coach rubs my back, the contractions stop for a short while."
3. "Each contraction feels like I'm wearing a very tight belt around my waist."
4. "The contractions seem more painful and stronger when I walk around."

Answer: 4

Rationale: True labor contractions continue and may get stronger with position changes; and ambulation. True labor contractions will progressively get longer and stronger; they will not stop with an intervention like massage and will be felt low in the abdomen.

Nursing process step: Diagnosis

Category of client need: Physiological integrity

Cognitive level: Analysis

Learning outcome 7-2: Discuss appropriate nursing actions for women who present for admission when in labor.

Test-taking tip: Choose answers that make the most sense when considering the physiology of the condition described.

---

3. Following a cervical examination of a laboring woman after spontaneous rupture of membranes, the nurse reports that the fetus remains ballotable. Cervical dilatation is 4 cm, cervical effacement is 70%. The most appropriate nursing intervention at this time is to:
1. Discuss the need for temporary bed rest.
2. Prepare the woman for immediate cesarean delivery.
3. Begin administration of Pitocin infusion.
4. Provide a light diet and encourage fluids.

Answer: 1

Rationale: A ballotable fetus is at risk for umbilical cord prolapse with the rupture of the membranes. The patient should remain on bed rest until the fetus is engaged and the risk of prolapse decreases. There is no need for a cesarean delivery or Pitocin at this time, and food and fluids would not be helpful to prevent cord prolapse.

Nursing process step: Planning

Category of client need: Physiological integrity

Cognitive level: Analysis

Learning outcome 7-1: Define key terms.

Test-taking tip: Look for the greatest risk given the client situation and for what is most appropriate to minimize those risks.

---

4. Which of the following situations during labor is most likely to lead to a cesarean delivery?
1. The fetus is in a longitudinal lie with a cephalic presentation.
2. Fetal position shows the occiput on the mother's right side.
3. The maternal pelvis is gynecoid and estimated fetal weight is 3,000 grams.
4. The fetus is head down with arms extended and fetal legs flexed.

Answer: 4

Rationale: When any part of the fetus is in extension, passage through the birth canal is more difficult and a vaginal birth may not be possible. A cephalic presentation, longitudinal lie, occiput anterior position, and gynecoid maternal pelvis would all enhance the possibility of a vaginal birth.

Nursing process step: Assessment

Category of client need: Health promotion and maintenance

Cognitive level: Analysis

Learning outcome 7-3: Describe variables affecting labor and delivery.

Test-taking tip: Know the definition of key terms so that when those terms are used in questions, the question will be easier to answer.

5. You are the nurse teaching a primigravida client about pain relief during labor. Effective pain relief during the transition phase of the first stage of labor may include which of the following? *Select all that apply.* 1. Pudendal block 2. Coached pushing 3. Patterned pace breathing 4. Epidural block 5. Effleurage	Answer: 3, 4 Rationale: Patterned pace breathing requires a lot of concentration in order to perform correctly, and so it will provide better pain relief during the most intense pain of labor. An epidural block is also appropriate to provide relief from the pain of transition. A pudendal block will only numb the vagina and the perineum, thus it would not be effective for first stage, transition. Effleurage and other forms of light touch will usually not be effective and may actually distract the client from the ability to focus. The cervix during transition is not fully dilated and pushing at this time may tear the cervix or cause it to swell and prolong labor. Nursing process step: Planning Category of client need: Physiological integrity Cognitive level: Application Learning outcome 7-4: Identify various methods of pain relief used during labor. Test-taking tip: Know the definition of key terms so that when those terms are used in questions, the question will be easier to answer.
6. A client has been in labor for about 8 hours and is now dilated to 6 cm, contraction duration is 60 seconds, and contraction frequency is 4–5 minutes. This represents: 1. Second stage labor 2. First stage labor, transition phase 3. First stage labor, active phase 4. First stage labor, latent phase	Answer: 3 Rationale: The active phase of fist stage of labor is when the cervix is dilated from 4–8 cm. Second stage labor is the stage from complete dilation of the cervix until the birth of the baby. Transition is when the cervix dilates from 8–10 cm, and the latent phase is when the cervix begins to dilate until 4 cm. Nursing process step: Assessment Category of client need: Physiological integrity Cognitive level: Analysis Learning outcome 7-5: Differentiate the stages of labor. Test-taking tip: If a question is asking about a process, know the milestones that define that process, such as the end points for the stages of labor.
7. The nurse completes an assessment of the laboring client in the second stage of labor and should notify the care provider that immediate delivery is expected when: 1. The cervix is dilated to 10 cm. 2. The woman expresses a strong urge to bear down. 3. Bright red blood is seen during a contraction. 4. The fetal head remains in view between contractions.	Answer: 4 Rationale: The fetal head that remains visible between contractions is crowning, and delivery will occur with just a few more pushes. Complete cervical dilation does not mean delivery is imminent since second stage may take from 30 minutes to several hours. The urge to push and bleeding may not be related to delivery. Nursing process step: Assessment Category of client need: Physiological integrity Cognitive level: Application. Learning outcome 7-5: Differentiate the stages of labor. Test-taking tip: Choose answers that make the most sense when considering the physiology of the condition described.
8. The following statements describe fetal position changes that occur as the fetus in a vertex presentation passes through the maternal pelvis. List them in the order they occur, with the earliest first. 1. The fetal occiput is even with the ischial spines 2. The fetal torso rotates to align the shoulder just beneath the symphysis pubis 3. The fetus stretches its neck and extends the head forward 4. The fetus flexes the chin to the chest and the knees are flexed to the abdomen	Answer: 1, 4, 3, 2 Rationale: The mechanisms of labor include engagement when the presenting part descends to the level of the ischial spines of the pelvis. Next, the fetal head flexes and the smallest diameter of the fetal head, the occiput, passes through the pelvic outlet. The fetus then rotates and extends so the head passes under the symphysis pubis. Finally, the fetus rotates to the posterior, allowing the shoulders to pass beneath the symphysis pubis and the body to be delivered. Nursing process step: Evaluation Category of client need: Physiological integrity Cognitive level: Analysis Learning outcome 7-6: Discuss the mechanisms of labor. Test-taking tip: If a question is asking about a process, know the milestones that define that process, such as the mechanisms of labor.

9. The nurse should notify the care provider when umbilical cord assessment immediately following delivery reveals:
1. The umbilical cord is clamped one inch from the abdomen.
2. The umbilical cord is pulsating.
3. The umbilical cord contains one artery.
4. The umbilical cord appears moist and rubbery.

Answer: 3
Rationale: The umbilical cord should contain 1 vein and 2 arteries. The presence of a single artery has been associated with genitourinary abnormalities. The other assessments are all normal for umbilical cord assessment immediately after birth.
Nursing process step: Assessment
Category of client need: Physiological integrity
Cognitive level: Analysis
Learning outcome 7-9: Describe important aspects of nursing care of the neonate immediately after birth.
Test-taking tip: Knowledge of anatomy will help to answer questions based on structure and function.

10. The nurse is concerned when which of the following occurs during the third stage of labor?
1. The amniotic sac remains attached to the placenta after the placenta is delivered.
2. The uterus continues to have contractions after the baby is delivered.
3. There is a sudden gush of bright red blood and the uterus appears rounded.
4. The placenta has not delivered in 30 minutes after the baby is delivered.

Answer: 4
Rationale: The placenta should deliver in about 20 minutes; if not, there may be an abnormal attachment. The uterus will not be able to contract and control bleeding if the placenta does not deliver. The amniotic sac should remain attached to the placenta, and contractions have to continue in order for the placenta to detach. A gush of blood and a change in uterine shape are expected signs of uterine detachment.
Nursing process step: Assessment
Category of client need: Physiological integrity
Cognitive level: Analysis
Learning outcome 7-7: Identify nursing diagnoses and nursing interventions to assist in the labor process.
Test-taking tip: If a question is asking about a process, know the milestones that define that process, such as second stage of labor.

11. Using a bulb syringe to clear a newborn's mouth and nose immediately after delivery is necessary to:
1. Provide a clear, patent airway.
2. Prevent aspiration of harmful organisms.
3. Stimulate the baby to begin to cry.
4. Elicit the sucking reflex before feeding.

Answer: 1
Rationale: Priority care for the newborn is to remove amniotic fluid and secretions and clear the airway. Aspiration prevention would require deeper suctioning of the oropharanyx. The bulb syringe may stimulate crying, but rubbing and stimulation work better to stimulate crying, and it is not necessary to stimulate the suck reflex prior to feeding.
Nursing process step: Implementation
Category of client need: Physiological integrity
Cognitive level: Application
Learning outcome 7-9: Describe important aspects of nursing care of the neonate immediately after birth.
Test-taking tip: Look for the answer that describes the simplest explanation for why nurses perform certain client care procedures.

12. The nurse initiates the following interventions to assist with temperature stabilization of the newborn. *Select all that are appropriate.*
1. Give the newborn a warm bath
2. Place the naked newborn on the mother's bare chest
3. Place a hat on the newborn's head
4. Dry the newborn with a warm blanket
5. Place the newborn under a radiant warmer

Answer: 2, 3, 4, 5
Rationale: One of the priorities of newborn stabilization is warming the infant. The newborn placed on the mother's chest will gain heat from the mother. Drying the newborn will prevent evaporative cooling, and a hat on the baby's head will conserve heat. The baby should not be bathed until the temperature has stabilized.
Nursing process step: Intervention
Category of client need: Physiological integrity
Cognitive level: Application
Learning outcome 7-8: Provide appropriate care for a client during labor and delivery
Test-taking tip: Look for the answer that describes the simplest explanation for why nurses perform certain client care procedures.

13. The nurse is preparing a client for electronic fetal monitoring. If the fetus is in the ROA position, fetal heart tones will best be heard in the:
1. Right upper quadrant.
2. Right lower quadrant.
3. Left upper quadrant.
4. Left lower quadrant.

Answer: 2
Rationale: The fetal heart tones are best heard over the shoulder. If the fetus is in ROA position, the fetal shoulder will be in the right lower quadrant and so heart tones will best be heard there.
Nursing process step: Intervention
Category of client need: Physiological integrity
Cognitive level: Analysis
Learning outcome 7-7: Identify nursing diagnoses and nursing interventions to assist in the labor process.
Test-taking tip: Know the definitions of key terms.

14. The nurse is assisting the client to practice different breathing techniques during the second stage of labor when the client reports numbness and tingling of her lips and fingers. The most appropriate nursing intervention at this time is to:

1. Provide oxygen at 6 L/min by mask.
2. Have the client breathe slowly while covering her mouth and nose.
3. Position the client on her left side and assess fetal heart tones.
4. Obtain vital signs and then notify the physician or midwife.

Answer: 2
Rationale: The client is hyperventilating and should either slow her breathing or re-breathe exhaled carbon dioxide in order to alleviate the symptoms. The other interventions would not help relieve the symptoms of hyperventilation.
Nursing process step: Implementation
Category of client need: Physiological integrity
Cognitive level: Analysis
Learning outcome 7-8: Provide appropriate care for a client during labor and delivery.
Test-taking tip: By understanding the physiology of common client problems, the nurse can plan appropriate interventions.

15. A newborn 5 minutes after birth has a heart rate of 100, is crying vigorously and shows some flexion of the arms and legs. The extremities are bluish in color. The head and chest are pale but pink. The best nursing intervention at this time is to:

1. Use a DeLee mucus trap and suction the nasopharnyx for 1–2 minutes.
2. Provide oxygen and prepare to assist ventilations with an Ambu bag.
3. Wrap the infant in a warm blanket and hand the baby to the parents.
4. Administer a vitamin K injection and place erythromycin ointment in each eye.

Answer: 3
Rationale: This situation describes a newborn with an APGAR score of 8 and the baby does not need resuscitation and so can be given to the parents to begin bonding. There is no indication that the newborn requires suctioning or oxygen. The vitamin K injection and erythromycin ointment should be delayed until the parents have an opportunity to bond with the newborn before the ointment obscures the newborn's vision.
Nursing process step: Implementation
Category of client need: Physiological integrity
Cognitive level: Analysis
Learning outcome 7-9: Describe important aspects of nursing care of the neonate immediately after birth.
Test-taking tip: Choose answers that make the most sense when considering the physiology of the condition described.

CHAPTER 8

1. Which of the following clients would be considered at the greatest risk during pregnancy?

1. The 19-year-old primigravida who lives in a mobile home and started prenatal care at 20 weeks.
2. The unmarried 36-year-old whose first child was born at 34 weeks gestation.
3. The 22-year-old bank teller who quit smoking when she found out she was pregnant.
4. The 28-year-old who is pregnant with a twin pregnancy following in vitro fertilization.

Answer: 2
Rationale: The greater the number of risk factors, the more the pregnancy is at risk. The correct answer shows risks related to age over 35, history of preterm delivery, and unmarried status. The other clients do not have as many risk factors.
Nursing process step: Assessment
Category of client need: Health promotion and maintenance
Cognitive level: Analysis
Learning outcome 8-2: Describe factors that put a woman at risk for complications of pregnancy.
Test-taking tip: Evaluate each risk for every client and choose the one with the most, not necessarily the single most, serious problem.

2. Fetal lung maturity can best be evaluated by:

1. The detection of phosphatidylglycerol (PG) in an amniocentesis sample
2. Measuring human chorionic gonadotropin levels in the amniotic fluid.
3. A biophysical profile score greater than 8.
4. A nonstress test that shows a reactive fetal heart rate.

Answer: 1
Rationale: Phosphatidylglycerol (PG) is the only listed test that deals with lung maturity. Human chorionic gonadotropin (hCG) is the hormone that sustains the pregnancy. A biophysical profile would show the overall well-being of the fetus, but not specifically related to lung maturity. The nonstress test determines fetal well-being, but is not specific to lung maturity.
Nursing process step: Planning
Category of client need: Physiological integrity
Cognitive level: Application
Learning outcome 8-3: Describe diagnostic tests commonly used during pregnancy.
Test-taking tip: The correct answer will be the answer that best fits with the question.

3. The following tests are all commonly preformed during the prenatal period. List them in the order they should be done during the pregnancy, starting with the earliest and ending with the last test completed.

1. Vaginal culture for group B *Streptococcus*
2. 1-hour glucose screen
3. Multiple marker screen, including alpha fetoprotein
4. Indirect Coomb's test

Answer: 3, 2, 4, 1
Rationale: The earliest test during a pregnancy may be the multiple marker (triple or quad screen) at 16 weeks, the 1-hour glucose screen at 24 weeks, the indirect Coomb's test at 28 weeks, and the vaginal culture for group B *Streptococcus* at 35 weeks.
Nursing process step: Planning
Category of client need: Health promotion and maintenance
Cognitive level: Application
Learning outcome 8-3: Describe diagnostic tests commonly used during pregnancy.
Test-taking tip: Look for the logical progression of the testing done from the start of the pregnancy to the end of the pregnancy.

4. You are obtaining an obstetric history for a client at 9 weeks gestation that includes the following: This is her fifth pregnancy. She had one baby at 28 weeks, followed by a spontaneous abortion at 12 weeks, another spontaneous abortion at 18 weeks, and most recently a pregnancy loss at 20 weeks. You anticipate her care will include:

1. Placement of a cerclage at 15–16 weeks.
2. Complete bed rest for the remained of the pregnancy.
3. Initiation of terbutaline therapy.
4. Weekly nonstress tests, starting at 22 weeks.

Answer: 1
Rationale: The question describes a situation of habitual abortion and incompetent cervix. Treatment includes a cerclage placement that sutures the cervix to prevent sudden dilation. Bed rest might be used in hypertensive disorders but may be of little value for an incompetent cervix. Terbutaline would not be initiated at this point in the pregnancy, and weekly nonstress tests would be appropriate at 32 weeks but not as early as 22 weeks.
Nursing process step: Implementation
Category of client need: Health promotion and maintenance
Cognitive level: Application
Learning outcome 8-4: Describe common complications of pregnancy, including symptoms, medical treatment, and nursing care.
Test-taking tip: Look for the answer that fits best with the client situation described and would be most effective to treat that problem.

5. A pregnant client at 37 weeks gestation presents with painless vaginal bleeding and no contractions. The most likely explanation for this is:

1. Ectopic pregnancy.
2. Placenta previa.
3. Placental abruption.
4. Preterm labor.

Answer: 2
Rationale: The symptoms of placenta previa include painless bleeding as the cervix begins to ready for labor. An ectopic pregnancy would not advance to 37 weeks but would cause complications during the middle of the first trimester. A placental abruption would be painful, and preterm labor is contractions that are often painful but without bleeding.
Nursing process step: Diagnosis
Category of client need: Physiological integrity
Cognitive level: Analysis
Learning outcome 8-1: Define key terms.
Test-taking tip: Choose answers that offer the broadest explanation to the problem as stated.

6. A pregnant client with a history of heart disease has come to the community-based prenatal clinic. Which of the following would indicate that the heart is not able to handle the additional workload of the pregnancy?

1. Blood pressure increase from 110/80 to 145/100
2. Capillary refill is less than 3 seconds
3. Feet and legs show significant swelling each evening
4. Crackles are heard in the lung bases

Answer: 4
The greatest risk for the pregnancy with cardiac disease is cardiac decompensation. Crackles, dyspnea, wet cough, and edema would all be found in the client experiencing heart failure. A blood pressure that increased from 110/80 to 145/100 would indicate hypertension and would need follow-up but is not a sign of heart failure. Capillary refill less than 3 seconds and edema in the lower extremities would be expected during pregnancy.
Nursing process step: Assessment
Category of client need: Physiological integrity
Cognitive level: Analysis
Learning outcome 8-4: Describe common complications of pregnancy, including symptoms, medical treatment, and nursing care.
Test-taking tip: The correct answer is one that is physiologically possible based on knowledge of anatomy and physiology.

7. A pregnant woman is being evaluated for hypertension. Her baseline pressure at the first prenatal visit at 8 weeks was 112/68. Other recorded pressures include 118/74 at 16 weeks, 122/70 at 20 weeks, and 146/92 at 24 weeks. She is now 28 weeks with a blood pressure of 152/96 and urine protein of 3+. This would be consistent with a classification of: 1. Chronic hypertension. 2. Gestational hypertension. 3. Pre-eclampsia. 4. Gestational eclampsia.	Answer: 3 Rationale: Pre-eclampsia is one of the hypertensive disorders of pregnancy that is diagnosed when the blood pressure is greater that 140/90 on two occasions and accompanied by proteinuria. Chronic hypertension would have shown before 20 weeks; gestational hypertension is hypertension without proteinuria; and eclampsia would include a seizure. Nursing process step: Diagnosis Category of client need: Physiological integrity Cognitive level: Analysis Learning outcome 8-1: Define key terms. Test-taking tip: By knowing the definitions to key terms, the student can choose the correct answer.
8. Which of the following criteria must be met if a client is to be considered as a candidate for vaginal birth after cesarean (VBAC)? 1. The previous cesarean was performed for a breech presentation 2. The client has not gained more than 30 pounds during the pregnancy 3. The client has not had more than 2 cesarean sections in the past 4. The client had a horizontal incision in the lower uterine segment	Answer: 4 Rationale: A horizontal incision is stronger than a vertical incision. A vertical incision could rupture during labor contractions. It does not matter if the previous section was for a breech presentation, and how much weight the client gained or the number of sections does not usually affect the decision for a VBAC. Nursing process step: Evaluation Category of client need: Physiological integrity Cognitive level: Analysis Learning outcome 8-4: Describe common complications of pregnancy, including symptoms, medical treatment, and nursing care. Test-taking tip: Look for answer choices that provide the safest possible environment for the client.
9. Which of the following lifestyle choices places the pregnant client at the greatest risk of developing toxoplasmosis? 1. The client has had no immunizations. 2. The client lives with three house cats. 3. The client uses IV drugs. 4. The client lives in a homeless shelter.	Answer: 2 Rationale: Toxoplasmosis is caused by a protozoan and increases a client's risk for stillbirth or preterm delivery. Toxoplasmosis can be carried by cat feces, and a pregnant woman can be exposed if she contacts cat feces, such as when cleaning a cat litter box. There is currently no immunization for toxoplasmosis. IV drug use and living in a homeless shelter would not increase the risk for toxoplasmosis. Nursing process step: Assessment Category of client need: Health promotion and maintenance Cognitive level: Application Learning outcome 8-4: Describe common complications of pregnancy, including symptoms, medical treatment, and nursing care. Test-taking tip: By knowing the characteristics of disease transmission, the student can choose the correct answer.
10. Preterm labor contractions may stop if the client is treated with: 1. Pitocin (oxytocin). 2. Prostoglandins (PGE). 3. Betamethasone (Celestone). 4. Terbutaline (Brethine).	Answer: 4 Rationale: Terbutaline (Brethine) is a smooth muscle relaxant that will prevent the uterus from contracting. Pitocin and prostaglandins are hormones used to stimulate labor, and betamethasone (Celestone) is a steroid that is used to promote fetal lung maturity. Nursing process step: Implementation Category of client need: Physiological integrity Cognitive level: Application Learning outcome 8-5: Describe common complications during labor and delivery, including symptoms, medical interventions, and nursing care. Test-taking tip: Look for the answer that is most different from the others.
11. A client in labor has just experienced the rupture of fetal membranes. If the nurse suspects a prolapsed cord and asks the LVN/LPN for assistance, the first priority should be to: 1. Start an IV fluid bolus. 2. Position the mother with knees to chest.	Answer: 2 Rationale: The priority for care is to decrease the pressure on the umbilical cord. The only intervention that would help to relieve the pressure is repositioning. An IV fluid bolus and oxygen administration would be appropriate, but unless the pressure on the cord is relieved, neither intervention would help the fetus. Vital signs would be important, but not the first priority. Nursing process step: Planning Category of client need: Physiological integrity

3. Obtain maternal vital signs.
4. Give oxygen 10 L/min by face mask.

Cognitive level: Analysis

Learning outcome 8-5: Describe common complications during labor and delivery, including symptoms, medical interventions, and nursing care.

Test-taking tip: Look for answer choices that provide the safest possible environment for the client.

---

12. The nurse should reposition a client if the fetal monitor strip is interpreted with the following:
1. Long-term variability.
2. FHR accelerations.
3. Early decelerations.
4. Variable decelerations.

Answer: 4

Rationale: Variable decelerations are the result of cord compression and repositioning can help to shift the weight of the baby from the cord and restore blood flow. Long-term variability, FHR accelerations, and early decelerations are all reassuring signs and no intervention would be necessary if they were seen on the fetal monitor strip.

Nursing process step: Diagnosis

Category of client need: Physiological integrity

Cognitive level: Analysis

Learning outcome 8-5: Describe common complications during labor and delivery, including symptoms, medical interventions, and nursing care.

Test-taking tip: By knowing the definitions to key terms, the student can choose the correct answer.

---

13. You are caring for a client with very heavy vaginal bleeding immediately after delivery. The placenta was examined and found to be complete. Fundal massage allows the uterus to become firm, but within minutes the uterus becomes boggy and the bleeding is heavy. You anticipate an initial intervention to be:
1. IV Pitocin or IM Methergine.
2. Surgical dilatation and curettage.
3. Blood transfusion and fluid bolus.
4. Magnesium sulfate administration.

Answer: 1

Rationale: Uterine atony can be treated with Pitocin or Methergine since both are uterine contraction stimulants. If the placenta were torn and causing the uterine atony, then the appropriate intervention might be for a dilatation and curettage. Blood transfusions and fluid boluses might be used but only after uterine tone was restored. Magnesium sulfate would cause uterine relaxation and would never be appropriate to treat heavy postpartum bleeding.

Nursing process step: Implementation

Category of client need: Physiological integrity

Cognitive level: Application

Learning outcome 8-6: Describe common complications during the postpartum period, including symptoms, medical interventions, and nursing care.

Test-taking tip: When a question is dealing with a crisis situation, such as bleeding or breathing, then look for the answer that would provide the most immediate result, and often that will be something a nurse could do at the bedside.

---

14. A treatment plan for mastitis most often will include which of the following? Select all that apply.
1. Moist heat
2. Antibiotics
3. Stopping breastfeeding
4. Surgical drainage of the lesion
5. Analgesics for pain

Answer: 1, 2, 5

Rationale: Mastitis is a breast infection often caused when a duct is not completely emptied during a feeding. Moist heat and analgesics will help with pain and promote healing. Antibiotics are also often part of the treatment. Breastfeeding will help to keep the milk ducts open and flush the organisms from the breast. The infection is often internal, and the duct can drain through the nipple pore. Surgical drainage is not appropriate.

Nursing process step: Planning

Category of client need: Physiological integrity

Cognitive level: Application

Learning outcome 8-6: Describe common complications during the postpartum period, including symptoms, medical interventions, and nursing care.

Test-taking tip: When answering a question with multiple answers, look for answers that are the most similar.

---

15. Which of the following clients is exhibiting signs of postpartum psychosis? The woman who:
1. Has not bathed for 2 days and skips meals.
2. Appears fatigued and sad, crying often.
3. Prays that God will protect her child.
4. Becomes agitated and mumbles when her baby cries.

Answer: 4

Rationale: Postpartum psychosis includes loss of reality orientation, hallucinations, and hyperactivity. The client who has not bathed or is fatigued and sad may have the postpartum blues. The client who asks God to protect her child is not demonstrating postpartum psychosis.

Nursing process step: Assessment

Category of client need: Psychosocial integrity

Cognitive level: Analysis

Learning outcome 8-6: Describe common complications during the postpartum period, including symptoms, medical interventions, and nursing care.

Test-taking tip: The nurse should know what symptoms are most common in differentiating between major depression, psychosis, and postpartum blues.

---

CHAPTER 9

1. Conduction heat loss in the newborn can be prevented by:
1. Drying the infant immediately after a bath.
2. Warming the stethoscope before touching the newborn.
3. Placing the newborn in a crib with isolette.
4. Placing the newborn under a warmer.

Answer: 2
Rationale: Conduction heat loss is when a baby is placed on a cold surface or something cold is placed on the baby. A wet infant loses heat by evaporation. An isolette would prevent convection heat loss, and a cap or warmer would prevent radiant heat loss.
Nursing process step: Implementation
Category of client need: Physiological integrity
Cognitive level: Application
Learning outcome 9-2: Discuss physiologic adaptation of the newborn.
Test-taking tip: The correct answer is one that is physiologically possible based on knowledge of thermoregulation.

2. You anticipate that a newborn will respond to a resuscitation of stimulation and oxygen if the APGAR score is:
1. 2.
2. 6.
3. 8.
4. 10.

Answer: 2
Rationale: The APGAR score demonstrates the need for resuscitation. An APGAR score of 6 (any score 4–7) indicates that stimulation and oxygen are necessary as an initial intervention. An APGAR score of 2 (any score 0–3) requires immediate resuscitation and advanced techniques would be anticipated. Newborns with APGARs of 8–10 would not require immediate resuscitation.
Nursing process step: Planning
Category of client need: Physiological integrity
Cognitive level: Application
Learning outcome 9-3: Discuss APGAR score.
Test-taking tip: By knowing the definitions to key terms, the student can choose the correct answer.

3. The nurse is most concerned when the assessment of a 4-hour-old newborn reveals:
1. A heart rate of 130.
2. A respiratory rate of 50.
3. An axillary temperature of 97.5.
4. That the newborn has not eaten for 2 hours.

Answer: 3
Rationale: A temperature of 97.5 is too low, and thermoregulation is one of the most critical adaptations a newborn must make in the transition to extrauterine life. The normal range for the heart rate is 110–160, and the normal range for the respiratory rate is 30–60. A newborn is expected to feed every 2–4 hours.
Nursing process step: Assessment
Category of client need: Physiological integrity
Cognitive level: Analysis
Learning outcome 9-4: Describe physical characteristics of the newborn.
Test-taking tip: Know the expected range of vital signs for any groups of clients.

4. Which of the following physical assessments is most consistent with a gestational age of 35 weeks? Select all that apply.
1. The newborn lies with arms and legs slightly flexed
2. The soles of the feet are covered with deep creases
3. The skin is dry and peeling
4. There is very little lanugo seen on the baby
5. The pinna of the ear springs back slowly when compressed

Answer: 1, 5
Rationale: A premature newborn will have decreased muscle mass and poor muscle tone and will rest with arms and legs extended. The ear will have soft cartilage that will remain compressed when the pinna of the ear is compressed. Deep foot creases, dry, peeling skin, and decreased lanugo are all signs of term and post-term newborns.
Nursing process step: Diagnosis
Category of client need: Physiological integrity
Cognitive level: Analysis
Learning outcome 9-4: Describe physical characteristics of the newborn.
Test-taking tip: Look for the answer that is most different from the others.

5. The nurse has assessed the weight and length of a 36-week gestation newborn. The results show growth in the 85th percentile. Which term best describes this newborn?
1. Full term
2. Preterm
3. Small for gestational age
4. Large for gestational age

Answer: 2
Rationale: A newborn at 36 weeks is preterm, and full term is greater than 38 weeks. Growth at the 85th percentile is normal, with less than 10th percentile being small for gestational age and greater than 90th being large for gestational age.
Nursing process step: Diagnosis
Category of client need: Physiological integrity
Cognitive level: Analysis
Learning outcome 9-1: Define key terms.
Test-taking tip: By knowing the definitions to key terms, the student can choose the correct answer.

6. Scalp edema that crosses the suture lines of the skull of a newborn is documented in the newborn's chart as: 1. Molding 2. Cephalohematoma 3. Cranial distention 4. Caput succedaneum	Answer: 4 Rationale: Since a caput seccedaneum is just superficial and beneath the scalp, the swelling can cross the suture lines. Molding is overriding of the cranial plates, and cephalohematoma does not cross the suture lines since it results when blood is trapped beneath the periosteum. Cranial distention is not a term used in newborn assessment. Nursing process step: Diagnosis Category of client need: Physiological integrity Cognitive level: Application Learning outcome 9-1: Define key terms. Test-taking tip: By knowing the definitions to key terms, the student can choose the correct answer.
7. When the nurse gently bumps the side of the infant's bed, the newborn suddenly extends both arms and legs with a tremor. The nurse knows that this response indicates: 1. The newborn has an intact neurologic system. 2. Opioids were given to the mother during labor. 3. The infant may be premature. 4. Birth trauma may have caused permanent damage.	Answer: 1 Rationale: The Moro reflex is a sign that the infant is neurologically intact. This is a normal response to movement. Opioids will depress the reflexes, and a premature newborn will have sluggish reflexes. The Moro reflex is not a sign of any injury. Nursing process step: Diagnosis Category of client need: Physiological integrity Cognitive level: Analysis Learning outcome 9-5: Describe neonatal reflexes. Test-taking tip: By knowing the definitions to key terms, the student can choose the correct answer.
8. Teaching parents proper home care for the umbilical cord should include: 1. The newborn may be bathed in the tub after the cord has dried completely. 2. A 1-inch circle at the base of the cord should be cleaned daily with alcohol. 3. The cord stump should fall off in about 3 days. 4. After the cord dries completely, the clamp may be removed.	Answer: 4 Rationale: The cord clamp may be removed after the cord is dry. It is easier to diaper the infant once the clamp is removed, so it should be removed as soon as possible. The newborn should not be immersed until the cord stump falls off. Applying alcohol to the skin is not appropriate. The cord stump should fall off in about a week. Nursing process step: Implementation Category of client need: Physiological integrity Cognitive level: Application Learning outcome 9-9: Discuss parent teaching related to care of the newborn. Test-taking tip: Look for answers that demonstrate safe nursing practice and follow accepted standards of care.
9. Newborn safety measures while in the hospital should include: 1. Matching the mother's and infant's fingerprints. 2. Encouraging the mother to sleep with the newborn in her bed. 3. Holding the baby in the football hold while moving the baby from room to room. 4. Teaching parents to observe the identification of staff who care for their newborn.	Answer: 4 Rationale: Parents should be aware of and always identify any personnel who provide care for their newborn. Mother and baby should have identification bands that match, but fingerprints are not matched as this is not a skill most nurses possess. The baby should always be placed in a bed for transport and never be transported in the nurse's arms. Nursing process step: Implementation Category of client need: Physiological integrity Cognitive level: Application Learning outcome 9-6: Describe nursery care for the newborn. Test-taking tip: Look for answer choices that provide the safest possible environment for the client.
10. Following a circumcision with a Plastibell, the nurse should include in the plan of care to: 1. Use A and D ointment or petroleum jelly at each diaper change. 2. Clean the glans with alcohol during the bath. 3. Apply an ice pack to reduce swelling. 4. Apply direct pressure if bleeding occurs.	Answer: 4 Rationale: Although bleeding is rare with a Plastibell circumcision, direct pressure should be applied immediately should bleeding occur. No ointment is needed with a Plastibell circumcision, and the glans should be cleaned with plain water only. An ice pack would be inappropriate care for a circumcision. Nursing process step: Planning Category of client need: Physiological integrity Cognitive level: Application Learning outcome 9-7 Discuss common procedures and screening tests for the newborn. Test-taking tip: When reviewing a procedure, the student should recognize how to react when complications occur.

11. Calculate the amount of 20-cal/ounce formula needed daily for an 8-pound newborn who needs 50 cal/pound each day.	Answer: 20 ounces ($8 \times 50/20$) Rationale: Multiply 8×50 to find daily caloric need—400 cal/day. With formula that has 20 cal per ounce, divide 400 by 20 to find that this baby should have 20 ounces per day. Nursing process step: Planning Category of client need: Physiological integrity Cognitive level: Application Learning outcome 9-8: Discuss the newborn's nutritional needs and how they can be met. Test-taking tip: Calculating formula needs for a newborn uses the same methods as other drug calculation problems.
12. Correct latch during breastfeeding includes: 1. The areola is visible at the edge of the infant's lips. 2. The mother reports a mild pinching during feeding. 3. The tongue should press gently on the tip of the nipple. 4. The infant's lips appear flared while the baby sucks.	Answer: 4 Rationale: The flaring of the lips represents a good latch and will assure proper nipple placement in the infant's mouth. The areola should not be visible during breastfeeding. Proper latch should be painless, and the tongue should press upward and press the nipple against the hard palate of the baby's mouth. Nursing process step: Evaluation Category of client need: Physiological integrity Cognitive level: Analysis Learning outcome 9-8: Discuss the newborn's nutritional needs and how they can be met. Test-taking tip: The correct answer is one that is physiologically possible based on knowledge of anatomy and physiology.
13. A parent may need additional teaching about newborn care when he or she states: 1. "If the baby is fussy, I can swaddle him securely in a clean blanket." 2. "After feeding I should place the baby on his side in the crib." 3. "I can expect 8–10 wet diapers and several stools each day." 4. "I should stop feeding and burp the baby ½ way through each feeding."	Answer: 2 Rationale: Parents should always place their infants on their backs to sleep. Babies like the security of swaddling and may be comforted by being tightly wrapped in a blanket. Normal output for a newborn would be 8–10 wet diapers and several stools. All babies should be burped, even breastfed babies. Nursing process step: Evaluation Category of client need: Health promotion and maintenance Cognitive level: Analysis Learning outcome 9-9: Discuss parent teaching related to care of the newborn. Test-taking tip: Look for an answer that describes appropriate nursing actions.
14. You are the LVN/LPN obtaining vital signs for a 6-hour-old newborn. Which of the following assessment findings indicate respiratory distress? 1. Respiratory rate of 50 2. Hands and feet are dark blue 3. The nostrils flare with each breath 4. Respirations are irregular and shallow	Answer: 3 Rationale: The flaring of the nostrils is a sign that the newborn is in respiratory distress and that the nurse should intervene. The normal respiratory rate is 30–60. Blue hands and feet, called acrocyanosis, are normal in the newborn. Respirations are typically irregular, and so the nurse should count respirations for one full minute. Nursing process step: Assessment Category of client need: Health promotion and maintenance Cognitive level: Analysis Learning outcome 9-10: Describe signs of respiratory distress in the newborn. Test-taking tip: Know the key assessments for each age group of clients.
15. Which of the following indicates the newborn is at risk for hemolytic disease? 1. The mother and baby have Rh negative blood 2. The mother with Rh negative blood and the baby with Rh positive blood 3. The mother and baby both have Rh positive blood 4. The mother has Rh positive blood and the baby has Rh negative blood	Answer: 2 Rationale: A newborn is at risk for hemolytic disease when the mother has Rh negative blood and the newborn has Rh positive blood. The other situations would not increase the risks. Nursing process step: Diagnosis Category of client need: Health promotion and maintenance Cognitive level: Analysis Learning outcome 9-11: Discuss conditions and treatment of the high-risk newborn. Test-taking tip: By knowing the definitions to key terms, the student can choose the correct answer.

CHAPTER 10

1. During the assessment of a postpartum client 24 hours after delivery, the nurse palpates the firm uterine fundus in the midline, at the level of the umbilicus. The nurse's first action should be to:
1. Massage the fundus.
2. Press the call bell and summon help.
3. Encourage the woman to void.
4. Let the client know that this is normal recovery.

Answer: 4
Rationale: A firm fundus in the midline at the level of the umbilicus is a normal assessment finding and the client should be reassured that this represents a normal recovery. No additional interventions are needed at this time.
Nursing process step: Diagnosis
Category of client need: Physiological integrity
Cognitive level: Analysis
Learning outcome 10-1: Describe physical changes in the mother during the postpartum period.
Test-taking tip: Know the normal assessment findings and look for deviations.

2. Which of the following assessment findings 6 hours after delivery requires immediate intervention?
1. Lochia is dark red and contains 2 nickel-sized clots
2. The episiotomy is slightly bruised
3. The breasts are secreting a thin yellowish fluid
4. The mother has not voided since delivery

Answer: 4
Rationale: The nurse should intervene to empty the bladder of a client who has not voided within 4 hours after delivery. The bladder fullness could contribute to uterine atony. Lochia that is dark red with small clots, a slightly bruised episiotomy, and the secretion of colostrum are all normal assessment findings at this time.
Nursing process step: Diagnosis
Category of client need: Physiological integrity
Cognitive level: Analysis
Learning outcome 10-1: Describe physical changes in the mother during the postpartum period.
Test-taking tip: Know the normal assessment findings and look for deviations.

3. A mother adapting to the role of motherhood is in the taking-in stage when she:
1. Inquires about the quality of her breast milk.
2. Eagerly participates in all aspects of newborn care.
3. Talks with visitors about the labor experience.
4. Plans to have friends visit her and the baby at home.

Answer: 3
Rationale: The taking-in phase is characterized by the need for the mother to resolve the labor experience. The mother has completed the taking-in phase when she is moving forward and participating in newborn care, improving the quality of care, and making plans for the future with her baby.
Nursing process step: Assessment
Category of client need: Psychosocial integrity
Cognitive level: Analysis
Learning outcome 10-2: Discuss psychological changes in the mother during the postpartum period.
Test-taking tip: Look for the answer that is most different from the others.

4. You are the nurse in the community-based clinic when a new mother brings her 1-week-old infant for a checkup. You suspect she is experiencing the postpartum blues when:
1. She becomes tearful and reports not sleeping well.
2. She jumps from her chair and moves quickly across the room as the baby cries.
3. She refuses to allow anyone else to hold the infant.
4. She describes the baby as looking exactly like the brother she remembers as a "difficult" child.

Answer: 1
Rationale: The postpartum blues are characterized by mild depressive symptoms such as crying and fatigue. The blues may be related to hormone levels and fatigue. Responding to a crying infant and refusing to let anyone hold the baby do not indicate depression. Identifying the baby with someone in a negative connotation may indicate a problem with bonding, but is not a sign of postpartum blues.
Nursing process step: Diagnosis
Category of client need: Psychosocial integrity
Cognitive level: Application
Learning outcome 10-2: Discuss psychological changes in the mother during the postpartum period.
Test-taking tip: By knowing the definitions to key terms, the student can choose the correct answer.

5. You are providing hourly postpartum assessments of a woman following the vaginal delivery of twins. Because of uterine overdistention, you are most concerned about:
1. Frequent urination.
2. 2+ patellar reflexes.
3. Shaking chills just after delivery.
4. A uterus that needs frequent massage.

Answer: 4
Rationale: Overdistention may place the client at risk for uterine atony, and an early sign of this may be the uterus that needs frequent massage. The other choices all represent normal assessment findings.
Nursing process step: Assessment
Category of client need: Physiological integrity
Cognitive level: Analysis
Learning outcome 10-3: Discuss important aspects of postpartum assessment and nursing care.
Test-taking tip: Know the normal assessment findings and look for deviations.

6. Which of the following assessments at 24 hours postpartum is the strongest indication of postpartum hemorrhage?
1. Perineal pad saturated every 4 hours
2. Fundus measures 1 FB below the umbilicus
3. Pulse is 120 and respirations are 24
4. Skin is warm, moist and the face is flushed

Answer: 3
Rationale: Following hemorrhage, the cardiovascular system will compensate for the decreased volume by increasing the pulse, so a pulse of 120 would indicate volume depletion. The other assessments are all normal findings during the first postpartum day.
Nursing process step: Diagnosis
Category of client need: Physiological integrity
Cognitive level: Analysis
Learning outcome 10-4: Describe the complications commonly seen during the postpartum period.
Test-taking tip: Know the normal assessment findings and look for deviations.

7. Postpartum teaching for the postpartum client should include:
1. Breastfeeding may increase "afterpains."
2. As the milk supply is established, breastfeeding clients may notice breast becoming hard and lumpy.
3. Lochia flow should remain red and heavy for about 24 hours and then will become pink and much lighter.
4. Most women will resume menstrual periods within 2 months after delivery.

Answer: 1
Rationale: Breastfeeding stimulates the release of oxytocin and will cause the uterus to contract. Afterpains will be stronger for the multigravida client. Breast should be firm but should not be hard and lumpy. Lochia should remain red or rubra for about 3 days and should not be heavy at any time. Most women will resume menstrual periods by the third month, not the second month after delivery.
Nursing process step: Evaluation
Category of client need: Physiological integrity
Cognitive level: Application
Learning outcome 10-5: Discuss topics for client teaching about self-care in the postpartum period.
Test-taking tip: The correct answer is one that is physiologically possible based on knowledge of anatomy and physiology.

8. Proper assessment of the postpartum uterine fundus should include (*select all that apply*):
1. Have the woman empty her bladder.
2. Begin at the symphysis pubis and palpate gently upward to the fundus.
3. The fundus should be about the size of a baseball and firm.
4. A boggy fundus should be massaged in a circular pattern.
5. Document fundal position relative to the umbilicus.

Answer: 1, 4, 5
Rationale: To determine proper uterine involution, the bladder should be empty. Massage should be gentle and follow a circular pattern. Correct documentation includes the distance between the fundus and the umbilicus measured by finger breadth (FB). The nurse should always palpate downward from just above the umbilicus to determine uterine height. The fundus should be about the size of a softball or small grapefruit.
Nursing process step: Implementation
Category of client need: Physiological integrity
Cognitive level: Analysis
Learning outcome 10-3: Discuss important aspects of postpartum assessment and nursing care.
Test-taking tip: When evaluating a procedure, review the procedure from start to finish and choose answers that most closely follow the procedure.

9. You are the LVN/LPN performing assessment of a postpartum client 2 hours after delivery. You find the fundus firm, midline and 3 FB above the umbilicus. Your next action is to:
1. Ask the mother to void.
2. Massage the fundus.
3. Document your findings.
4. Notify the supervising RN.

Answer: 4
Rationale: A firm uterus that is larger than expected could be full of clots and may need massage to evacuate the clots. This may not be within the scope of practice for the LPN/LVN and represents a significant variation from normal, so the supervising RN should be notified. If woman needed to void, the fundus would likely be deviated to the side. Massage would not be an effective intervention at this time and documentation without intervention would not be an appropriate course of action.
Nursing process step: Implementation
Category of client need: Physiological integrity
Cognitive level: Analysis
Learning outcome 10-4: Describe the complications commonly seen during the postpartum period.
Test-taking tip: Look for the answer that is most different from the others when considering a deviation from the normal.

10. Perineal assessment is best performed with the woman in what position?
1. Supine with knees flexed
2. With the head of the bed elevated 30 degrees

Answer: 3
Rationale: The left lateral Sims position allows for the best and most complete visualization of the perineum. The other positions as described would not allow for complete visualization. The supine visualization would not allow for complete

3. Left Sims with the head resting on a small pillow
4. Side lying with the legs and knees extended

visualization of the posterior perineum, and side lying with extended legs and knees would not allow complete visualization of the anterior perineum.

Nursing process step: Implementation

Category of client need: Health promotion and maintenance

Cognitive level: Application

Learning outcome 10-3: Discuss important aspects of postpartum assessment and nursing care.

Test-taking tip: Look for an answer that describes appropriate nursing actions.

---

11. Which of the following client situations should the LVN/LPN report to the supervisory RN or physician for further assessment? *Select all that are appropriate.*
1. The breastfeeding client at 72 hours postpartum with very firm, warm breasts
2. The client at 48 hours postpartum who reports pain in one leg when the nurse dorsiflexes the foot
3. The client 12 hours after a cesarean section with hypoactive bowel sounds
4. The client on IV magnesium sulfate 24 hours after delivery who appears flushed and complains of fatigue
4. The client 2 hours after delivery with continuous lochia flow who has saturated 3 pads since delivery

Answer: 2, 5

Rationale: Pain with dorsiflexion of the foot indicates a positive Homan's sign, and the client should be evaluated for a deep vein thrombosis. The client who saturates more than one pad per hour or has continuous lochia flow should be evaluated for a laceration. The client with warm, firm breasts has established a milk supply. Hypoactive bowel sounds after a cesarean section, and the client on magnesium sulfate with fatigue and flushed skin are both expected findings and would not need immediate intervention.

Nursing process step: Evaluation

Category of client need: Safe, effective care environment

Cognitive level: Analysis

Learning outcome 10-4: Describe the complications commonly seen during the postpartum period.

Test-taking tip: Look for answer choices that provide the safest possible environment for the client.

---

12. Which of the following should be included in the discharge teaching plan for the client following a cesarean delivery?
1. A warm tub bath may help relieve incisional pain
2. The perineum should be rinsed with clear, warm water after each voiding
3. Steristrips should be removed from the incision on the fifth post operative day
4. Sexual intercourse should be delayed until at least 2 weeks after delivery

Answer: 2

Rationale: Rinsing the perineum with clear, warm water will reduce the risk of infection for all postpartum clients, including those that had a cesarean delivery. The client should avoid a tub bath because of exposure of the surgical incision to the bath water could increase infection risks. Steristrips should be allowed to fall off in the first two weeks after delivery. Sexual intercourse should be delayed for 6 weeks after delivery.

Nursing process step: Implementation

Category of client need: Physiological integrity

Cognitive level: Application

Learning outcome 10-5: Discuss topics for client teaching about self-care in the postpartum period.

Test-taking tip: Know the best self-care practices for clients who have had surgery or procedures.

---

13. Your postpartum client asks when she can begin to exercise to "get back into shape." Your best response is:
1. "You can begin walking any time after delivery."
2. "You should wait 2 weeks before beginning any exercise program."
3. "If you do not experience pain, there are no restrictions to exercise."
4. "Abdominal exercises will help the uterus return to its former size and shape."

Answer: 1

Rationale: Walking is safe and will help in the recovery process. Gradually beginning an exercise program can start with gentle stretches the first day after delivery, so it is not necessary to wait for 2 weeks for this type of exercise. Strenuous exercises should not be initiated until two weeks after delivery. Abdominal exercises will not help promote uterine involution.

Nursing process step: Planning

Category of client need: Health promotion and maintenance

Cognitive level: Application

Learning outcome 10-5: Discuss topics for client teaching about self-care in the postpartum period.

Test-taking tip: Know the best self-care practices for clients who have had surgery or procedures.

---

14. You are the LVN/LPN providing care to a client immediately after she returns to her room following a cesarean section. You note that when the baby is

Answer: 4

Rationale: Touch that begins with fingertip touching and progresses to stroking with the whole hand to enfolding of the newborn is normal. This is not a sign of rejection, the postpartum blues, or pain.

---

placed in her arms for the first time, she touches him with her fingertips only. You recognize this as:
1. An early sign of rejection.
2. A symptom of postpartum blues.
3. Evidence that the mother is in pain.
4. Normal bonding progression.

Nursing process step: Diagnosis
Category of client need: Health promotion and maintenance
Cognitive level: Analysis
Learning outcome 10-3: Discuss important aspects of postpartum assessment and nursing care.
Test-taking tip: Know the normal assessment findings and look for deviations.

---

15. Which of the following clients would be most at risk for postpartum hemorrhage?
1. The client who labored for 15 hours with a 45-minute second stage
2. The client who delivered twins by cesarean section
3. The client who has a temperature of 100.1°F just after delivery
4. The client who delivered a preterm infant at 34 weeks gestation

Answer: 2
Rationale: A condition such as delivering twins and a procedure such as a cesarean section will increase the risk for postpartum hemorrhage. A 15-hour labor with a 45-minute second stage is a normal expectation for labor. Prolonged labor would increase the risk for hemorrhage. A temperature of 100.1°F just after delivery is a normal finding and would not increase the risk for hemorrhage. A preterm delivery would not be a risk for hemorrhage since the uterus would not have been overdistended.
Nursing process step: Diagnosis
Category of client need: Physiological integrity
Cognitive level: Analysis
Learning outcome 10-4: Describe the complications commonly seen during the postpartum period.
Test-taking tip: Know what risks the client faces given a diagnosis or procedure.

CHAPTER 11

1. Which of the following situations represents an expected pattern of development (*select all that apply*)?
1. 1-month-old who easily and frequently turns from stomach to back
2. 2-month-old who holds his bottle during every feeding
3. 7-month-old who can transfer an object from one hand to the other
4. 12-month-old who walks unsteadily across the room (a distance of 14 feet)
5. 15-month-old who can take off her own shoes and socks

Answer: 3, 4, 5
Rationale: The child at 7 months has the hand-eye coordination to transfer objects from one hand to the other. A 12-month-old who can walk alone may be unsteady, but walking across the room would be normal development. At 15-months of age, most children are beginning to undress themselves but cannot be expected to dress themselves. The ability to turn from stomach to back should be developed by 5 months of age, although a 1-month-old may accidentally turn from back to front, so parents should be cautioned to not leave the child unattended. A 4-month-old child would be expected to hold a bottle. A 2-month-old child would not have the ability to hold a bottle.
Nursing process step: Assessment
Category of client need: Health promotion and maintenance
Cognitive level: Analysis
Learning outcome 11-7: Describe the usual physical development for each age group.
Test-taking tip: Avoid answers that include absolute terms, such as *frequently* or "during *every* feeding."

---

2. Which of the following best illustrates Piaget's preoperational level of cognitive development?
1. The child who asks how words are spelled and writes them letter by letter
2. The newborn who cries when hungry and then falls asleep in the mother's arms after feeding
3. The school-age child who insists on sitting on the same seat on the school bus every day
4. The teenager who runs 2 miles daily during summer vacation in order to play on the soccer team in the fall

Answer: 1
Rationale: The preoperational level involves learning language and symbols. The sensorimotor level represents only reflex responses, and a child operating in the concrete operational level will see everything as black and white, with routines being very important. The formal operations level shows maturity and recognizes the effects of actions and planning ahead for desired goals.
Nursing process step: Evaluation
Category of client need: Health promotion and maintenance
Cognitive level: Analysis
Learning outcome 11-3: Describe Piaget's stages of cognitive development.
Test-taking tip: Look for answers that are possible. The *pre*operational stage is the only stage that involves early conscious thought.

---

3. The 8-year-old child who becomes upset with playmates because they are not "following the rules" is operating at which of Piaget's levels of cognitive development?
1. Sensorimotor
2. Preoperational
3. Concrete operational
4. Formal operational

Answer: 3
Rationale: A child functioning in the concrete operational level would see rules as very important and would become upset if others were not following the rules. "Sensorimotor" refers to reflex responses and would apply primarily to infants. The preoperational child would not be bound by rules and so would not become upset with playmates not following the rules. Formal operations allow for the abstract, and the child will begin to see flexibility in rules and exceptions.
Nursing process step: Assessment
Category of client need: Health promotion and maintenance
Cognitive level: Application
Learning outcome 11-3: Describe Piaget's stages of cognitive development.
Test-taking tip: By knowing the characteristics of Piaget's different stages, the child's behavior should fit with the description.

4. Which of the following statements regarding growth and development is true?
1. Growth is primarily determined by heredity, race, and gender
2. Even though traditional family roles have changed, the rate a child develops has remained the same for many generations
3. Culture can influence child development through diversity of gender roles, dietary practices, and family structure
4. Child development refers to the physical growth of a body as the child increases in size and is strongly based in genetics

Answer: 3
Rationale: Culture can influence how a child will view and interact with the world. Growth can also be influenced by nutrition, environment, and general health. Child development has changed based on changes in traditional family roles, structure, and values. Child development refers to social and cognitive development as well as physical growth.
Nursing process step: Evaluation
Category of client need: Health promotion and maintenance
Cognitive level: Analysis
Learning outcome 11-1: Differentiate growth from development.
Test-taking tip: Avoid answers that include absolutes and very specific terms. The more general terms often are the most realistic when the question is dealing with a wide range of responses or patterns, such as with growth and development.

5. Which of the following children is expected to learn to trust their caregivers before they can move into the next stage of development as described by Erickson?
1. The newborn
2. The toddler
3. The school-age child
4. The adolescent

Answer: 1
Rationale: Newborns learn to trust that their needs will be met by their caregivers (trust vs. mistrust). Toddlers should learn autonomy to develop confidence (autonomy vs. shame and doubt). School-age children learn that work well done can provide inner satisfaction (industry vs. inferiority). Adolescents should develop peer relationships and begin to separate from their parents (identity vs. role confusion).
Nursing process step: Evaluation
Category of client need: Health promotion and maintenance
Cognitive level: Application
Learning outcome 11-4: Describe Erikson's levels of psychosocial development.
Test-taking tip: Choose the answer that is most realistic based on the question.

6. Which of the following teenagers is demonstrating appropriate behaviors for achieving the developmental task associated with Erickson's stage of adolescence (*select all that apply*)?
1. The 15-year-old who talks on the phone to friends for several hours each day
2. The 19-year-old who goes away to college and plans on living in a dormitory
3. The 17-year-old who spends most of his or her free time alone playing video games
4. The 14-year-old who does not want to go on a family vacation
5. The 16-year-old single mother who lives with her parents and must work after school

Answer: 1, 2, 4
Rationale: The developmental task for teenagers is identity versus role confusion, and it is appropriate behavior for a 16-year-old to develop peer relationships. Separation from parents is necessary to achieve a sense of identity, and adolescents prefer peer relationships to family time. A 17-year-old who spends most of his or her time alone might not have peer support, which could lead to a delay in the development of identity. Teen mothers are at risk for developmental stagnation if they do not develop a sense of identity before they have the responsibilities of parenting.
Nursing process step: Assessment
Category of client need: Health promotion and maintenance
Cognitive level: Analysis
Learning outcome 11-4: Describe Erikson's levels of psychosocial development.
Test-taking tip: Look for answers that are reasonable and possible.

7. A potty-trained child who insists on using diapers after a new baby is brought into the home is demonstrating which of the following defense mechanisms?
1. Regression
2. Repression
3. Rationalization
4. Fantasy

Answer: 1
Rationale: Regression involves the reemergence of past behaviors. Repression is the inability to recall painful situations. Rationalization involves providing a reason for behaviors. Fantasy involves creating an imaginary solution for fears.
Nursing process step: Diagnosis
Category of client need: Health promotion and maintenance
Cognitive level: Analysis
Learning outcome 11-5: Describe Freud's stages of psychosexual development.
Test-taking tip: Choose answers that fit the definition required by the question.

8. At which age should a child be expected to start to develop a conscience?
1. 2
2. 5
3. 10
4. 14

Answer: 3
Rationale: A 10-year-old is in the conventional stage and recognizes the importance of rules and will start to develop a conscience. Moral development as described by Kohlberg does not begin at age 2. A 5-year-old will avoid punishment and may lie without remorse. A 14-year-old should already have a conscience and is learning ethical and moral responsibilities.
Nursing process step: Assessment
Category of client need: Health promotion and maintenance
Cognitive level: Application
Learning outcome 11-6: Describe Kohlberg's levels of moral development.
Test-taking tip: Often the correct answer to questions that involve numbers is in the middle of the range and not the highest or lowest number choices.

9. Which of the following conclusions is correct regarding the child who is at the 70th percentile for weight and the 90th percentile for height? The child is:
1. Taller than 89% of other children.
2. Overweight for the height recorded.
3. Average for both height and weight.
4. Growing slower than most children the same age.

Answer: 1
Rationale: A child at the 90th percentile for height is taller than 89% of other children and shorter than 10 % of the population of the same age. The child would be underweight for the height given, average for weight, and above average for height. This child would be growing faster than most children the same age.
Nursing process step: Diagnosis
Category of client need: Health promotion and maintenance
Cognitive level: Analysis
Learning outcome 11-7: Describe the usual physical development for each age group.
Test-taking tip: A nurse should be able to interpret assessment data.

10. Which of the following would be important to teach the parents of a newborn about expected growth during the first year of life?
1. The baby should double the birth weight by 2 months of age
2. The baby should double the birth length by one year of age
3. The baby's head will grow faster than the torso and limbs
4. Teeth begin to erupt at about the sixth month

Answer: 4
Rationale: Teeth do begin to erupt at about 6 months of age. Normal growth patterns include doubling of birth weight by 5 months of age; length would increase about 12 inches in the first year of life. The growth of the head slows and the body grows faster to become more proportional.
Nursing process step: Assessment
Category of client need: Health promotion and maintenance
Cognitive level: Application
Learning outcome 11-9: Provide some guidelines for age-appropriate teaching to each age group.
Test-taking tip: Normal growth and development parameters are guidelines for nursing assessment and teaching.

11. Which of the following would indicate a deviation from the expected developmental milestones for a toddler?
1. The toddler wants to try to feed themselves
2. The toddler is able to identify the urge to urinate or defecate
3. The toddler is expected to form sentences of 6–8 words
4. The toddler may play beside other children, not with them

Answer: 3
Rationale: Toddlers are expected to form simple sentences of 3–5 words. Wanting to feed themselves, an interest in toilet training, and parallel play are all normal toddler activities and behaviors.
Nursing process step: Assessment
Category of client need: Health promotion and maintenance
Cognitive level: Application
Learning outcome 11-8: Describe characteristic milestones and deviations from the norm for each age group.
Test-taking tip: Choose the answer that is most unlike the others when looking for an answer to a question that is asking about an exception.

12. Which of the following toys would be most appropriate for a hospitalized 3-year-old? 1. Card games 2. Puzzles 3. Board games 4. Pull toys	Answer: 2 Rationale: Puzzles are good for toddlers because they have developed fine motor coordination and enjoy completing tasks. Most toddlers will not play well with others, so card games are not appropriate. Board games require too much concentration and too much attention to rules for a 3-year-old to enjoy. Pull toys are more appropriate choices for younger children. Nursing process step: Intervention Category of client need: Health promotion and maintenance Cognitive level: Application Learning outcome 11-8: Describe characteristic milestones and deviations from the norm for each age group. Test-taking tip: The correct answer will often be the most reasonable answer.
13. Which of the following children is using the defense mechanism of regression to deal with a situation? 1. A child who communicates only with an imaginary friend. 2. A child who cannot remember witnessing an automobile accident. 3. A potty-trained child who begins to have frequent episodes of wetting. 4. The child who broke a sibling's toy because "she hit me."	Answer: 3 Rationale: Regression is returning to a previous stage of behavior, as with the child who no longer demonstrates potty training skills. A child with an imaginary friend is demonstrating the use of fantasy as a defense mechanism. Children can repress hurtful situations to protect themselves emotionally and children will rationalize bad behavior by placing blame on others. Nursing process step: Diagnosis Category of client need: Health promotion and maintenance Cognitive level: Analysis Learning outcome 11-8: Describe characteristic milestones and deviations from the norm for each age group. Test-taking tip: Normal growth and development parameters are guidelines for nursing diagnosis.
14. Which of the following young adults is demonstrating successful completion of the appropriate developmental stage? 1. The 22-year-old attending college and living with parents 2. The 25-year-old who has full responsibility for aging parents 3. The 28-year-old who is married and expecting a first child 4. The 30-year-old who lives alone and is financially independent	Answer: 3 Rationale: A young adult who is married and having children is developing long-term relationships. Attending school is appropriate, but the young adult needs to separate from parents. Young adults should be focusing on establishing their own family and developing lasting relationships. Financial independence is only part of the developmental stage that young adults should complete; they also should develop intimate relationships. Nursing process step: Evaluation Category of client need: Health promotion and maintenance Cognitive level: Application Learning outcome 11-8: Describe characteristic milestones and deviations from the norm for each age group. Test-taking tip: Choose answers that are the most general; often very specific answers give extra information to distract the student.
15. Older adults experience normal physical changes such as: 1. Increasing memory losses from peripheral circulation changes. 2. Hardening of the lens of the eye causing cataracts. 3. Difficulty urinating from frequent bladder and prostate infections. 4. Bone density decreases may cause high calcium levels and arrhythmias.	Answer: 1 Rationale: Increased short-term memory loss may occur as circulation declines. Cataracts are clouding of the lens; hardening of the lens will result in farsightedness. Prostate enlargement may cause difficulty urinating. Infection is not usually a contributing factor. Bone density decreases may lead to increased fractures. Nursing process step: Assessment Category of client need: Health promotion and maintenance Cognitive level: Application Learning outcome 11-8: Describe characteristic milestones and deviations from the norm for each age group. Test-taking tip: Choose answers that are the most general, as very specific answers often give extra information to distract the student.

1. The nurse who works with clients in teaching and evaluating learning should be aware that good educational practices enhance learning. Which of the following would best help a client to learn?
1. Include the client, parents, and any family that will be present in the household.
2. Utilize instructional techniques specific to the client's age, developmental stage, and culture.
3. Use only written instructions so clients will have proof they understood what was said.
4. Refer any client questions to the nurse supervisor.

Answer: 2
Rationale: Teaching methods should be adapted to the client, including age, development, and culture. The teaching environment should be limited only to the client and caregivers to avoid confusion. Written instructions are only one part of the teaching process, and the nurse providing the teaching should answer questions, unless the nurse needs more information.
Nursing process step: Implementation
Category of client need: Safe, effective care environment
Cognitive level: Analysis
Learning outcome 12-1: Describe techniques for client/family teaching.
Test-taking tip: Answers that promote nursing care that adapts to changing client situations are often the right choice.

2. The best example of a nurse acting as a good role model for clients is:
1. Calling for an interpreter when the family speaks a different language from the nurse.
2. Demonstrating good health practices, such as not smoking and maintaining a healthy weight.
3. Performing nursing interventions in a timely manner.
4. Attending continuing education courses and joining professional organizations.

Answer: 2
Rationale: A good role model will set a good example, such as not smoking and maintaining a healthy weight. Use of an interpreter, demonstrating good time management, and professional development are important parts of good nursing practice but do not meet the definition of a role model.
Nursing process step: Implementation
Category of client need: Health promotion and maintenance
Cognitive level: Application
Learning outcome 12-1: Describe techniques for client/family teaching.
Test-taking tip: Look for answers that provide a reasonable response to the definition described in the question.

3. Which of the following is a primary prevention activity?
1. Hearing test for the preschool child
2. Applying dental sealants to teeth
3. Testing a newborn for sickle cell disease
4. Dietary teaching for a child just diagnosed with diabetes mellitus

Answer: 2
Rationale: Primary prevention involves preventing problems from occurring, such as providing sealants to prevent cavities. Hearing testing of a preschool child and newborn testing for sickle cell disease are secondary prevention activities, and dietary teaching for a diabetic is a tertiary prevention activity.
Nursing process step: Intervention
Category of client need: Health promotion and maintenance
Cognitive level: Analysis
Learning outcome 12-2: Describe illness prevention activities.
Test-taking tip: When one choice is very different from the others, it is likely that the different choice is the correct answer.

4. Checking each child in a classroom for head lice is an example of:
1. Primary prevention.
2. Secondary prevention.
3. Tertiary prevention.
4. Health promotion.

Answer: 2
Rationale: Secondary prevention activities include those activities that involve early detection of problems, so a classroom screening for head lice would be a secondary prevention activity. Primary prevention is preventing an occurrence. Tertiary prevention is rehabilitation, and health promotion does not involve an infestation like a lice outbreak.
Nursing process step: Intervention
Category of client need: Health promotion and maintenance
Cognitive level: Analysis
Learning outcome 12-2: Describe illness prevention activities.
Test-taking tip: Look for choices that provide the best choice related to the definition of the key terms.

5. Tertiary prevention activities would include:
1. Rubella and varicella immunizations.
2. Lead and vision screenings.

Answer: 4
Rationale: Tertiary prevention involves restoration of maximum functioning, such as rehabilitation after a leg fracture. Prevention of motor vehicle injuries would be primary prevention, and immunizations and screenings are secondary prevention activities.

3. Wearing a seat belt and using infant car seats. 4. Range of motion exercises after a leg fracture.	Nursing process step: Intervention Category of client need: Health promotion and maintenance Cognitive level: Analysis Learning outcome 12-2: Describe illness prevention activities. Test-taking tip: Look for choices that provide the best choice related to the definition of the key terms.
6. The child who learns to eat a healthy diet, exercise regularly, and limit alcohol consumption is practicing: 1. Health promotion. 2. Environmental safety. 3. Self-discipline. 4. Self-regulation.	Answer: 1 Rationale: Health promotion activities are those that maximize functioning, such as healthy eating, exercise, and limiting alcohol and tobacco use. None of the activities listed are related to environmental safety, self-discipline, or self-regulation. Nursing process step: Intervention Category of client need: Health promotion and maintenance Cognitive level: Application Learning outcome 12-3: Describe health promotion activities for children in each age group. Test-taking tip: By learning the definition of terms, you can eliminate some choices and pick the correct choice.
7. A client's immunization might be delayed if (*select all that apply*): 1. The client is currently taking antibiotics. 2. The client had a serious reaction to a previous immunization. 3. The client has a temperature of 101° F. 4. The client might be pregnant. 5. The client has been exposed to an infectious disease.	Answer: 2, 3, 4 Rationale: All reactions to immunizations should be investigated and, if the reaction was serious, then the immunization may need to be deferred or delayed. A client who has a temperature of 101°F should delay immunizations until they are well, and some immunizations should be withheld during pregnancy. The other choices are not reasons to defer or delay an immunization. Nursing process step: Intervention Category of client need: Health promotion and maintenance Cognitive level: Application Learning outcome 12-2: Describe illness prevention activities. Test-taking tip: Look for choices that might affect the immune response or place the client at risk should the activity occur.
8. Proper preparation and administration of immunizations requires the nurse to: 1. Obtain school immunization records to avoid overdose of vaccines. 2. Provide parents with a copy of the National Childhood Vaccine Injury Act. 3. Record the vaccine lot number and site of administration. 4. Notify the local health department of vaccine administration.	Answer: 3 Rationale: Documentation is one of the rights of medication administration, so record keeping regarding immunizations is a priority. It is not possible to overdose on vaccines. The parents should receive an immunization information sheet and sign an informed consent but would not routinely receive a copy of the National Childhood Vaccine Injury Act. It is not mandatory to notify the local health department about vaccine administration. Nursing process step: Intervention Category of client need: Safe, effective care environment Cognitive level: Analysis Learning outcome 12-2: Describe illness prevention activities. Test-taking tip: Always look for interventions that follow the safe administration of medications.
9. An acceptable form of discipline for a toddler would include: 1. Canceling social activities. 2. Spanking. 3. A "timeout" period. 4. Restricting television watching.	Answer: 3 Rationale: Toddlers should be placed in an area free from distractions and their activity limited while they think about their actions. Toddlers need immediate reinforcement for their negative behavior and canceling social activities would delay the consequences; thus the toddler may not relate the negative behavior to the loss of activities. Spanking is controversial, with most experts agreeing that other methods should be tried first. Restricting television watching is a form of discipline more appropriate for school-age children. Nursing process step: Implementation Category of client need: Health promotion and maintenance Cognitive level: Application Learning outcome 12-3: Describe health promotion activities for children in each age group. Test-taking tip: Look for choices that are age appropriate when dealing with a pediatric population.

10. Teaching a parent correct preparation and use of infant formula should include: 1. Formula should be used for 12 months, then a gradual switch to cow's milk. 2. Formula should always be prepared with boiled or sterile water, then placed in sterilized bottles. 3. Heating a bottle in the microwave should occur in 30-second increments and the bottle stirred between heatings. 4. Formula left over after a feeding should be frozen or discarded. Frozen formula may be kept for up to 6 months.	Answer: 1 Rationale: Delaying the introduction of cow's milk until after 12 months of age has been shown to decrease the development of allergies. It is not necessary to sterilize water or bottles for infants. Bottles should never be heated in the microwave, since they may heat unevenly. Formula should be discarded if exposed to bacteria in the infants mouth but does not need to be frozen. Nursing process step: Intervention Category of client need: Health promotion and maintenance Cognitive level: Application Learning outcome 12-4: Discuss important aspects of nutrition for each age group. Test-taking tip: Always consider client safety; the correct answer is often the most conservative and safest.
11. A good choice for a finger food for a toddler would be (*select all that apply*): 1. Raisins. 2. Grapes. 3. Hot dog slices. 4. Peanuts. 5. Cheerios.	Answer: 1, 5 Rationale: Raisins and Cheerios are safe choices for toddlers. Grapes, hot dog slices, and peanuts could cause a toddler to choke and should be avoided. Nursing process step: Intervention Category of client need: Health promotion and maintenance Cognitive level: Application Learning outcome 12-4: Discuss important aspects of nutrition for each age group. Test-taking tip: Normal growth and development parameters are guidelines for nursing assessment and teaching.
12. A child weighs 32 pounds. Teaching the parents about car seat safety for this child should include: 1. Recline the car seat in the front facing position for 45 degrees or less. 2. Always place the car seat in the rear seat of the vehicle. 3. Move the child to a larger seat when the top of the head is 2 inches below the car seat top. 4. If the child falls asleep, the child may be secured by a lap belt to prevent neck injuries.	Answer: 2 Rationale: The car seat should always be placed in the rear seat of the vehicle. If the car seat faces forward, it should be upright and not inclined to 45 degrees. The car seat should be replaced when the child's head is at the top of the car seat. Even though the child is asleep, they should remain in the car seat. Nursing process step: Intervention Category of client need: Health promotion and maintenance Cognitive level: Application Learning outcome 12-3: Describe health promotion activities for children in each age group. Test-taking tip: Always consider client safety; the correct answer is often the most conservative and safest.
13. Preschool children will learn to get along with others by engaging in play activities that include: 1. Exploring the environment alone. 2. Playing alongside other children. 3. Working on projects and learning to share. 4. Organized games and sports.	Answer: 3 Rationale: Preschool children need to begin to socialize and learn to share by working on projects at the same time. Infants explore the environment alone, toddlers participate in parallel play, and school-age children and adolescents socialize with organized sports and games. Nursing process step: Assessment Category of client need: Health promotion and maintenance Cognitive level: Application Learning outcome 12-3: Describe health promotion activities for children in each age group. Test-taking tip: Look for age appropriate behaviors when asked about growth and development.
14. Which of the following behaviors indicates a readiness for toilet training? 1. The child can lift the toilet lid and look inside 2. The child can tell the caregiver that they have soiled their diaper	Answer: 2 Rationale: Awareness of bodily functions is necessary before toilet training can begin. Physical and verbal skills are not as important as the recognition of urges and responses. Nursing process step: Assessment Category of client need: Health promotion and maintenance Cognitive level: Application

3. The child can sit without support on the toilet 4. The child can say the family words for urination and defecation	Learning outcome 12-3: Describe health promotion activities for children in each age group. Test-taking tip: Look for age-appropriate behaviors when asked about growth and development.
15. The nurse whose role is to teach parents about child care issues should be aware that auditory learners will learn best by: 1. Reading prepared materials. 2. Discussing the content after it is presented. 3. Physically manipulating any tools or equipment. 4. Games and role-playing activities.	Answer: 2 Rationale: Auditory learners prefer to listen and verbalize the content to fully integrate the new knowledge into their understanding. Visual learners benefit from reading prepared materials, and kinesthetic learners learn by using their hands and through touch. An accommodator is a flexible learner and will learn through games and role-playing. Nursing process step: Evaluation Category of client need: Health promotion and maintenance Cognitive level: Analysis Learning outcome 12-1: Describe techniques for client/family teaching. Test-taking tip: Look for clues to the correct answer in the definition of terms.

CHAPTER 13

1. When conducting physical assessment of a 3-year-old, the nurse performs this physical assessment: 1. In head to toe order. 2. By listening to heart and lungs last. 3. By moving from the least invasive to the most invasive. 4. By removing the child from the parent's lap and laying the child on the examination table.	Answer: 3 Rationale: Unlike adults, the assessment of the child is not usually done in a head to toe manner. It is easiest to listen to heart and lungs when the child is quiet, so it may be easier to do that part of the exam first. Looking in the child's ears may make the child cry, so it would be best to examine the child's ears last. Much of the assessment can be done while the child is sitting in the parent's lap. Nursing process step: Planning Category of client need: Safe, effective care environment Cognitive level: Application Learning outcome 13-3: Identify specific adaptations for selected procedures in the care of children. Test-taking tip: The student must be familiar with the growth and development of the child to determine the order for assessment.
2. Body mass index (BMI): 1. Is not useful in children. 2. Determines an infant's risk for obesity. 3. Does not need to be age or gender specific. 4. Can be used to determine a child's risk of obesity.	Answer: 4 Rationale: BMI can be used in children age 2 years through adolescence. It is age specific, and gives an indication of whether a child is underweight, overweight, or at risk for being overweight. Body fat changes as children grow and also changes according to gender. Nursing process step: Assessment Category of client need: Health promotion and maintenance Cognitive level: Application Learning outcome 13-1: Define key terms. Test-taking tip: Knowledge of body mass index and the relationship to children and gender is necessary to correctly answer this question.
3. A nurse is assessing an 18-month-old female for a well-child check-up at the pediatrician's office. The weight of this child is 25 pounds, length is 32 inches, head circumference is 18.5 inches, and chest circumference is 18.75 inches. At this age, the nurse recognizes this chest circumference is: 1. Normal. 2. Too large. 3. Too small. 4. Not pertinent information at this age.	Answer: 1 Rationale: Head circumference is equal to or 2 cm greater than chest circumference until the age of 2. Nursing process step: Implementation Category of client need: Physiological integrity Cognitive level: Application Learning outcome 13-3: Identify specific adaptations for selected procedures in the care of children. Test-taking tip: Recognize normal growth patterns for children.
4. Following a cleft lip and palate reconstructive surgery on a 2-year-old, the nurse recognizes which of the following restraints may be necessary	Answer: 1 Rationale: Sleeve restraints will keep a young child from bending his or her arms. This is useful to prevent the child from playing with tubes, dressing, and incisions of the arms, head, and chest. Mummy and papoose restraints restrict total body

to prevent the child from pulling at the suture lines:
1. Sleeve restraints.
2. Mummy restraints.
3. Papoose restraints.
4. Should not need restraints if parents are with the child.

movement. Even if parents are present, the child still can reach suture lines before a parent can stop them.
Nursing process step: Implementation
Category of client need: Safe, effective care environment
Cognitive level: Application
Learning outcome 13-3: Identify specific adaptations for selected procedures in the care of children.
Test-taking tip: Understanding normal growth and development and postoperative care of a small child will help the student choose the correct answer.

---

5. A 6-year-old with a history of cerebral palsy has had a tracheostomy since he was a toddler. This child has been admitted to the pediatric floor with a diagnosis of pneumonia. The nurse knows when suctioning this tracheostomy tube he or she must:
1. Apply suction for no more than 15 seconds.
2. Use clean gloves when suctioning the client.
3. Advance the suction catheter 0.5 cm beyond the end of the tracheostomy tube opening.
4. Insert the suction catheter until resistance is met before withdrawing the catheter.

Answer: 3
Rationale: The suction catheter should be inserted no more than 0.5 cm below the opening of the trach. The maximum amount of time for suction to be applied is 5–10 seconds at any given time. Suctioning a tracheostomy tube is a sterile procedure.
Nursing process step: Implementation
Category of client need: Safe, effective care environment
Cognitive level: Application
Learning outcome 13-2: Describe why procedures need to be adapted in the care of children.
Test-taking tip: The correct response for this question is the one that denotes the safest care for the client.

---

6. When placing a small child in a mist tent, the nurse should:
1. Monitor the child closely for hyperthermia due to the warm air inside the tent.
2. Monitor the child for hypothermia due to the cool air inside the tent.
3. Leave the tent open for periods of time while the child has family visitors.
4. Be careful not to tuck the edges of the mist tent under the child's mattress.

Answer: 2
Rationale: The cool humidity inside the tent causes condensation on everything inside the tent. This cool, moist air can cause the child to chill. The edges of the tent must be secured to deliver the prescribed amount of oxygen and prevent escape of oxygen.
Nursing process step: Planning
Category of client need: Physiological integrity
Cognitive level: Application
Learning outcome 13-4: Discuss the role of the LPN/LVN in adapting procedures in the care of children.
Test-taking tip: Knowledge of oxygen devices is needed for this question.

---

7. When administering otic medications to a 6-year-old, the nurse should:
1. Pull the pinna down and back.
2. Pull the pinna up and back.
3. Instill without moving the pinna.
4. Place the dropper in the ear canal to instill the proper amount of solution.

Answer: 2
Rationale: When administering ear drops to a child over 3 year of age, the pinna is pulled up and back. In a child younger than 3, the pinna should be pulled down and back. Hold the ear dropper above the ear to instill the prescribed number of drops, so the dropper is not contaminated by touching the ear.
Nursing process step: Implementation
Category of client need: Physiological integrity
Cognitive level: Application
Learning outcome 13-4: Discuss the role of the LPN/LVN in adapting procedures in the care of children.
Test-taking tip: Knowing proper medication administration is vital for safe care of the child.

---

8. A 9-month-old is seen in the physician's office and is diagnosed with a urinary tract infection. The mother asks the physician to give the child an injection of antibiotic instead of an oral antibiotic. When giving an IM injection to this child, the nurse knows:
1. The ventrogluteal muscle is the preferred site.

Answer: 2
Rationale: Intramuscular injections are given to the infant in the vastus lateralis muscle. Once the child has walked for at least one year, injections can be given in the ventrogluteal muscle, though the preferred site remains the vastus lateralis. The deltoid is not used for antibiotic injections. Antibiotics are given to infants via the intramuscular route.
Nursing process step: Planning
Category of client need: Physiological integrity

---

2. The vastus lateralis muscle is the preferred site.
3. Intramuscular antibiotics are not given to children under 1 year old.
4. The deltoid muscle is the preferred site.

Cognitive level: Application
Learning outcome 13-3: Identify specific adaptations for selected procedures in the care of children.
Test-taking tip: Knowledge of safe medication administration is vital in the care of children.

---

9. In establishing a relationship with a child in the hospital, the nurse needs to:
1. Not be concerned with her own body language.
2. Always maintain a nurse-focused relationship with child.
3. Have an understanding of the child's growth and development, height, and weight.
4. Recognize that the child's vocabulary, psychomotor abilities, and emotional state will have an impact on what the child is able to hear or understand.

Answer: 4
Rationale: When communicating with a child, a nurse should speak to the child in language and terms the child can understand. Developmental levels influence how a child learns, but height and weight do not impact the child's ability to form a relationship. The nurse must be very aware of his or her body language when communicating with a child. Nonverbal communication conveys more than 80% of our message. The relationship must be client-focused, not nurse-focused.
Nursing process step: Planning
Category of client need: Psychosocial integrity
Cognitive level: Analysis
Learning outcome 13-4: Discuss the role of the LPN/LVN in adapting procedures in the care of children.
Test-taking tip: The answer that is most inclusive of a child's needs is the correct answer.

---

10. The physician has ordered a nasogastric feeding tube insertion for a 3-year-old child who has not been eating while in the hospital. Number the following steps in the correct order for safe insertion of a nasogastric tube for this client:
1. Apply lubricant to the tip of the catheter.
2. Aspirate a small amount of gastric content.
3. Place the child in semi-Fowler's position.
4. Test the pH of the gastric contents using litmus paper.
5. Measure the tube from the tip of the nose to the tragus of the ear to the xiphoid process.
   1. 1, 3, 5, 2, 4
   2. 3, 5, 1, 2, 4
   3. 3, 5, 2, 4, 1
   4. 1, 3, 1, 2, 4

Answer: 2
The correct order in this procedure is: Place the child in a semi-Fowler's position. This utilizes gravity when inserting the tube and helps minimize aspiration of fluid. Measure the nasogastric tube from the tip of the child's nose to the tragus of the ear, then to the xiphoid process. This determines the length of the nasogastric tube to be inserted. Apply lubricant to tip of the tube for easier insertion. Aspirate a small amount of gastric content. Test the pH of the gastric contents using litmus paper. A pH of 3 or less indicates gastric contents and therefore proper placement.
Nursing process step: Planning
Category of client need: Physiological integrity
Cognitive level: Application
Learning outcome 13-4: Discuss the role of the LPN/LVN in adapting procedures in the care of children.
Test-taking tip: Knowledge of correct procedures in a child is necessary for safe client care.

---

11. The physician has ordered Tylenol (acetaminophen) for a 14-kg client. The safe therapeutic dose range of Tylenol is 10–15 mg/kg. The nurse knows a safe, therapeutic dose for this client is:
1. 180 mg.
2. 120 mg.
3. 240 mg.
4. 360 mg.

Answer: 1
Rationale: The safe dose range is 10 mg $\times$ 14 kg = 140 mg and 15 mg $\times$ 14 kg = 210 mg. The only dose listed that falls between these two numbers is 180 mg. The dose of 120 mg is too low to be therapeutic. The 240 mg and 360 mg doses are too high.
Nursing process step: Implementation
Category of client need: Safe, effective care environment
Cognitive level: Analysis
Learning outcome 13-3: Identify specific adaptations for selected procedures in the care of children.
Test-taking tip: Knowledge of safe medication administration is vital for the safety of the child.

---

12. When performing an assessment of a pediatric client receiving intravenous therapy, what must be included? *Select all that apply.*
1. The rate of infusion.

Answer: 1, 3, 4
Rationale: The rate of infusion is how much fluid the child is actually receiving, usually ordered by the hour. The condition of the IV site is important to note, for if the IV is infiltrated, the client may have damage to tissues and is not getting the prescribed amount of fluid, and client care is compromised. The client's intake

---

2. The size of the intravenous bag.
3. The condition of the intravenous site.
4. Intake and output of the client.

and output allow the nurse to keep track of what the client is actually taking in compared to what the child is excreting. The size of the intravenous bag will not directly affect the fluid status of the client.
Nursing process step: Evaluation
Category of client need: Safe, effective care environment
Cognitive level: Analysis
Learning outcome 13-4: Discuss the role of the LPN/LVN in adapting procedures in the care of children.
Test-taking tip: Recognize safe intravenous infusion principles in the child.

13. A 4-year-old child is postoperative after a tonsillectomy. He is crying and wanting his mother to hold him. In assessing this child's behavior, the nurse knows that:
1. Children do not experience the same amount of pain as an adult.
2. Nonpharmacological measures are not helpful in small children.
3. Pain can be expressed in young children by crying and regressive behavior.
4. The child is overreacting to the operative experience and will calm done once left alone with his family.

Answer: 3
Rationale: Pain in the toddler can be expressed by crying and aggressive or regressive behavior. Studies show children do experience pain similar to an adult. Nonpharmacological measures, such as distraction, positioning, and soothing music, complement pain relief methods. The child's pain must be addressed before leaving the child alone with his parents.
Nursing process step: Assessment
Category of client need: Physiological integrity
Cognitive level: Analysis
Learning outcome 13-3: Identify specific adaptations for selected procedures in the care of children.
Test-taking tip: Recognize the symptoms of pain in a child.

14. The nurse recognizes the following as important in the art of communication with children (*select all that apply*):
1. Displaying empathy.
2. Never saying, "I don't know."
3. Speaking with enthusiasm and energy.
4. Changing the subject when a child starts to talk about toys or cartoons.

Answer: 1, 3
Rationale: Displaying empathy includes recognizing the child's needs and acknowledging the child is real. Speaking with energy and enthusiasm allows the nurse to communicate a message effectively. The nurse should not be afraid to say, "I don't know," for it is imperative to be honest with a child. Children can see through dishonesty. The nurse must listen attentively to what the child says, even if the child is talking about cartoons or toys.
Nursing process step: Implementation
Category of client need: Psychosocial
Cognitive level: Analysis
Learning outcome 13-2: Describe why procedures need to be adapted in the care of children.
Test-taking tip: Recognizing the most effective means of communication with children will enhance nurse-client relationships.

15. A 15-year-old who is hospitalized after a motor vehicle accident is admitted to the pediatric floor. Which of the following vital signs would the nurse want to report to the charge nurse or physician?
1. P 58, R 18, BP 110/74
2. P 90, R 15, BP 122/84
3. P 50, R 20, BP 108/70
4. P 50, R 16, BP 88/48

Answer: 4
Rationale: Normal vital signs for a 15-year-old are: P 50–90, R 15–20, and BP 120/80. A blood pressure of 88/48 falls out of this range.
Nursing process step: Evaluation
Category of client need: Physiological integrity
Cognitive level: Analysis
Learning outcome 13-3: Identify specific adaptations for selected procedures in the care of children.
Test-taking tip: Recognize normal range of vital signs for the child.

CHAPTER 14

1. A 6-year-old has had a tonsillectomy at an outpatient center. The mother asks the nurse, "What do I need to do for my child at home?" The discharge instructions provided to the mother should include (*select all that apply*):
1. Nutrition and fluids.
2. Medications.

Answer: 1, 2, 3, 4
Rationale: It is important for the nurse to make sure the mother understands the importance of nutrition, fluids, medications, possible complications, and when the child can resume normal activity.
Nursing process step: Planning
Category of client need: Physiological integrity
Cognitive level: Analysis

3. Symptoms of complications. 4. When the child can return to school.	Learning outcome 14-7: Describe the role of the LPN/LVN in caring for children with acute or chronic disorders. Test-taking tip: Recognize expected home care for a child after outpatient surgery.
2. Some pediatric units have child life specialists. The role of these professionals is to: 1. Give nursing care in a playful way. 2. Talk with parents about pediatric life issues. 3. Play with siblings while the child is in the treatment room for a procedure. 4. Utilize distraction and give praise while the nurse starts a 2-year-old's intravenous line.	Answer: 4 Rationale: The child life specialist is trained to utilize age-appropriate activities and distractions to help the child work through their feelings about hospitalization. In this case, the child life specialist makes an invasive procedure a little less threatening. Child life specialists are not nurses and do not do nursing care. Though they may talk with parents about the child's hospitalization, they do not address life and death issues. It is possible they could be utilized to watch siblings, though this is not the main purpose and role for child life specialists. Nursing process step: Implementation Category of client need: Psychosocial integrity Cognitive level: Application Learning outcome 14-2: Describe how to prepare children for hospitalization. Test-taking tip: Recognize the role of other specialists on the pediatric healthcare team.

3. An 8-month-old is admitted to the hospital. The parents must leave to care for other children at home. If this child experiences separation anxiety, the child will most likely experience which stages of separation (*select the appropriate responses and put in order of occurrence*):
1. Despair stage.
2. Protest stage.
3. Forgiveness stage.
4. Detachment stage.
    1. 1, 2, 3
    2. 2, 1, 3
    3. 2, 1, 4
    4. 2, 4, 1
	Answer: 3
	Rationale: The child first experiences the protest stage, which leads to the despair stage; the third stage is the detachment stage. Forgiveness is not one of the stages.
	Nursing process step: Assessment
	Category of client need: Psychosocial integrity
	Cognitive level: Analysis
	Learning outcome 14-3: Describe how to prepare parents for their child's hospitalization.
	Test-taking tip: Recognize normal growth and development in children. Note the plural stages.

4. A preoperative x-ray has been ordered for a 2-year-old client. Considering the developmental age and safety of the client, which of the following is the best mode of transportation to the procedure area? 1. In the nurse's arms. 2. In a crib with side rails up. 3. On a stretcher with side rails up. 4. In a wheelchair with the strap fastened.	Answer: 2 Rationale: The safest way to transport a small child is in a crib with the side rails all the way up. The side rails on a stretcher are not designed to hold small children, and the bars are too far apart. The strap in the wheelchair would be too big to secure a child safely. The nurse could potentially drop the child, or stumble while carrying the child, so that is not a safe way to transport a small child. Nursing process step: Planning Category of client need: Safe, effective care environment Cognitive level: Application Learning outcome 14-4: Describe the preoperative and postoperative care of children. Test-taking tip: Choose the answer that is safest for the child.
5. EMLA cream is often used in children prior to a painful procedure. In administering EMLA before starting an intravenous, the nurse knows the time involved to numb the targeted site is: 1. 15–30 minutes. 2. 30–45 minutes. 3. 45–60 minutes. 4. 60–90 minutes.	Answer: 3 Rationale: It takes 45–60 minutes for EMLA cream to anesthetize the skin to start an IV. If it is for an intramuscular injection, it may take more time. This is an example of atraumatic care. Nursing process step: Implementation Category of client need: Safe, effective care environment Cognitive level: Application Learning outcome 14-2: Describe how to prepare children for hospitalization. Test-taking tip: Recognize atraumatic care in children.

6. One of the most important means of assuring client safety while undergoing a procedure under conscious sedation is:
1. Having a nurse at the bedside.
2. Keeping an emergency cart close by.
3. Placing an artificial airway in the child.
4. Taking the client's vital signs every 20 minutes.

Answer: 2
Rationale: The safest care for a child under conscious sedation is to have the code cart close by in case the child becomes so sedated an airway is needed. The nurse at the bedside is certainly important also. The vital signs need to be monitored more often than every 20 minutes. A child under conscious sedation usually would not tolerate an artificial airway because the child is not sedated deeply enough.
Nursing process step: Planning
Category of client need: Physiological integrity
Cognitive level: Application
Learning outcome 14-4: Describe the preoperative and postoperative care of children.
Test-taking tip: Choose the safest answer for the child.

7. A 7-year-old sickle cell client has been admitted to the hospital in sickle cell crisis. When should the preparation for discharging this child from the hospital begin?
1. Admission
2. Day before discharge
3. 24 hours after admission
4. As soon as the physician writes the discharge order

Answer: 1
Rationale: Preparation for discharge needs to begin at admission of the child to the hospital.
Nursing process step: Planning
Category of client need: Safe, effective care environment
Cognitive level: Application
Learning outcome 14-5: Describe how to prepare parents and children for discharge.
Test-taking tip: Recognize the importance of discharge instructions in a hospitalized child.

8. Hospitalization of a child is very disruptive to the whole family system. The most appropriate nursing diagnosis for the hospitalized child is:
1. Ineffectual coping related to fatigue.
2. Interrupted family processes related to shift of health status of family member.
3. Sleep pattern disturbances related to hospitalized child.
4. Fear related to hospitalization.

Answer: 4
Rationale: The only nursing diagnosis related specifically to the child is fear. The rest of the diagnoses are more related to the family situation.
Nursing process step: Evaluation
Category of client need: Health promotion and maintenance
Cognitive level: Application
Learning outcome 14-7: Describe the role of the LPN/LVN in caring for children with acute or chronic disorders.
Test-taking tip: Read the question carefully and note to whom the question is referring.

9. The physician has written an order for a 2-month-old hospitalized infant to receive ampicillin (Marcillin), 180 mg every 6 hours intravenously. The nurse must prepare this solution for injection. The vial has 250 mg in 2 mL once the diluent has been added. The correct amount of ampicillin the nurse should prepare is:
1. 1.4 mL.
2. 0.8 mL.
3. 1.8 mL.
4. 2.4 mL.

Answer: 1
Rationale: The formula for calculating a drug dose is to divide the dose ordered by the dose on hand, times the quantity: 180 mg/250 mg = 0.72 × 2 = 1.44 mL
Nursing process step: Implementation
Category of client need: Physiological integrity
Cognitive level: Application
Learning outcome 14-7: Describe the role of the LPN/LVN in caring for children with acute or chronic disorders.
Test-taking tip: Know the formula for calculating drug doses in children.

10. When developing a plan of care for a 3-year-old who has had abdominal surgery, the nurse knows fluids by mouth are usually resumed:
1. Immediately.
2. Once pain is under control.
3. Once bowel sounds are present.
4. Once the child has had a bowel movement.

Answer: 3
Rationale: Once bowel sounds have returned, the physician usually writes an order for the nurse to start clear liquids.
Nursing process step: Planning
Category of client need: Physiological integrity
Cognitive level: Application
Learning outcome 14-4: Describe the preoperative and postoperative care of children.
Test-taking tip: Recognize expectations of routine postoperative care.

11. A 3-year-old with sickle cell anemia is admitted to the hospital with a respiratory illness. This child would be considered to have a/an:
1. Congenital condition.
2. Hereditary condition.
3. Condition of mental retardation.
4. Acute condition.

Answer: 2
Rationale: Sickle cell anemia is a hereditary condition because it is caused from a genetic inheritance from the parents.
Nursing process step: Evaluation.
Category of client need: Physiological integrity
Cognitive level: Analysis
Learning outcome 14-1: Define key terms.
Test-taking tip: Recognize key terms.

12. An individualized education plan (IEP) has been received at the elementary school for a new child entering the second grade. The nurse knows this plan:
1. Is the same for all students.
2. Is an interdisciplinary plan that is aimed at the special needs of a particular student.
3. Lets the school know which buses a particular child will ride.
4. Lets the school know the particular classes and experiences this child has had at the last school.

Answer: 2
Rationale: An IEP is an interdisciplinary plan that pinpoints the special education needs of a particular student.
Nursing process step: Planning
Category of client need: Health promotion and maintenance
Cognitive level: Application
Learning outcome 14-6: Describe the important aspects of care for the chronically ill child and the family.
Test-taking tip: Know possible adaptations needed for a child.

13. A 5-year-old has been returned to her room after a tonsillectomy. The child's vital signs were HR 68, RR 18, and BP 98/54 preoperatively. The nurse would expect her vital signs postoperatively to be:
1. Similar to the preoperative vital signs.
2. Higher than the preoperative vital signs.
3. Lower than the preoperative vital signs.
4. Preoperative and postoperative vital signs can vary and have no relation to each other.

Answer: 1
Rationale: The postoperative vital signs should be in the range of the preoperative vital signs. The preoperative vital signs are a guide for what the nurse should expect postoperatively.
Nursing process step: Evaluation
Category of client need: Safe effective care environment
Cognitive level: Analysis
Learning outcome 14-4: Describe the preoperative and postoperative care of children.
Test-taking tip: Recognize appropriate care of the postoperative client.

14. A 2-year-old is hospitalized with a severe respiratory infection. This child is not taking fluids by mouth, so the physician orders an intravenous (IV) line to be inserted by the nurse. The nurse realizes it will be less traumatic to start the child's IV in which of the following locations?
1. The playroom.
2. The treatment room.
3. The client's bed.
4. The client's room, but not in the bed.

Answer: 2
Rationale: Overall, the least traumatic place to have the IV started for the child is the treatment room; then the child will not associate his room or bed with painful procedures. Nothing painful should ever happen to the child in the playroom. This must always be a safe place for the child.
Nursing process step: Planning
Category of client need: Safe, effective care environment
Cognitive level: Analysis
Learning outcome 14-7: Describe the role of the LPN/LVN in caring for children with acute or chronic disorders.
Test-taking tip: Setting priorities to lessen a child's fears.

15. A 16-year-old has been transferred to a rehabilitation hospital after a hospitalization for a serious head injury. The purpose of this transfer is to (*select all that apply*):
1. Help the adolescent regain independence.
2. Transition the adolescent from hospital to home.
3. Give the family time off from care of this adolescent.
4. Help the adolescent and family adjust to new care and routines.

Answer: 1, 2, 4
Rationale: The rehabilitation center would help the teenager adapt to new circumstances, help him regain independence, allow the family to adjust to new routines, and be a transition form the intense care of the hospital to the more limited care at home. Clients are not admitted to rehabilitation hospitals to give parents a rest.
Nursing process step: Evaluation
Category of client need: Health promotion and maintenance
Cognitive level: Application
Learning outcome 14-8: Discuss how to care for children in the home or in long-term care settings.
Test-taking tip: Know resources available to children and families outside of the hospital.

1. A newborn is admitted to the hospital after having 12 diarrhea stools a day. The physician is concerned about fluid balance in this baby because:
1. 45% of a newborn's weight is water.
2. 55% of a newborn's weight is water.
3. 65% of a newborn's weight is water.
4. 75% of a newborn's weight is water.

Answer: 4
Rationale: Seventy-five percent of a newborn's weight is water.
Nursing process step: Assessment
Category of client need: Health promotion and maintenance
Cognitive level: Application
Learning outcome 15-1: Discuss fluid and electrolyte balance in children.
Test-taking tip: Recognize what is normal for a newborn.

2. In the child, homeostasis is the goal to maintain health and well-being. Homeostasis is influenced by (*select all that apply*):
1. Osmosis.
2. Fluid output.
3. Active transport.
4. Hormonal regulation.

Answer: 1, 2, 3, 4
Rationale: Osmosis and active transport are part of the process of the movement of fluids and electrolytes, which affects homeostasis. Homeostasis is also affected by fluid output and hormonal regulation.
Nursing process step: Evaluation
Category of client need: Physiological integrity
Cognitive level: Application
Learning outcome 15-1: Discuss fluid and electrolyte balance in children.
Test-taking tip: Know key terms in relation to fluid balance in children.

3. A 6-month-old has been admitted with gastroenteritis. The most accurate means of monitoring the baby's fluid balance is through:
1. Daily weights.
2. Weighing diapers.
3. Monitoring CBC labs.
4. Monitoring electrolyte counts.

Answer: 1
Rationale: Daily weights are the most accurate way to monitor fluid balance. Weighing diapers is a good way to measure output, but parents might forget and throw diapers away, so that particular output would not be counted. Lab studies may give some indication of fluid status, but do not give the most information.
Nursing process step: Implementation
Category of client need: Physiological integrity
Cognitive level: Application
Learning outcome 15-1: Discuss fluid and electrolyte balance in children.
Test-taking tip: Sometimes the simplest answer is the correct one.

4. A 2-year-old with a fever is admitted to the hospital for pneumonia. The child is not taking in fluids by mouth, so the physician orders intravenous (IV) fluids to be given. This child weighs 16 kg. The amount of fluid this child should receive per hour is:
1. 35 mL/hour.
2. 48 mL/hour.
3. 54 mL/hour.
4. 62 mL/hour.

Answer: 3
Rationale: A 16 kg child should receive 1,000 mL plus 50 mL/kg for each kg over 10. The formula for this child is: $1,000 + 300 (50 \text{ mL} \times 16 \text{ kg} = 300 \text{ mL}) = 1300 \text{ mL/day}$. To figure out the hourly amount, divide 1,300 by 24 hours, which equals 54 mL/hour.
Nursing process step: Evaluation
Category of client need: Physiological integrity
Cognitive level: Analysis
Learning outcome 15-4: Describe appropriate assessment and interventions related to fluid and electrolyte and acid-base imbalances.
Test-taking tip: Know the formula for calculating daily fluid requirements for children.

5. A newly diagnosed type I diabetic child is admitted to the pediatric intensive care unit with a blood sugar of 823. This has led to dehydration. The nurse knows this type of dehydration is caused by:
1. More sodium is lost than fluid.
2. More fluid is lost than sodium.
3. More fluid than potassium is lost.
4. More potassium than fluid is lost.

Answer: 2
Rationale: Hypertonic dehydration is caused when more fluid is lost than sodium; it is seen in diabetes, in which an excess of salt is left in the body. When more sodium is lost than fluid, it is called hypotonic dehydration, as seen in burns and renal disease. If an equal amount of fluid and sodium is lost, it is isotonic dehydration. Potassium is not directly related to dehydration.
Nursing process step: Evaluation
Category of client need: Physiological integrity
Cognitive level: Analysis
Learning outcome 15-3: Identify alterations in fluid and electrolyte and acid-balance in children.
Test-taking tip: Recognize it is fluid and sodium that causes the shift in dehydration.

6. A hospitalized 5-year-old, who has just returned from surgery, is restless, has a blood pressure of 72/40, heart rate of 110, respiratory rate of 29, and a capillary

Answer: 3
Rationale: Symptoms of impending shock are rapid pulse, decreased blood pressure, capillary refill greater than 3 seconds, and restless behavior. Respiratory rate increases with shallow breaths. Symptoms of fluid overload also include edema, rales in the lung fields.

refill of greater than 3 seconds. In this client, these symptoms may indicate:
1. Hyponatremia.
2. Fluid overload.
3. Impending shock.
4. Respiratory alkalosis.

Nursing process step: Assessment
Category of client need: Physiological integrity
Cognitive level: Analysis
Learning outcome 15-3: Identify alterations in fluid and electrolyte and acid-base balance in children.
Test-taking tip: Choose the answer that matches all of the symptoms.

---

7. A 9-month-old is seen by the physician due to vomiting for the last 2 days. The physician suspects dehydration. Which of the following laboratory values would confirm this diagnosis?
1. Increased hemoglobin and decreased BUN
2. Decreased hemoglobin and increased BUN
3. Increased creatinine and increased glucose
4. Decreased creatinine and decreased hematocrit

Answer: 3
Rationale: Loss of fluid as seen in dehydration causes concentration of the solutes within the plasma; therefore creatinine and glucose levels are elevated.
Nursing process step: Evaluation
Category of client need: Physiological integrity
Cognitive level: Analysis
Learning outcome 15-1: Discuss fluid and electrolyte balance in children.
Test-taking tip: Know the physiology of dehydration in children.

---

8. The nurse is weighing a 6-month-old client who weighed 17 pounds at the last visit. After repeated episodes of vomiting and diarrhea, the client now weighs 14 pounds. The percentage of weight loss is:
1. 10%.
2. 13%.
3. 15%.
4. 18%.

Answer: 4
Rationale: To figure the percentage of weight loss, subtract 14 from 17, which equals 3. Now divide 3 by the original weight of 17 pounds to find the percentage. $17 - 14 = 3$. $3/17 = 0.176$
Nursing process step: Evaluation
Category of client need: Physiological integrity
Cognitive level: Application
Learning outcome 15-4: Describe appropriate assessment and interventions related to fluid and electrolyte and acid-base imbalances.
Test-taking tip: Know the formula for finding weight loss as a percentage.

---

9. The nurse is teaching the mother of a 2-year-old how to give oral rehydration fluids. This child has mild dehydration, and the physician would like to keep the child out of the hospital. This 2-year-old weighs 12 kg. The amount of oral rehydration for this child is:
1. 100 mL/hr.
2. 125 mL/hr.
3. 150 mL/hr.
4. 175 mL/hr.

Answer: 3
Rationale: To figure the amount to rehydrate a child with mild dehydration, multiply 50 mL $\times$ 12 kg = 600 mL. This should be given over 4 hours, so hourly this child needs 150 mL of oral rehydration solution. This needs to be given in small amounts at a time.
Nursing process step: Evaluation
Category of client need: Health promotion and maintenance
Cognitive level: Analysis
Learning outcome 15-4: Describe appropriate assessment and interventions related to fluid and electrolyte and acid-base imbalances.
Test-taking tip: Know the formula for oral rehydration replacement in children.

---

10. A 6-year-old child has been hospitalized with a diagnosis of pneumonia. This child has been receiving intravenous fluids and antibiotics. The nurse checks the child's vital signs and finds the heart rate is 98 and bounding, respiratory rate is 32, and the client is restless and diaphoretic. His urine specific gravity is 1.000. These symptoms indicate:
1. Dehydration.
2. Hyperkalemia.
3. Hyponatremia.
4. Hypervolemia.

Answer: 4
Rationale: The specific gravity is decreased (normal $1.010-1.030$) and the child is exhibiting symptoms of pulmonary edema and volume overload. The nurse needs to know the symptoms of restlessness, tachypnea, and bounding pulse may be signs of pulmonary edema.
Nursing process step: Assessment
Category of client need: Physiological integrity
Cognitive level: Analysis
Learning outcome 15-3: Identify alterations in fluid and electrolyte and acid-base balance in children.
Test-taking tip: The question does not give any information about electrolyte balance, so those answers can be omitted.

11. The physician has started a 4-year-old on calcium because of a dairy allergy. When providing education to the client's mother, which of the following instructions must be included?
1. Give with milk.
2. Give before meals.
3. Give with orange juice.
4. Give one hour after meals.

Answer: 4
Rationale: Calcium should be given with milk, or 1 hour after meals. Because this child has a milk allergy, it must be given one hour after meals and not with milk.
Nursing process step: Implementation
Category of client need: Safe, effective care environment
Cognitive level: Application
Learning outcome 15-3: Identify alterations in fluid and electrolyte and acid-base balance in children.
Test taking tip: Read the stem carefully and take into consideration all of the information offered.

12. A 17-year-old has been on a ventilator in the intensive care unit after a motor vehicle accident. The last blood gases show this client is in respiratory acidosis. Which of the following blood gas reports confirm respiratory acidosis?
1. pH 7.33, $PaCO_2$ 50, HCO_3 20
2. pH 7.31, $PaCO_2$ 42, HCO_3 22
3. pH 7.49, $PaCO_2$ 43, HCO_3 28
4. pH 7.51, $PaCO_2$ 33, HCO_3 25

Answer: 1
Rationale: Respiratory acidosis is an accumulation of carbon dioxide. As carbon dioxide builds, pH decreases. The pH and $PaCO_2$ values move in opposite directions when the client has a respiratory condition. The pH and HCO_3 values move in the same direction when the client has a metabolic condition.
Nursing process step: Evaluation
Category of client need: Physiological integrity
Cognitive level: Analysis
Learning outcome 15-2: Discuss acid-base balance in children.
Test-taking tip: Know the normal limits of blood gas values will help to select the right answer.

13. A 3-year-old with tetralogy of Fallot takes Lasix (furosemide) to help prevent complications of congestive heart failure. The nurse teaches this mother it is important to offer a diet that will help to counteract the side effects of the diuretic. The nurse helps the mother choose which of the following foods from the menu for this child?
1. Hamburger and peaches
2. Apple slices and spinach
3. Carrots and mashed potatoes
4. Yogurt and whole wheat bread

Answer: 3
Rationale: Potassium can be lost from taking a diuretic. Carrots, potatoes, dairy products, meat, and spinach are high in potassium. The rest of the foods listed are not helpful in counteracting the side effects of a diuretic.
Nursing process step: Implementation
Category of client need: Health promotion and maintenance
Cognitive level: Analysis
Learning outcome 15-4: Describe appropriate assessment and interventions related to fluid and electrolyte and acid-base imbalances.
Test-taking tip: Recognize the side effects of diuretic use.

14. A 14-year-old with anorexia bulimia has been hospitalized due to continued weight loss. The nurse knows anorexic clients often have which one of the following imbalances?
1. Hyponatremia
2. Hypokalemia
3. Hypernatremia
4. Hypercalcemia

Answer: 2
Rationale: Hypokalemia is low potassium and can be related to both anorexia nervosa and bulimia. Potassium is depleted by repeat vomiting, diarrhea, and inappropriate use of diuretics. The other imbalances are not seen in anorexic clients.
Nursing process step: Assessment
Category of client need: Physiological integrity
Cognitive level: Application
Learning outcome 15-4: Describe appropriate assessment and interventions related to fluid and electrolyte and acid-base imbalances.
Test-taking tip: Recognize the pathophysiology in eating disorders.

15. Which of the following symptoms would be found in dehydration of a 20-month-old (*select all that apply*)?
1. Rapid pulse
2. Sunken fontanel
3. Periorbital edema
4. Tenting of skin on abdomen

Answer: 1, 4
Rationale: Rapid, weak pulse and poor skin turgor with tenting on the abdomen are seen in dehydration. A 20-month-old has a closed fontanel. Periorbital edema is seen with fluid overload.
Nursing process step: Assessment
Category of client need: Physiological integrity
Cognitive level: Application
Learning outcome 15-3: Identify alterations in fluid and electrolyte and acid-base balance in children.
Test-taking tip: Recognize the signs of dehydration. Know normal growth and development.

1. A 13-month-old is admitted to the pediatric unit with failure to thrive (FTT). The nurse is taking the child's vital signs and notes the anterior fontanel is open. The nurse knows this fontanel usually closes by:
1. 2 months.
2. 6–12 months.
3. 12–18 months.
4. 18–24 months.

Answer: 4
Rationale: The anterior fontanel closes at 18–24 months of age. The posterior fontanel closes around 2 months.
Nursing process step: Assessment
Category of client need: Health promotion and maintenance
Cognitive level: Application
Learning outcome 16-1: Discuss the anatomy and physiology of the pediatric neurological system.
Test-taking tip: Know the physiology of normal development in an infant and toddler.

2. A nurse is admitting an infant who the parents report fell off of a changing table. The nurse uses the Glasgow coma scale to assess the infant's neurological status. The infant's score is 3. This score indicates:
1. This scale is not useful in infants.
2. Normal neurological function.
3. Neurological unresponsiveness.
4. Infant arouses, but goes back to sleep when not stimulated.

Answer: 3
Rationale: Scoring 3 on the Glasgow coma scale is the lowest possible score and means the infant is totally unresponsive. The Glasgow coma scale is used for infants.
Nursing process step: Assessment
Category of client need: Physiological integrity
Cognitive level: Analysis
Learning outcome 16-6: Discuss clinical manifestations, diagnostic procedures, medical management, and nursing interventions related to neurological trauma.
Test-taking tip: Know the rating scales of the Glasgow coma scale.

3. A newborn is found to have a myelomeningocele at birth. The plan is to take this baby to surgery as soon as possible. In the meantime, the nurse knows the position for this newborn is:
1. Prone.
2. Supine.
3. In a sling.
4. Side-lying.

Answer: 1
Rationale: The newborn must be placed in a prone position to keep pressure off of the myelomeningocele.
Nursing process step: Implementation
Category of client need: Safe, effective care environment
Cognitive level: Application
Learning outcome 16-3: Explain appropriate nursing interventions for children with neurological disorders.
Test-taking tip: Understand the pathology of a myelomeningocele and the safety of an infant with this condition.

4. A 4-year-old 18-kg child is admitted to the pediatric unit postoperatively after a ventriculoperitoneal shunt repair. The child was becoming increasingly lethargic at home and was diagnosed with a shunt blockage. The nurse would question which of the following physician post-op orders?
1. Semi-Fowler position
2. IV solution of D5.45NS at 40 cc/hr
3. Neurological checks every 2 hours
4. Morphine sulfate 0.1–0.2 mg IV every 2 hours as needed for pain

Answer: 1
Rationale: In the immediate postoperative period, the child needs to lie flat to prevent a rapid decrease in cerebral spinal fluid (CSF) drainage. The rest of the physician orders are reasonable for this child.
Nursing process step: Evaluation
Category of client need: Safe, effective care environment
Cognitive level: Analysis
Learning outcome 16-3: Explain appropriate nursing interventions for children with neurological disorders.
Test-taking tip: Understand the principles of CSF fluid and gravity.

5. A 2-year-old with a history of febrile seizures is admitted to the hospital with a febrile illness. The nurse expects the physician will order for this child (*select all that apply*):
1. Frequent vital signs.
2. Seizure precautions.
3. Alcohol compresses.
4. Anticonvulsant therapy.

Answer: 1, 2
Rationale: Frequent vital signs and seizure precautions are appropriate therapy. The American Academy of Pediatrics (AAP) does not recommend long-term anticonvulsant therapy for febrile seizures. Alcohol is no longer used to help bring down a child's fever.
Nursing process step: Implementation
Category of client need: Physiological integrity
Cognitive level: Analysis
Learning outcome 16-2: Describe neurological disorders, including seizures, cerebral palsy, meningitis, spina bifida, hydrocephalus, and Guillain-Barré syndrome.
Test-taking tip: Safety of the client must always be a priority.

6. The nurse is walking by the hospital room of a 5-year-old, and hears the mother yell, "My son is having a seizure." The nurse's first response is to: 1. Restrain the child. 2. Check the child's pupils. 3. Establish a safe environment. 4. Get something in the child's mouth.	Answer: 3 Rationale: The nurse must first make sure the child is safe and that the head and extremities are protected from hitting the floor, side rails, or furniture. A seizing child should never be restrained or have anything placed in their mouth. Pupils will need to be checked after the seizure. Nursing process step: Implementation Category of client need: Safe, effective care environment Cognitive level: Analysis Learning outcome 16-3: Explain appropriate nursing interventions for children with neurological disorders. Test-taking tip: Utilize Maslow's hierarchy.
7. Signs of increased intracranial pressure in a 2-year-old are (*select all that apply*): 1. Vomiting. 2. Irritability. 3. Bulging fontanel. 4. Decreasing level of consciousness.	Answer: 1, 2, 4 Rationale: Vomiting, irritability, and decreasing level of consciousness all can be present with increased intracranial pressure. The fontanels in a 2-year-old are closed. Nursing process step: Evaluation Category of client need: Physiological integrity Cognitive level: Application Learning outcome 16-2: Describe neurological disorders, including seizures, cerebral palsy, meningitis, spina bifida, hydrocephalus, and Guillain-Barré syndrome. Test-taking tip: Know the pathopsysiology of intracranial pressure.
8. In the postictal portion of a seizure, the nurse expects to see: 1. An aura. 2. Tremors. 3. Confusion. 4. Unresponsiveness.	Answer: 3 Rationale: The postictal period follows a seizure and is a period of confusion, sleepiness, slurred speech, poor coordination, or headache. An aura is seen before a seizure. Tremors and unresponsiveness can be seen during the seizure. Nursing process step: Assessment Category of client need: Psychosocial integrity Cognitive level: Application Learning outcome 16-2: Describe neurological disorders, including seizures, cerebral palsy, meningitis, spina bifida, hydrocephalus, and Guillain-Barré syndrome. Test-taking tips: Recognize expected outcomes in seizure disorders.
9. Care of the child with a concussion includes: 1. Keep the child awake. 2. Awaken the child every 2 hours. 3. Watch carefully for 12 hours after injury. 4. Tylenol (acetaminophen) as needed for pain.	Answer: 2 Rationale: The child can be allowed to sleep, but must be awakened every 2 hours to check level of consciousness. Analgesics such as Tylenol should not be given, for it could mask symptoms. The child must be watched for 24–72 hours after a head injury. Nursing process step: Implementation Category of client need: Physiological integrity Cognitive level: Application Learning outcome 16-3: Explain appropriate nursing interventions for children with neurological disorders. Test-taking tip: Recognize the priorities in the care of the client with a head injury.
10. A child with Down syndrome often presents with which of the following characteristics? 1. Nystagmus 2. Kernicterus 3. Simian crease 4. "Setting sun" eyes	Answer: 3 Rationale: A child with Down syndrome often will have a simian crease. Kernicterus is associated with infantile hyperbilirubinemia. "Setting sun" eyes are seen in children with hydrocephalus. Nystagmus is involuntary movement of the eyes and is not associated with Down syndrome. Nursing process step: Assessment Category of client need: Physiological integrity Cognitive level: Application Learning outcome 16-2: Describe neurological disorders, including seizures, cerebral palsy, meningitis, spina bifida, hydrocephalus, and Guillain-Barré syndrome. Test-taking tip: Recognize the characteristics of a child with Down syndrome.
11. In teaching the parent of a child with conjunctivitis to prevent the spread of this infection, it is important to stress that the child (*select all that apply*): 1. Avoid rubbing eyes. 2. Wash hands frequently.	Answer: 1, 2, 4 Rationale: It is important to use ophthalmic drops as ordered, wash hands frequently, and avoid rubbing eyes. The child should not go to school or day care while infection is present. Nursing process step: Implementation Category of client need: Physiological integrity Cognitive level: Analysis

3. May return to day care.
4. May use ophthalmic drops as ordered.

Learning outcome 16-5: Explain appropriate nursing interventions for children with disorders of the eye and ear.

Test-taking tip: Know the manner in which infections are passed in small children.

---

12. A child who is experiencing unco-ordinated eye muscles and fails to main-tain proper eye alignment has:
1. Esotropia.
2. Exotropia.
3. Strabismus.
4. Hypertrophia.

Answer: 3

Rationale: Strabismus is commonly known as cross-eye, which occurs when eye muscles are uncoordinated and fail to maintain proper eye alignment. Esotropia is the turning of the eye inward. Exotropia is the turning outward of the eye. Hyper-trophia is a vertical deviation of one of the eyes.

Nursing process step: Assessment

Category of client need: Health promotion and maintenance

Cognitive level: Application

Learning outcome 16-4: Describe disorders of the eye and ear in children.

Test-taking tip: Know the pathopsysiology of eye disorders in children.

---

13. The eustachian tube in a young child is different than in an adult. The young child's eustachian tube is:
1. Longer than an adult's.
2. Shorter than an adult's.
3. Narrower than an adult's.
4. More rigid than an adult's.

Answer: 2

Rationale: The eustachian tube in a young child is shorter, wider, more horizontal, and more flaccid than an adult's.

Nursing process step: Assessment

Category of client need: Health promotion and maintenance

Cognitive level: Application

Learning outcome 16-1: Discuss the anatomy and physiology of the pediatric neu-rological system.

Test-taking tip: Recognize the differences between adult and child ear physiology.

---

14. A 9-month-old is diagnosed with oti-tis media. The mother asks the nurse if there is a way to prevent otitis media in her child. The nurse answers:
1. Burp the baby often.
2. Pacifier use is recommended.
3. Let the baby lie down flat for feedings.
4. Do not expose the baby to second-hand smoke.

Answer: 4

Rationale: Secondhand smoke can cause respiratory infections in children, and this can lead to otitis media. Burping a baby does not impact otitis media. Babies should not be flat for feedings. Pacifiers are not recommended because it raises the soft palate and alters the direction of the eustachian tube.

Nursing process step: Evaluation

Category of client need: Health promotion and maintenance

Cognitive level: Analysis

Learning outcome 16-5: Explain appropriate nursing interventions for children with disorders of the eye and ear.

Test-taking tip: This question is about safe care of the child.

---

15. A 21-kg child is admitted to the hos-pital and started on phenytoin (Dilantin). The safe range of this drug is 15–20 mg/kg/day in 2 divided doses. The safe dose for this child is:
1. 315–420 mg/day.
2. 250–310 mg/day.
3. 120–160 mg/dose.
4. 56–102 mg/dose.

Answer: 1

Rationale: 21 kg $\times$ 15 mg = 315 mg/day. 21 kg $\times$ 20 mg = 420 mg/day.

Nursing process step: Implementation

Category of client need: Physiological integrity

Cognitive level: Application

Learning outcome 16-3: Explain appropriate nursing interventions for children with neurological disorders.

Test-taking tip: Know the formula to calculate safe drug doses in children.

CHAPTER 17

1. A 2-week old newborn is brought to the pediatrician's office for a routine checkup. The nurse, while getting the in-fant ready to see the physician, weighs the infant and then performs the Ortolani-Bar-low maneuver. The nurse notices some re-sistance and feels a click with movement bilaterally. The nurse's responsibility is to:
1. Tell the mother everything is fine.
2. Inform the pediatrician of the findings.
3. Take a history from the mother be-cause abuse is suspected.
4. The Ortolani-Barlow maneuver is never done on a newborn.

Answer: 2

Rationale: The Ortolani-Barlow maneuver is done to assess the newborn for par-tial or complete dislocation of the hip joint. The finding of resistance and/or clicking may be indicative of developmental dysplasia of the hip. The abnormality may be in the femoral head or the acetabulum.

Nursing process step: Assessment

Category of client need: Health promotion and maintenance

Cognitive level: Application

Learning outcome 17-1: Discuss the anatomy and physiology of the pediatric musculoskeletal system.

Test-taking tip: Recognize abnormalities of the musculoskeletal system.

---

2. A 2-year-old toddler is brought to the physician's office for a physical. The mother is concerned about the toddler's mobility. She states the child was slow to learn to walk and he falls down often. Mother is worried about the toddler's coordination. The nurse notes a waddling gait in the toddler and observes him walking on his toes. The nurse suspects this toddler may have:
1. Kyphosis.
2. Lordosis.
3. Legg–Calvé–Perthes disease.
4. Duchenne's muscular dystrophy.

Answer: 4

Rationale: Duchenne's muscular dystrophy is seen in children in the first 3 to 4 years of life. It is characterized by waddling gait, frequent falls, slow to learn to walk, and walking on toes. Kyphosis is excessive concave curvature of the thoracic spine. Lordosis is excessive concave curvature of the lumbar spine. In Legg–Calvé–Perthes disease, the femoral head dies from lack of blood supply and is exhibited by hip and thigh pain and a limp.

Nursing process step: Evaluation
Category of client need: Health promotion and maintenance
Cognitive level: Application
Learning outcome 17-2: Describe musculoskeletal disorders, including developmental hip dysplasia, scoliosis, muscular dystrophy, osteomyelitis, osteosarcoma, and musculoskeletal injuries.
Test-taking tip: Look for answer that is consistent with the symptoms.

---

3. A nurse is caring for a child postoperatively after an open reduction internal fixation of the radius. The nurse notes the plaster cast feels damp and cool and needs to be placed on pillows for elevation. The nurse knows to move this cast, she must:
1. Not move the cast until it is fully dry.
2. Only use the tips of her fingers to move the cast.
3. Use only the palms of the hands to move the cast.
4. Lift the child's arm by the fingers to avoid touching the damp cast.

Answer: 3

Rationale: Handle the damp cast only with palms of the hand. Fingertips can make indentations in the cast and result in pressure areas where skin breakdown could occur. It is imperative to elevate the limb postoperatively, so not moving the cast is not an option. Lifting on the child's fingers would cause pressure on the newly repaired fracture.

Nursing process step: Planning
Category of client need: Safe, effective care environment
Cognitive level: Analysis
Learning outcome 17-4: Explain appropriate nursing interventions for children with musculoskeletal disorders.
Test-taking tip: Know safe care of a cast in a child.

---

4. A middle school child is recovering in the pediatric ward after a bike accident. His left leg is in a cast and is elevated on two pillows. The client is sleeping much of the time because of the Lortab elixir that he has been receiving every 4–5 hours. The nurse is checking his vital signs and notes the toes on his left foot are pale, cool, and capillary refill is four seconds. He is complaining of pain in his left leg, and his last dose of Lortab was four hours ago. The first action of the nurse is:
1. Call the physician.
2. Do nothing; this is an expected finding.
3. Give the client his dose of pain medication.
4. Watch the extremity to see if there are changes.

Answer: 1

Rationale: The nurse should notify the physician. The toes on the left foot should be warm, pink, with a capillary refill less than two seconds. The child may also be experiencing an increased amount of pain due to possible decreased circulation to his toes.

Nursing process step: Assessment
Category of client need: Physiological integrity
Cognitive level: Analysis
Learning outcome 17-4: Explain appropriate nursing interventions for children with musculoskeletal disorders.
Test-taking tip: This question is asking for setting priorities. When the solution is not a nursing function, call the physician.

---

5. Cast care of a plaster cast is often done in the home. In reinforcing discharge instructions to the family of a child with a cast, the nurse must inform the caregiver to (*select all that apply*):
1. Use lotion without alcohol under the cast.
2. Report unusual odor of the cast or unexplained fever.
3. The area under the cast, toes, and fingers can be cleaned with alcohol.
4. The child may go swimming if the cast is covered with a plastic bag.

Answer: 2, 3

Rationale: Alcohol may be used under the cast and on the fingers. Water must be avoided. If the caregiver notices a foul odor coming from the cast and/or unexplained fever, he or she needs to call and report this finding to the physician. Though the cast may be covered with a plastic bag for bathing, a prolonged event in the water, such as swimming, would likely dissolve the plaster cast. Lotion and powders under the cast should be avoided because they could cause skin irritation.

Nursing process step: Planning
Category of client need: Safe, effective care environment
Cognitive level: Application
Learning outcome 17-4: Explain appropriate nursing interventions for children with musculoskeletal disorders.
Test-taking tip: Know safe care of a cast in a child.

---

6. Instructing a client on the use of crutches may be the responsibility of the office nurse. If the child is ambulating using crutches with his neck flexed, the nurse knows:

1. The crutches are too long.
2. The crutches are too short.
3. The crutches are at the appropriate height.
4. It is difficult to assess the position of the crutches with the information given.

Answer: 2

Rationale: If the child's neck is flexed when using his crutches, the crutches are too short. Crutches should fit comfortably under the axillae. The child should not have to stoop to use crutches.

Nursing process step: Evaluation

Category of client need: Health promotion and maintenance

Cognitive level: Analysis

Learning outcome 17-3: Discuss clinical manifestations, diagnostic procedures, and medical management related to musculoskeletal disorders.

Test-taking tip: To choose the correct answer, try to visualize what each of the answers looks like.

---

7. A 12-year-old boy is two days post-op after an above-the-knee amputation of the right leg due to osteosarcoma. He is complaining of pain and heaviness in the right foot. The nurse knows the child is actually:

1. Disoriented from pain medications.
2. Experiencing normal side effects of the radiation he received.
3. Experiencing phantom pain, which would be considered normal for this client.
4. Using this as an attention-seeking behavior and is in denial of his circumstances.

Answer: 3

Rationale: It is normal to experience pain and heaviness after an amputation. The other behaviors would not be appropriate to this situation.

Nursing process step: Assessment

Category of client need: Physiological integrity

Cognitive level: Analysis

Learning outcome 17-3: Discuss clinical manifestations, diagnostic procedures, and medical management related to musculoskeletal disorders.

Test-taking tip: Recognize the possible clinical manifestations of amputation.

---

8. A nurse is caring for a school-age child in skeletal traction. The priority in the care of this client is:

1. Allow school friends to visit.
2. Provide high-protein meals and snacks.
3. Provide diversional activities for the child.
4. Check the child's temperature every four hours.

Answer: 4

Rationale: In skeletal traction, the pin is placed through the extremity, so it is a site where microorganisms can enter and cause infection. Sterile pin care must be performed according to institutional policy. Adequate nutrition, diversion, and school friends are important, but assessing for infection is the priority.

Nursing process step: Implementation

Category of client need: Safe, effective care environment

Cognitive level: Analysis

Learning outcome 17-4: Explain appropriate nursing interventions for children with musculoskeletal disorders.

Test-taking tip: This question is asking for a priority of nursing care.

---

9. In the nursing care of children with musculoskeletal disorders, a priority of the pediatric nurse is:

1. Monitor cardiac function.
2. Assess respiratory function.
3. Seek to promote independence.
4. Encourage age-appropriate play.

Answer: 2

Rationale: Respiratory function is first in the ABCs of assessment. The other three answers are important, but the respiratory system is the priority.

Nursing process step: Planning

Category of client need: Safe, effective care environment

Cognitive level: Application

Learning outcome 17-4: Explain appropriate nursing interventions for children with musculoskeletal disorders.

Test-taking tip: Priority question dealing with the ABCs.

---

10. The following signs, if noted in a 16-year-old with a musculoskeletal disorder, may indicate the teen is experiencing body image disturbance (*select all that apply*).

1. Hiding the affected body part
2. Feelings of shame and/or guilt
3. Refusal to touch the affected body part
4. Overexposure of the affected body part

Answer: 1, 2, 3, 4

Rationale: Hiding the affected body part, feelings of shame and/or guilt, refusal to touch the affected body part, and overexposure of the affected body part are all signs of disturbed body image.

Nursing process step: Evaluation

Category of client need: Psychosocial integrity

Cognitive level: Analysis

Learning outcome 17-2: Describe musculoskeletal disorders, including developmental hip dysplasia, scoliosis, muscular dystrophy, osteomyelitis, osteosarcoma, and musculoskeletal injuries.

Test-taking tip: Recognize normal development of a teen and importance of body image.

---

11. Indications of compartment syndrome in a 7-year-old child with a newly applied synthetic cast are (*select all that apply*):
1. Pulselessness and paralysis.
2. Pain and pressure.
3. Paresthesia and pallor.
4. Petechiae and pain.

Answer: 1, 2, 3
Rationale: Symptoms of compartment syndrome include paresthesia, pain, pallor, paralysis, and pulselessness. This is caused from increased pressure in a limited space, so circulation is compromised and nerve damage can occur.
Nursing process step: Assessment
Category of client need: Safe, effective care environment
Cognitive level: Analysis
Learning outcome 17-4: Explain appropriate nursing interventions for children with musculoskeletal disorders.
Test-taking tip: Recognize the symptoms of compromised circulation.

---

12. Petaling a child's cast is done to protect the child's skin from the rough edges of the cast. Appropriate material for this procedure is:
1. Gauze.
2. Moleskin.
3. Synthetic cast material.
4. Waterproof plastic material.

Answer: 2
Rationale: Moleskin is soft and effective to keep the rough edges of the cast away from a child's skin. Synthetic cast material could still leave rough edges next to the child's skin, and gauze alone would not stick to the cast. Plastic waterproof material is a good protection for the cast when there is a chance of the cast getting wet, but would not be a soft covering of the rough edges.
Nursing process step: Implementation
Category of client need: Physiological integrity
Cognitive level: Application
Learning outcome 17-4: Explain appropriate nursing interventions for children with musculoskeletal disorders.
Test-taking tip: Know safe care of a cast in a child.

---

13. The office nurse received a call from a mother who stated, "My child has fallen, her foot is crooked, and the bone is sticking out of her ankle." The nurse would realize this child has experienced a:
1. Spiral fracture.
2. Open depressed fracture.
3. Open compound fracture.
4. Closed comminuted fracture.

Answer: 3
Rationale: Open compound fracture is when a bone protrudes through he skin. In a depressed fracture, the bone is pressed inward. A spiral fracture is a jagged break due to a twisting force. A comminuted fracture is when the bone is fragmented into many pieces.
Nursing process step: Evaluation
Category of client need: Physiological integrity
Cognitive level: Application
Learning outcome 17-2: Describe musculoskeletal disorders, including developmental hip dysplasia, scoliosis, muscular dystrophy, osteomyelitis, osteosarcoma, and musculoskeletal injuries.
Test-taking tip: Look for answer that is consistent with the symptoms.

---

14. The nurse knows lumber lordosis and a protruding abdomen in a 15-month-old toddler is:
1. An early sign of scoliosis.
2. Normal growth and development.
3. Signs the client may need a Pavlik harness.
4. An early symptom seen in children with muscular dystrophy.

Answer: 2
Rationale: This is normal growth and development because an infant's posture changes from a straight spine to a protruding abdomen and lumbar lordosis at 10–15 months of age. Scoliosis is diagnosed in school-age children. This is not indicative of muscular dystrophy or of a required correction with a Pavlik harness.
Nursing process step: Assessment
Category of client need: Health promotion and maintenance
Cognitive level: Application
Learning outcome 17-1: Discuss the anatomy and physiology of the musculoskeletal system.
Test-taking tip: Know normal growth and development of a toddler.

---

15. Gower's maneuver is characteristic of a child with:
1. Scoliosis.
2. Genu valgum.
3. Muscular dystrophy.
4. Osgood-Schlatter disease.

Answer: 3
Rationale: Gower's maneuver is seen in children with muscular dystrophy. This maneuver is used when a child with muscular dystrophy gets up from the floor. The child first maneuvers to a position supported by arms and legs before pushing off the floor to rest on hands and knees. The child then pushes the body up straight. Scoliosis is a deviation of the spine to the left. Genus valgum is knock-knees. Osgood-Schlatter disease is found in school-age children participating in sports that involve running, such as soccer.
Nursing process step: Assessment
Category of client need: Physiological integrity
Cognitive level: Analysis
Learning outcome 17-3: Discuss clinical manifestations, diagnostic procedures, and medical management related to musculoskeletal disorders.
Test-taking tip: Recognize and describe the key terms of this chapter.

---

1. The child has conchae frond in the respiratory tract. The nurse knows the conchae are:
1. Openings into the sinus cavities.
2. Masses of lymphatic tissue found in the nasal pharynx.
3. Auditory canals from the middle ear opening into the nasal pharynx.
4. Structures that increase the surface area for warming and humidifying air.

Answer: 4
Rationale: The conchae are mucous-membrane-covered structures that increase the surface area for warming and humidifying air and trapping foreign particles. Openings into the sinus cavities are named according to the sinus it opens into: frontal, sphenoidal, ethmoidal, and maxillary. The auditory canals are the eustachian canals. Masses of lymphatic tissue in the nasal pharynx are the adenoids.
Nursing process step: Assessment
Category of client need: Health promotion and maintenance
Cognitive level: Application
Learning outcome 18-1: Discuss the anatomy and physiology of the pediatric respiratory system.
Test-taking tip: Describe key terms in the respiratory tract.

2. The anatomy of the respiratory system is similar in an adult and a child. The main difference in these two systems is:
1. The trachea is longer in a child.
2. The tonsils are larger in the adult.
3. The pharynx is shorter in the child.
4. The airway diameter is smaller in a child.

Answer: 4
The main difference in the two structures is the smaller diameter of the child's airway. The size of the child's trachea approximates the diameter of the child's small finger. Tonsils in the adult are atrophied and so are smaller than a child's. The child's trachea is shorter than an adult.
Nursing process step: Evaluation
Category of client need: Health promotion and maintenance
Cognitive level: Application
Learning outcome 18-1: Discuss the anatomy and physiology of the pediatric respiratory system.
Test-taking tip: Know the difference between an adult's and a child's airway.

3. In assessing the breathing patterns of a 3-month-old infant, the nurse knows (*select all that apply*):
1. Respirations are irregular.
2. Infants are nose breathers.
3. Normal respiratory rate is shallow.
4. Infants use abdominal muscles to breathe.

Answer: 1, 2, 4
Rationale: In infants, respiratory pattern is irregular. Infants are nose breathers until they are approximately 6 months old. Infants use abdominal muscles to breathe. Normal respirations are not shallow.
Nursing process step: Assessment
Category of client need: Health promotion and maintenance
Cognitive level: Application
Learning outcome 18-1: Discuss the anatomy and physiology of the pediatric respiratory system.
Test-taking tip: Know the physiology of the airway and breathing in an infant.

4. In auscultating lungs in a 10-month-old, the nurse hears rhonchi. The nurse knows rhonchi are:
1. Fine, dry sounds.
2. Coarse, wet sounds.
3. High-pitched inspiratory crowing.
4. Musical sounds noted with inspiration and expiration.

Answer: 2
Rationale: Rhonchi are coarse, wet sounds. Fine, dry sounds are called crackles. A high-pitched inspiratory crowing is called stridor. Wheezes are musical sounds noted on inspiration and/or expiration.
Nursing process step: Assessment
Category of client need: Physiological integrity
Cognitive level: Application
Learning outcome 18-2: Describe respiratory disorders, including upper respiratory infections, tracheoesophageal fistula, cystic fibrosis, asthma, and lower respiratory infections.
Test-taking tip: Recognize abnormal lung sounds.

5. Epistaxis is common in school-age children. Epistaxis can be caused by (*select all that apply*):
1. Trauma.
2. Allergies.
3. High humidity.
4. Foreign body.

Answer: 1, 2, 4
Rationale: Epistaxis or nosebleeds can be caused by trauma, allergies, and/or a foreign body. Nosebleeds also can be caused by low humidity that causes drying of the mucous membranes.
Nursing process step: Evaluation
Category of client need: Safe, effective care environment
Cognitive level: Analysis
Learning outcome 18-4: Discuss clinical manifestations, diagnostic procedures, medical management, and nursing interventions related to respiratory trauma.
Test-taking tip: Know key terms.

6. The nurse teaches a mother the treatment for a nosebleed in a child. This treatment consists of (*select all that apply*):
1. Place a cold cloth on the forehead.
2. Have the child hold his head slightly up and back.
3. Have the child blow his nose to clear the nasal passages of blood.
4. Hold pressure by pushing the outer side of the nares against the nasal septum.

Answer: 1, 4
Rationale: Placing a cold cloth on the forehead and holding pressure on the nose will help to stop a nosebleed. Having the child hold his head up and back will cause blood to go down the throat into the stomach, possibly causing nausea and vomiting. Once the nosebleed stops, the child should not blow his nose for several hours.
Nursing process step: Implementation
Category of client need: Health promotion and maintenance
Cognitive level: Analysis
Learning outcome 18-4: Discuss clinical manifestations, diagnostic procedures, medical management, and nursing interventions related to respiratory trauma.
Test-taking tip: Select the answer that best addresses the question.

7. If an air leak occurs in a child with a chest tube, the nurse should:
1. Suction the child.
2. Discontinue the chest tubes.
3. Clamp the tubes as close to the client as possible.
4. Do nothing; chest tubes are supposed to have air leaks.

Answer: 3
Rationale: If a chest is leaking air, the tube(s) must be clamped with large hemostats as close to the client as possible and the charge nurse and doctor must be notified immediately.
Nursing process step: Implementation
Category of client need: Physiological integrity
Cognitive level: Analysis
Learning outcome 18-4: Discuss clinical manifestations, diagnostic procedures, medical management, and nursing interventions related to respiratory trauma.
Test-taking tip: Recognize normal functioning of chest tubes.

8. A 5-year-old is returned to her room in the outpatient center after a tonsillectomy and adenoidectomy (T & A). The postoperative care for this child involves:
1. Give aspirin as needed for pain.
2. Watching for excessive swallowing.
3. Gargling with salt water to promote healing.
4. Drinking milk products for the protein needed for healing.

Answer: 2
Rationale: Excessive swallowing may be indicative of bleeding. Aspirin would never be used after a T&A because of the chance of bleeding. Gargling with salt water is not recommended due to the risk of bleeding. Milk is avoided because it can cause an increase in mucous production.
Nursing process step: Implementation
Category of client need: Physiological integrity
Cognitive level: Analysis
Learning outcome 18-4: Discuss clinical manifestations, diagnostic procedures, medical management, and nursing interventions related to respiratory trauma.
Test-taking tip: Recognize abnormal postoperative symptoms.

9. The nurse is reviewing the physician's orders for a newly admitted child with suspected epiglottitis. The order the nurse should question is:
1. Obtain a throat culture.
2. Stat lateral x-ray of the neck.
3. Start an IV with normal saline.
4. Allow child to maintain position of comfort.

Answer: 1
Rationale: Visual inspection or culture of the throat is contraindicated due to a danger of triggering laryngospasm and obstruction of the airway. The other physician's orders are appropriate for this child.
Nursing process step: Implementation
Category of client need: Physiological integrity
Cognitive level: Analysis
Learning outcome 18-3: Explain appropriate nursing interventions for children with respiratory disorders.
Test taking tip: Know safe interventions when dealing with an airway problem.

10. Cystic fibrosis is an inherited recessive disorder of the exocrine glands. Parents who are known carriers for this disease have a:
1. 1 in 4 chance of having a child with cystic fibrosis.
2. 1 in 4 chance of having a child with the cystic fibrosis trait.
3. 1 in 2 chance of having a child with cystic fibrosis.
4. 1 in 2 chance of having a child with cystic fibrosis trait.

Answer: 1
Rationale: Known carriers have a 1 in 4 chance of having a child with cystic fibrosis.
Nursing process step: Evaluation
Category of client need: Health promotion and maintenance
Cognitive level: Application
Learning outcome 18-2: Describe respiratory disorders, including upper respiratory infections, tracheoesophageal fistula, cystic fibrosis, asthma, and lower respiratory infections.
Test-taking tip: Know the pathophysiology of cystic fibrosis.

11. An 11-year-old with cystic fibrosis is admitted to the pediatric unit with a respiratory infection. Care for this child entails (*select all that apply*):
1. Vitamins A, B, D, and E.
2. Pancreatic enzymes.
3. Postural drainage.
4. Antibiotics by mouth.

Answer: 2, 3
Rationale: Treatment of this disorder includes pancreatic enzymes and postural drainage. Vitamins A, D, E, and K are given. Antibiotics would be administered intravenously to a child with cystic fibrosis who is hospitalized.
Nursing process step: Planning
Category of client need: Safe, effective care environment
Cognitive level: Analysis
Learning outcome 18-2: Describe respiratory disorders, including upper respiratory infections, tracheoesophageal fistula, cystic fibrosis, asthma, and lower respiratory infections.
Test-taking tip: Recognize pathophysiology of cystic fibrosis so that treatment can match symptoms.

---

12. A 2-month-old infant is admitted to the pediatric unit with respiratory syncytial virus (RSV). The nurse knows to properly care for this infant, she must (*select all that apply*):
1. Monitor vital signs.
2. Monitor oxygenation saturation.
3. Monitor level of consciousness.
4. Give the infant no fluids by mouth.

Answer: 1, 2, 3
Rationale: Vital signs will help the nurse identify changes in respiration and heart rate. Monitoring oxygen saturation will alert the nurse if the infant's condition is deteriorating. Level of consciousness may be the first indication that the infant's status is changing for the worse. The infant may be able to tolerate fluids by mouth, depending on his or her respiratory condition.
Nursing process step: Planning
Category of client need: Safe, effective care environment
Cognitive level: Analysis
Learning outcome 18-3: Explain appropriate nursing interventions for children with respiratory disorders.
Test-taking tip: Know the pathophysiology of RSV so that treatment can match symptoms.

---

13. The nurse knows the symptoms of croup are:
1. Wheezing on expiration.
2. Rapid onset of drooling.
3. Increased mucous production.
4. A barking cough and hoarseness.

Answer: 4
Rationale: Croup is characterized by a barking "seal-like" cough and hoarseness. Rapid onset of drooling is seen in a child with acute epiglottitis. Increased mucous production is not a symptom related to croup, but may be seen with upper respiratory infections or cystic fibrosis. Wheezing on expiration is seen in a child with asthma.
Nursing process step: Assessment
Category of client need: Safe, effective care environment
Cognitive level: Analysis
Learning outcome 18-2: Describe respiratory disorders, including upper respiratory infections, tracheoesophageal fistula, cystic fibrosis, asthma, and lower respiratory infections.
Test-taking tip: Know the pathophysiology so treatment can match symptoms.

---

14. A child is admitted with a diagnosis of tuberculosis. The nurse would expect to see which laboratory test as a definitive diagnosis?
1. Blood culture
2. Mantoux test
3. CBC with differential
4. Electrolytes and sedimentation rate

Answer: 2
Rationale: A positive Mantoux test (PPD) is a definitive sign of tuberculosis. Although other tests may be utilized, the Mantoux test is the most specific.
Nursing process step: Evaluation
Category of client need: Physiological integrity
Cognitive level: Application
Learning outcome 18-2: Describe respiratory disorders, including upper respiratory infections, tracheoesophageal fistula, cystic fibrosis, asthma, and lower respiratory infections.
Test-talking tip: Recognize pertinent laboratory tests for the child with tuberculosis.

---

15. In a child who has known asthma, exercise is:
1. Not recommended.
2. Done in bursts of activity and rest.
3. Done whenever possible in cold air.
4. Allowed, with the child taking prescribed medication 15 minutes before exercising.

Answer: 4
Rationale: Exercise is recommended and the child must use prescribed medication fifteen minutes before exercising to avoid an asthma attack. Cold air can exacerbate an asthma attack.
Nursing process step: Planning
Category of client need: Health promotion and maintenance
Cognitive level: Application
Learning outcome 18-2: Describe respiratory disorders, including upper respiratory infections, tracheoesophageal fistula, cystic fibrosis, asthma, and lower respiratory infections.
Test-taking tip: Recognize plan of care for a child with asthma.

---

1. The LPN is assessing a newborn immediately after delivery. Which symptom would lead the nurse to suspect the newborn had a transposition of the great arteries?
1. Hypoxia that does not improve with oxygen administration
2. Blood pressure greater in the arms than in the legs
3. Hypoxia that improves with oxygen administration
4. Cyanosis that is relieved when the newborn is placed in a knee-chest position

Answer: 1
Rationale: Hypoxia that does not improve with oxygen administration is indicative of transposition of the great arteries. Blood pressure that is greater in the arms than in the legs is indicative of coarctation of the aorta. Hypoxia that improves with oxygen administration is characteristic of most cardiac anomalies except transposition of the great arteries. Cyanosis that is relieved when a newborn is placed in a knee-chest position is typical of tetralogy of Fallot.
Nursing process step: Assessment
Category of client need: Physiological integrity
Cognitive level: Application
Learning outcome 19-2: Describe cardiovascular disorders, including both congenital and acquired disorders.
Test-taking tip: Recognize abnormal circulation in the newborn.

2. A 4-year-old client is seen at the pediatrician's office for a regular checkup. The mother reports that this child does not seem to have much energy, still needs two naps a day, and is the smallest child in his preschool class. While taking the child's vital signs, the nurse notes a soft systolic heart murmur. His weight and height are in 3% range. These symptoms may be indicative of:
1. Normal growth and development of a 4-year-old.
2. Patent ductus arteriosus.
3. Coarctation of the aorta.
4. Atrial septal defect.

Answer: 4
Rationale: Symptoms of atrial septal defect (ASD) include a soft systolic murmur, fatigue, and delayed growth. This is not normal growth and development for a 4-year-old. Normal growth falls between the 5th and 95th percentile on the growth chart. Patent ductus arteriosus defects are noted to have a continuous systolic murmur and a pulmonic thrill.
Nursing process step: Assessment
Category of client need: Health promotion and maintenance
Cognitive level: Analysis
Learning outcome 19-2: Describe cardiovascular disorders, including both congenital and acquired disorders.
Test-taking tip: Recognize symptoms of heart defects in children.

3. The pediatric nurse suspects a mucocutaneous lymph node syndrome in a child who exhibits (*select all that apply*):
1. Fever.
2. Carditis.
3. Swelling in hands.
4. Conjunctival hyperemia.

Answer: 1, 3, 4
Rationale: Conjunctival hyperemia, fever, and swelling in the hands and feet are associated with the acute phase of mucocutaneous lymph node syndrome (Kawasaki disease). Carditis and Sydenham chorae (St. Vitus's dance) are seen in the course of rheumatic fever.
Nursing process step: Evaluation
Category of client need: Physiological integrity
Cognitive level: Application
Learning outcome 19-3: Discuss clinical manifestations, diagnostic procedures, medical management, and nursing interventions related to cardiovascular disorders.
Test-taking tip: Recognize symptoms consistent with the disease process.

4. In caring for a child with congestive heart failure, the nurse recognizes which of the following is essential in the care for this client?
1. Aspirin
2. Antibiotics
3. Daily weights
4. Diet high in protein and carbohydrates

Answer: 3
Rationale: Daily weights are important to assess the status of fluid balance, especially fluid retention. Aspirin and antibiotics are not routinely used in the diagnosis of congestive heart failure. The recommended diet for children with congestive heart failure is one that is adequate in protein and vitamins and low in sodium and fat.
Nursing process step: Assessment
Category of client need: Safe, effective care environment
Cognitive level: Analysis
Learning outcome 19-4: Explain appropriate nursing interventions for children with cardiovascular disorders.
Test-taking tip: Knowing the pathophysiology of congestive heart failure allows the student to recognize the proper intervention.

5. A 6-year-old child is seen by the pediatrician and diagnosed with hypertension. The nurse knows this may be related to a history of:
1. Frequent urinary tract infections.
2. Frequent bouts of otitis media.

Answer: 1
Rationale: Hypertension in children is often secondary to kidney disease. Frequent bouts of otitis media are not related to hypertension. Frequent respiratory infections are commonly seen in children with patent ductus arteriosus. Staphylococcal infection is not related to hypertension.
Nursing process step: Evaluation

3. Frequent respiratory infections.
4. Staphylococcal infection.

Category of client need: Physiological integrity

Cognitive level: Analysis

Learning outcome 19-3: Discuss clinical manifestations, diagnostic procedures, medical management, and nursing interventions related to cardiovascular disorders.

Test-taking tip: Know the effect kidneys may have on the vascular system.

---

6. A small child has been diagnosed with a cardiac defect with increased pulmonary blood flow. Which of the following symptoms would alert the nurse to suspect early congestive heart failure in this child?
1. Increased BUN
2. Bulging fontanel
3. Clubbing of the fingers
4. Capillary refill greater than 4 seconds

Answer: 4

Rationale: Slow capillary refill is indicative of congestive failure. Increased BUN may be found in children with hypertension. A small child's fontanel is closed. Clubbing of the fingers is associated with prolonged hypoxia, as seen in children with cardiac disorders causing cyanosis.

Nursing process step: Evaluation

Category of client need: Safe, effective care environment

Cognitive level: Analysis

Learning outcome 19-4: Explain appropriate nursing interventions for children with cardiovascular disorders.

Test-taking tip: Know the priority of onset of symptoms.

---

7. It is desirable to keep a patent ductus arteriosus open in a newborn diagnosed with transposition of the great arteries. In order to do this, the physician will most likely prescribe:
1. Inderal.
2. Indomethacin.
3. Prostaglandin E$_1$.
4. Nonsteroidal anti-inflammatory prostaglandin inhibitor.

Answer: 3.

Rationale: Prostaglandin E$_1$ is used to maintain patency of the patent ductus arteriosus prior to surgical intervention. Indomethacin and nonsteroidal anti-inflammatory prostaglandin inhibitors are used to stimulate closure of the patent ductus arteriosus. Inderal is a beta-adrenergic antagonist used in the treatment of hypertension.

Nursing process step: Planning

Category of client need: Physiological integrity

Cognitive level: Application

Learning outcome 19-3: Discuss clinical manifestations, diagnostic procedures, medical management, and nursing interventions related to cardiovascular disorders.

Test-taking tip: Recognize specific cardiac medications and their function.

---

8. Which of the following would lead a nurse to suspect a cardiac anomaly in a 4-month-old infant?
1. Abdominal breathing
2. Frequent rests during feeding
3. Frequent respiratory infections
4. Waking at night to be fed

Answer: 2

Rationale: Feeding difficulties and fatigue are consistent with congenital heart disease in infants. Abdominal breathing and waking at night for feeding are normal in a 4-month-old infant. Frequent respiratory infections are not exclusive to a diagnosis of cardiac anomaly.

Nursing process step: Assessment

Category of client need: Health promotion and maintenance

Cognitive level: Analysis

Learning outcome 19-1: Discuss the anatomy and physiology of the cardiovascular system.

Test-taking tip: Recognize how the circulatory system affects other systems.

---

9. A 2-year-old child is returned to the pediatric floor after a cardiac catheterization to repair his ventricular septal defect. The immediate priority in his care is:
1. Take his temperature.
2. Start fluids slowly by mouth.
3. Check for bleeding.
4. Allow him to go to the playroom.

Answer: 3

Rationale: A child who has had a cardiac catherization is at risk for bleeding from the catheter insertion site. Checking the temperature of the child and starting fluids by mouth are routine post-procedure care as long as the child is not experiencing bleeding. The child must be kept quiet until any risk of bleeding is passed, so he or she would not be allowed to go to the playroom.

Nursing process step: Implementation

Category of client need: Safe, effective care environment

Cognitive level: Analysis

Learning outcome 19-4: Explain appropriate nursing interventions for children with cardiovascular disorders.

Test-taking tip: Recognize side effects of common cardiac procedures.

---

10. A cardiac defect should be suspected in an infant with:
1. Frequent vomiting and weak cry.
2. Slow heart rate and circumoral pallor.
3. Growth retardation and dyspnea.
4. Feeding difficulties and crying with bowel movements.

Answer: 3

Growth retardation, dyspnea, feeding difficulties, weak cry, and circumoral pallor are found in children with cardiac defects. Vomiting, slow heart rate, and crying with bowel movements are not associated with cardiac problems.

Nursing process step: Evaluation

Category of client need: Physiological integrity

Cognitive level: Analysis

Learning outcome 19-2: Describe cardiovascular disorders, including both congenital and acquired disorders.

Test-taking tip: Recognize cardiac anomalies and the pertinent symptoms in children.

---

11. In caring for a 22-kg child with Kawasaki disease, the physician has ordered 2,200 mg of aspirin to be given daily. The normal dose ordered is 80–100 mg/kg/day. This dose of aspirin is:

1. Too low, not therapeutic.
2. Within the safe range for this child.
3. Never used in children with this disease.
4. Too high, out of the safe range for this child.

Answer: 2

Rationale: The safe dose of aspirin for a child with Kawasaki disease is 80–100 mg/kg/day. 2,200 mg is 100 mg/kg for this child, so it is in the safe range. Aspirin is the drug of choice in Kawasaki disease.

Nursing process step: Planning

Category of client need: Safe, effective care environment

Cognitive level: Analysis

Learning outcome 19-3: Discuss clinical manifestations, diagnostic procedures, medical management, and nursing interventions related to cardiovascular disorders.

Test-taking tip: Know drug calculations related to care of the child.

---

12. In a toddler with a left to right shunt, the nurse would expect to find:

1. Cyanosis.
2. Clubbing of fingers.
3. Pulmonary stenosis.
4. Normal growth and development.

Answer: 4

Rationale: A toddler with a left to right shunt may be asymptomatic. In a left to right shunt, oxygenated blood is shunted to the right side of the heart to be returned to the lungs, so cyanosis is not seen. Pulmonary stenosis is seen with tetrology of Fallot. Clubbing of the fingers is found in cardiac defects that cause cyanosis.

Nursing process step: Assessment

Category of client need: Physiological integrity

Cognitive level: Analysis

Learning outcome 19-2: Describe cardiovascular disorders, including both congenital and acquired disorders.

Test-taking tip: Recognize cardiac anomalies and the pertinent symptoms in children.

---

13. An adolescent with known hypertension is admitted to the hospital. In helping the client choose appropriate lunch selections from the menu, the nurse would encourage the client to choose:

1. Whole milk.
2. Bag of potato chips.
3. Chicken noodle soup.
4. Grilled chicken sandwich.

Answer 4

Rationale: Grilled chicken sandwich is both low in fat and low in sodium. The whole milk is high in fat. The potato chips and chicken noodle soup are high in sodium.

Nursing process step: Planning

Category of client need: Safe, effective care environment

Cognitive level: Analysis

Learning outcome 19-4: Explain appropriate nursing interventions for children with cardiovascular disorders.

Test-taking tip: Know the recommended dietary guidelines for a child with a cardiac diagnosis.

---

14. A mother of an 8-year-old has brought her child to the pediatric cardiologist for a routine checkup. In discussing the child's condition, the mother questions whether the child would benefit from a supplement of vitamin E. The physician recommends which of the following foods as good sources of vitamin E?

1. Oranges and asparagus
2. Almonds and peanut butter
3. Egg whites and chicken
4. Green leafy vegetables and potatoes

Answer: 2

Rationale: The only foods listed high in vitamin E are almonds and peanuts.

Nursing process step: Planning

Category of client need: Safe, effective care environment

Cognitive level: Analysis

Learning outcome 19-3: Discuss clinical manifestations, diagnostic procedures, medical management, and nursing interventions related to cardiovascular disorders.

Test-taking tip: Know the recommended dietary guidelines for a child with a cardiac diagnosis.

---

15. The nurse is reinforcing discharge instructions for a child who was admitted with a diagnosis of acute rheumatic fever. Which of the following statements, if made by the mother, would indicate to the nurse that the mother did understand the discharge instructions for this child? *Select all that apply.*

1. "I will continue to give my child aspirin every time she starts to run a fever."
2. "I will let my dentist know about this hospitalization in case he wants to prescribe prophylactic antibiotics."

Answer: 2, 4

Rationale: It is imperative for the mother to understand the importance of prophylactic antibiotics when her child sees a dentist, and equally important to treat any additional case of strep throat with antibiotics. Aspirin is not recommended for children with a fever, due to the relationship of aspirin and Reye's syndrome. The client recovering from rheumatic fever must have limited activity.

Nursing process step: Implementation

Category of client need: Health promotion and maintenance

Cognitive level: Application

Learning outcome 19-3: Discuss clinical manifestations, diagnostic procedures, medical management, and nursing interventions related to cardiovascular disorders.

3. "I am glad my child can go back to softball practice tomorrow. She has already missed two games."
4. "I will bring my child back to the doctor if she develops a sore throat and fever."

Test-taking tip: Recognize follow-up care for a child with rheumatic heart disease.

CHAPTER 20

1. In caring for children with hematological disorders, the nurse should understand hematopoiesis, which is:
1. The process of destroying red blood cells to cleanse the hematologic system of waste.
2. The body's mechanism to store blood cells in the spleen until they are needed.
3. The process of producing blood cells by the bone marrow for carrying oxygen and fighting infection.
4. The process of transporting oxygen by the blood to the tissues for nourishment and oxygenation.

Answer: 3
Rationale: Hematopoiesis is the process of producing blood cells in the bone marrow. Destroying red blood cells is called hemolysis.
Nursing process step: Evaluation
Category of client need: Physiological integrity
Cognitive level: Application
Learning outcome 20-1: Describe the anatomy and physiology associated with the hematologic system.
Test-taking tip: Know the anatomy and physiology associated with the hematological system.

2. The primary tissues of the hematological system are (select all that apply):
1. Liver, spleen, and brain.
2. Spleen, heart, and kidneys.
3. Kidneys, liver and spleen.
4. Bone marrow, liver and spleen.

Answer: 4
Rationale: The tissues of the hematological system are the liver, spleen, and bone marrow. The liver produces coagulants. The spleen produces RBCs, filters RBCs, and stores lymphocytes, monocytes, and platelets. The bone marrow produces blood cells. The kidneys have no role in the production or storage of blood or blood cells.
Nursing process step: Assessment
Category of client need: Physiological integrity
Cognitive level: Application
Learning outcome 20-1: Describe the anatomy and physiology associated with the hematologic system.
Test-taking tip: Know the anatomy associated with the hematological system.

3. The LPN is caring for a child after removal of lymph nodes due to cancer. The nurse understands the purpose of these lymph nodes was to:
1. Filter lymph fluid.
2. Filter red blood cells.
3. Act as a duct and collect lymph fluid.
4. Return lymph fluid to the intravascular system.

Answer: 1
Rationale: The lymph fluid flows through the lymph nodes, which act as a filter. The right lymphatic duct drains the lymph fluid from upper body; the thoracic duct drains the lymph fluid from the lower body. All lymph is returned to the intravascular system. Lymph nodes have no function in filtering RBCs.
Nursing process step: Assessment
Category of client need: Physiological integrity
Cognitive level: Application
Learning outcome 20-2: Describe the anatomy and physiology associated with the lymphatic system.
Test-taking tip: Recognize the functions of the lymphatic system.

4. In reviewing the lab reports of a child with hemophilia, the nurse would expect to see:
1. Decreased platelet count.
2. Prolonged thrombin time (TT).
3. Prolonged prothrombin time (PT).
4. Prolonged activated partial thromboplastin time (APPT).

Answer: 4
Rationale: The APPT is prolonged, while the PT, TT, and platelet counts are within normal limits in a child with hemophilia.
Nursing process step: Assessment
Category of client need: Physiological integrity
Cognitive level: Application
Learning outcome 20-4: Discuss medical management of disorders of the hematologic and lymphatic system.
Test-taking tip: Recognize pertinent laboratory tests.

5. A 5-year-old with hemophilia is admitted to the pediatric floor. The nurse knows the care of this client involves bleeding precautions, so the nurse should avoid:

1. Intravenous access.
2. Careful hand washing.
3. Rectal suppositories.
4. Any venipuncture.

Answer: 3

Rationale: Rectal suppositories can cause bleeding in children. Intravenous access and some venipuncture are necessary in the care of a child hospitalized with hemophilia, though venipuncture should be limited.

Nursing process step: Implementation

Category of client need: Physiological integrity.

Cognitive level: Analysis

Learning outcome 20-5: Discuss nursing considerations related to disorders of the hematologic and lymphatic system.

Test-taking tip: Recognize safe care of the hemophiliac child.

---

6. A 10-year-old is being discharged from the hospital with a diagnosis of idiopathic thrombocytopenic purpura (ITP). In reinforcing discharge instructions with this mother, the nurse knows the mother does not understand when she replies:

1. "I will get a soft toothbrush for my child."
2. "I won't let my child go back to soccer practice until next week."
3. "I will call the physician immediately if my son's stools turn black."
4. "I will use pressure if my child has a nosebleed."

Answer: 2

Rationale: A child with ITP must avoid all contact sports due to the risk of bleeding.

Nursing process step: Implementation

Category of client need: Safe, effective care environment

Cognitive level: Analysis

Learning outcome 20-4: Discuss medical management of disorders of the hematologic and lymphatic system.

Test-taking tip: Eliminate all the right answers.

---

7. In children with anemia, the nurse knows which of the following foods will aid in the absorption of iron:

1. Cheeseburger and milk.
2. Grilled chicken and corn.
3. Scrambled eggs and whole wheat toast.
4. Raisin bran cereal and a glass of orange juice.

Answer: 4

Rationale: Foods containing vitamin C can increase the absorption of iron when ingested at the same time. Raisin bran is a fortified cereal and orange juice is high in vitamin C. The other foods listed do not contain vitamin C.

Nursing process step: Planning

Category of client need: Health promotion and maintenance

Cognitive level: Analysis

Learning outcome 20-5: Discuss nursing considerations related to disorders of the hematologic and lymphatic system.

Test-taking tip: Know vitamin C rich foods.

---

8. Rapid identification and treatment is vital for the child with sickle cell disease. The nurse knows a crisis may be avoided if the child is taught to (*select all that apply*):

1. Avoid exercise.
2. Drink plenty of fluids.
3. Rest between activities.
4. Report immediately pain in a localized area.

Answer: 2, 3, 4

Rationale: Dehydration and fatigue may bring on a crisis. Localized pain may indicate an occlusion. Exercise is allowed, though the child must drink plenty of fluids and be aware of the importance of rest and fluids.

Nursing process step: Planning

Category of client need: Safe, effective care environment

Cognitive level: Application

Learning outcome 20-5: Discuss nursing considerations related to disorders of the hematologic and lymphatic system.

Test-taking tip: Know the pathophysiology of sickle cell disease.

---

9. A child in sickle cell crisis has been admitted to the pediatric unit. The physician orders a blood transfusion to help relieve the anemia and sickling. The LPN knows this transfusion may cause hemosiderosis, which can be treated with (*select all that apply*):

1. Vitamin K.
2. Vitamin C.
3. Heparin.
4. An iron-chelating agent.

Answer: 2, 4

Rationale: Hemosiderosis is a buildup of iron in the tissues and organs of a child receiving frequent blood transfusions. An iron-chelating agent, such as deferoxamine, is given to bind to the iron so it can be excreted by the kidney. Vitamin C also may promote iron excretion. Vitamin K and heparin have no role in treating excess iron.

Nursing process step: Planning

Category of client need: Physiological integrity

Cognitive level: Analysis

Learning outcome 20-4: Discuss medical management of disorders of the hematologic and lymphatic system.

Test-taking tip: Know the pathophysiology involved with the treatment of children with sickle cell.

10. A 15-year-old is admitted to the pediatric unit for a round of chemotherapy to treat his Hodgkin's lymphoma. It is important for the nurse and caregivers of this client to know that most antineoplastic agents are excreted:
1. In the stool.
2. In the urine.
3. In all body fluids.
4. Through the skin in the form of sweat.

Answer: 2
Rationale: Most antineoplastic agents are excreted unchanged in the urine.
Nursing process step: Planning
Category of client need: Safe, effective care environment
Cognitive level: Application
Learning outcome 20-4: Discuss medical management of disorders of the hematologic and lymphatic system.
Test-taking tip: Safety is the correct choice.

---

11. In a child with hemophilia, bleeding can be stopped by (*select all that apply*):
1. Applying ice.
2. Applying heat.
3. Apply pressure.
4. Elevating the site.

Answers: 1, 3, 4
Rationale: Ice, elevation, and pressure all are useful in stopping bleeding. Warmth will bring more blood to the site and may increase bleeding.
Nursing process step: Implementation
Category of client need: Safe, effective care environment
Cognitive level: Application
Learning outcome 20-5: Discuss nursing considerations related to disorders of the hematologic and lymphatic system.
Test-taking tip: Recognize appropriate care to stop bleeding.

---

12. Bone marrow depression in the child who is receiving chemotherapy may be evidenced by:
1. Fatigue.
2. Alopecia.
3. Frequent infections.
4. Idiopathic thrombocytopenia purpura (ITP).

Answer: 3
Rationale: Frequent infections are directly related to bone marrow suppression of white blood cells. Fatigue and alopecia are seen in clients undergoing chemotherapy, but can be related to other factors, such as damage to the hair follicles and fatigue related to altered nutrition. A healthy diet and adequate fluid intake are essential for combating fatigue. ITP is not related to chemotherapy because the thrombocytopenia is not idiopathic.
Nursing process step: Assessment
Category of client need: Physiological integrity
Cognitive level: Analysis
Learning outcome 20-4: Discuss medical management of disorders of the hematologic and lymphatic system.
Test-taking tip: Recognize the side effects of chemotherapy.

---

13. A 4-year-old is admitted to the pediatric unit with a diagnosis of cancer. The nurse knows the most common cancer seen in this age group is:
1. Hodgkin's lymphoma (HL)
2. Nonhodgkin's lymphoma (NHL)
3. Acute myelogenous leukemia (AML)
4. Acute lymphoblastic leukemia (ALL)

Answer: 4
Rationale: Acute lymphoblastic leukemia is the most common cancer affecting children under 5 years old.
Nursing process step: Assessment
Category of client need: Physiological integrity
Cognitive level: Application
Learning outcome 20-3: Discuss the clinical manifestations of disorders of the hematologic and lymphatic system.
Test-taking tip: Recognize the differences in various leukemias.

---

14. Ferosal (ferrous sulfate) is given to children for treatment of iron deficiency anemia. The nurse knows to reinforce with a child's caregiver the importance of giving this medication properly. In administering iron preparations to children, the nurse knows:
1. Iron should be given with milk.
2. Liquid iron can cause staining of the teeth.
3. Diarrhea is a common side effect of iron.
4. Tablets should be crushed if the child is unable to swallow pills.

Answer: 2
Rationale: Liquid iron preparations can cause staining of the teeth and should be given to the child with a straw. Iron should be given with a vitamin C preparation, not milk. Constipation is a side effect, not diarrhea. Do not crush iron tablets.
Nursing process step: Implementation
Category of client need: Physiological integrity
Cognitive level: Application
Learning outcome 20-5: Discuss nursing considerations related to disorders of the hematologic and lymphatic system.
Test-taking tip: Know safe drug administration.

15. Fatigue is often seen in children who are being treated for cancer. Ways to decrease fatigue in these clients include (*select all that apply*):
1. Eat larger meals.
2. Prioritize essential activities.
3. Encourage physical activity.
4. Drink plenty of sugary fluids.

Answer: 2, 3
Rationale: Prioritize activities, and do these when the child has the most energy. Physical activities actually can promote energy. Meals should be small and frequent. Large meals can increase fatigue. Drinking sugary fluids only gives temporary energy and eventually decreases the overall energy level.
Nursing process step: Evaluation
Category of client need: Safe, effective care environment
Cognitive level: Analysis
Learning outcome 20-5: Discuss nursing considerations related to disorders of the hematologic and lymphatic system.
Test-taking tip: Recognize nursing interventions to make the child more comfortable.

CHAPTER 21

1. A 3-year-old is seen at the physician's office for repeated ear infections, failure to thrive, and chronic diarrhea. Mother was HIV positive when she gave birth to this child. This child has had a recent HIV test, which was positive. The next step for this child is:
1. Start the child on zidovudine (AZT) because he has been diagnosed with HIV.
2. Refer the client and mother to the chaplain for work on issues concerning death.
3. Repeat the enzyme-linked immunosorbent assay (ELISA) test.
4. Tell the mother to watch the child; he is too young to take zidovudine (Retrovir).

Answer: 3
Rationale: HIV is confirmed after two positive tests. Zidovudine is used in infants and children. This parent and child may need support, as in chaplain and/or support groups, but the HIV test must be repeated to confirm the diagnosis of HIV.
Nursing process step: Planning
Category of client need: Physiological integrity
Cognitive level: Analysis
Learning outcome 21-3: Discuss clinical manifestations, diagnostic procedures, medical management, and nursing interventions related to immunological disorders.
Test-taking tip: Recognize correct protocol for the diagnosis of HIV.

2. A child with juvenile rheumatoid arthritis (JRA) has come to the pediatrician for an exacerbation of her JRA. The physician recommends (*select all that apply*):
1. Advil (ibuprofen).
2. Tylenol (acetaminophen).
3. Ice to the affected joints.
4. Warm compresses to the affected joints.

Answer: 1, 4
Rationale: Nonsteroidal anti-inflammatory drugs like ibuprofen are used to reduce pain in JRA. Warm compresses are used to relieve discomfort and swelling. Ice and acetaminophen are not recommended in the treatment of JRA.
Nursing process step: Implementation
Category of client need: Physiological integrity
Cognitive level: Application
Learning outcome 21-3: Discuss clinical manifestations, diagnostic procedures, medical management, and nursing interventions related to immunological disorders.
Test-taking tip: Know the symptoms of JRA so that the correct responses can be chosen.

3. A 3-year-old with end-stage cardiomyopathy received a heart transplant 3 months ago and has been discharged to home on immunosuppressive drug therapy. When the child experiences weight gain, dyspnea, and tachycardia, the nurse knows the child may be experiencing:
1. Organ rejection.
2. A period of rapid growth.
3. Normal side effects of immunosuppressive therapy.
4. Symptoms not related to the transplanted organ.

Answer: 1
Rationale: Organ rejection can occur within days to months after a transplant. In the case of a heart transplant, the child would begin to exhibit symptoms of cardiac dysfunction, such as weight gain, dyspnea, and tachycardia. Weight gain can signal both a period of growth and can be a side effect of immunosuppressive therapy, but dyspnea and tachycardia are not related to growth or drug therapy.
Nursing process step: Assessment
Category of client need: Physiological integrity
Cognitive level: Analysis
Learning outcome 21-4: Describe the care of children requiring organ transplants.
Test-taking tip: Recognize expected outcomes of organ transplantation.

4. A 6-month-old has been diagnosed with his first case of otitis media and is started on amoxicillin (Polycillin). The mother is surprised to know her baby has an ear infection because he has

Answer: 2
Rationale: Reactions to an allergen do not occur until repeated exposure has taken place, so the rash could not be allergic at the first exposure of amoxicillin. Acetaminophen does not treat rashes or allergies. A rash is not commonly associated with amoxicillin.

never been sick before. After the first dose of amoxicillin, the baby develops a fine rash all over his trunk. The nurse would advise the mother:
1. Stop the antibiotic, for he may be allergic to this medication.
2. Continue the medication as ordered.
3. It is common to experience a rash when taking amoxicillin.
4. Give the baby acetaminophen (Tylenol) because the rash may be from the otitis media.

Nursing process step: Evaluation
Category of client need: Safe, effective care environment
Cognitive level: Analysis
Learning outcome 21-2: Describe immunological disorders, including HIV, AIDS, juvenile rheumatoid arthritis, and allergies.
Test-taking tip: Recognize the characteristics of an allergic reaction.

---

5. A breastfeeding mother is alarmed because her 2-month-old has started spitting up large feedings of breast milk and seems to have abdominal pain after eating. The mother is calling the pediatrician's office because she thinks her baby has developed an allergy to the breast milk. The nurse should explain:
1. Babies are commonly allergic to breast milk, so the mother should switch her baby to formula.
2. The baby may be reacting to something the mother has eaten, so the mother can begin a food diary and eliminate foods she is eating to see if the baby improves.
3. This is perfectly normal, and expected at this age of development.
4. Infants at this age cannot have allergies; their immune system is too immature.

Answer: 2
Rationale: Food allergies can be identified by removing foods one at a time and observing for allergic reactions. Babies are not allergic to breast milk, though they may react to something the mother has eaten. Spitting up can be normal in a baby, but most likely would not just begin at 2 months of age.
Nursing process step: Implementation
Category of client need: Health promotion and wellness
Cognitive level: Application
Learning outcome 21-1: Discuss the anatomy and physiology of the pediatric immunological system.
Test-taking tip: Recognize the properties of breast milk in relation to the infant.

---

6. An 18-month-old is receiving DPT and IPV immunizations. These are an example of:
1. Acquired immunity.
2. Natural immunity.
3. Passive immunity.
4. Secondary immunity.

Answer: 1
Rationale: Immunizations provide children with active immunity. Natural immunity is present at birth and lasts for 3–6 months. Passive immunity is achieved through the administration of immunoglobulins to protect children against diseases to which they may have been exposed already. Secondary immunity occurs when a child is exposed to an antigen in the future.
Nursing process step: Evaluation
Category of client need: Health promotion and wellness
Cognitive level: Application
Learning outcome 21-1: Discuss the anatomy and physiology of the pediatric immunological system.
Test-taking tip: Recognize how the child responds to various exposures in enhancing the immune system.

---

7. A 4-year-old with HIV is hospitalized with an overwhelming infection. This child is not allowed to go to the playroom due to reverse isolation. The nurse knows appropriate toys for a child at this age are:
1. Board games so the child can play interactively with her family.
2. A musical mobile over the bed.
3. Stuffed dog and cat from the playroom.
4. A coloring book and crayons.

Answer: 4
Rationale: Paper for drawing or coloring, crayons, and tracing paper are appropriate developmental toys for a 4-year-old. Board games are not appropriate at this age, a musical mobile is not enough stimulation for this child, and stuffed animals from the playroom may carry organisms to a child in reverse isolation.
Nursing process step: Planning
Category of client need: Psychosocial integrity
Cognitive level: Analysis
Learning outcome 21-3: Discuss clinical manifestations, diagnostic procedures, medical management, and nursing interventions related to immunological disorders.
Test-taking tip: Describe normal growth and development of children.

---

8. A 12-year-old with systemic lupus erythematosus (SLE) has been on Prednisone for 1 month. Her mother is alarmed because she has started to gain weight, is not sleeping well, and is developing acne. The nurse advises the mother:
1. This is normal at this age.
2. This is most likely due to the SLE.
3. Start the child on a 1,500-calories per day diet.
4. This is a common side effect of this drug.

Answer: 4
Rationale: Prednisone can cause hunger leading to weight gain, mood changes, worsening acne, jitteriness, and insomnia. It would not be appropriate to change the child's diet at this time.
Nursing process step: Evaluation
Category of client need: Physiological integrity
Cognitive level: Analysis
Learning outcome 21-3: Discuss clinical manifestations, diagnostic procedures, medical management, and nursing interventions related to immunological disorders.
Test-taking tip: Recognize common side effects of drugs used in treatment of SLE.

9. A 9-year-old with a noted history of allergy to wasp stings has just been stung by a wasp on the right hand while on the playground. He is experiencing swelling of his lips and a rash. The nurse knows the priority of care for this child is:
1. Inform his mother of the incident.
2. Place an ice pack on his lips and right hand.
3. Give him a dose of epinephrine from his EpiPen.
4. Watch him carefully, though no intervention is needed at this time.

Answer: 3
Rationale: The priority is to administer a dose of epinephrine to the child as quickly as possible. The swelling of the lips can be a sign of anaphylactic shock, which is a systemic reaction that can lead to respiratory distress and death.
Nursing process step: Implementation
Category of client need: Physiological integrity
Cognitive level: Application
Learning outcome 21-3: Discuss clinical manifestations, diagnostic procedures, medical management, and nursing interventions related to immunological disorders.
Test-taking tip: The nursing priority is the safest choice for this child.

10. A teenager is being discharged from the hospital after a diagnosis of rheumatoid arthritis. The nurse knows the mother understands the discharge instructions when she tells the nurse:
1. "I am glad to hear my teenager won't be limited in activity because she is a cheerleader and already has missed three football games."
2. "We are going to stop on the way home and pick up some eggplant and cheese to help decrease her joint inflammation."
3. "I hope my child falls into the 30% who can have complete remission from this disease."
4. "I will encourage my child to eat pineapple and salmon for joint health."

Answer: 4
Rationale: Pineapple is associated with natural anti-inflammatory properties and salmon contains omega-3 fatty acids, which relieve joint stiffness and pain. Activity is limited due to pain and swelling, so cheerleading would not be an appropriate activity. Eggplant and cheese are not recommended for clients with RA because these foods can cause increased swelling in the joints. Seventy percent of children with RA will experience permanent remission by adulthood.
Nursing process step: Evaluation
Category of client need: Health promotion and maintenance
Cognitive level: Analysis
Learning outcome 21-2: Describe immunological disorders, including HIV, AIDS, juvenile rheumatoid arthritis, and allergies.
Test-taking tip: Recognize the role of nutrients in children with immunological disorders.

11. The risk for transmission of HIV in teens is worrisome to parents. The nurse reinforces the teaching that HIV can be spread through:
1. Hugging and kissing.
2. Sneezing and coughing.
3. Sharing hairbrushes.
4. Sharing toothbrushes.

Answer: 4
Rationale: Sharing toothbrushes can pass HIV if the infected person is experiencing bleeding of the gums. HIV is not passed through hugging, kissing, sneezing, coughing, or sharing hairbrushes.
Nursing process step: Planning
Category of client need: Safe, effective care environment
Cognitive level: Application
Learning outcome 21-2: Describe immunological disorders, including HIV, AIDS, juvenile rheumatoid arthritis, and allergies.
Test-taking tip: Understand that HIV is passed through body fluids.

12. Cultural sensitivity is required when talking to parents about possible organ donation of their child's organs. The nurse should recognize that some cul-

Answer: 1, 2, 3, 4
Rationale: All of the religious groups listed will consent to organ donation.
Nursing process step: Planning
Category of client need: Psychosocial integrity

tures may forbid such donations. The following religious groups consider organ donation a matter of individual choice (*select all that apply*):
1. Baptists.
2. Hindus.
3. Christian Scientists.
4. Seventh-Day Adventists.

Cognitive level: Application
Learning outcome 21-4: Describe the care of children requiring organ transplants.
Test-taking tip: Recognize the influence of culture when addressing sensitive issues with families.

---

13. The nurse suspects a young child may be having an infusion reaction to a platelet infusion. The priority of care for this child would be:
1. Call the physician.
2. Give IV Benadryl and continue the infusion.
3. Stop the platelets and remove the intravenous tubing.
4. Stop the platelets and run normal saline through the intravenous line.

Answer: 3
Rationale: Immediately stop the platelets and remove the tubing so the client does not receive any more platelets. Then call the physician for additional orders.
Nursing process step: Implementation
Category of client need: Safe, effective care environment
Cognitive level: Analysis
Learning outcome 21-2: Describe immunological disorders, including HIV, AIDS, juvenile rheumatoid arthritis, and allergies.
Test-taking tip: The question asks for a nursing priority, what is the safest action for the client.

---

14. Immmunoglobulins are vital in the role of immunity in all children. The nurse would expect a child with a history of environmental allergies who has clear rhinitis and itchy eyes to have an increase in:
1. IgM.
2. IgE.
3. IgG.
4. IgA.

Answer: 2
Rationale: Levels of IgE are primarily responsible for the symptoms of an allergic reaction. IgM mediates cytotoxic response and complement. IgA prevents binding of viruses to cells of respiratory and GI tracts. IgG is active against bacteria, toxins, and viruses and activates complement.
Nursing process step: Assessment
Category of client need: Physiological integrity
Cognitive level: Application
Learning outcome 21-2: Describe immunological disorders, including HIV, AIDS, juvenile rheumatoid arthritis, and allergies.
Test-taking tip: Understand the role of individual immunoglobulins.

---

15. Tuberculin testing is required for teenagers who are getting ready to enter college. The nurse recognizes that this form of testing consists of the following allergic reaction:
1. Delayed.
2. Tissue specific.
3. Localized.
4. Immune complex.

Answer: 1
Rationale: TB testing is a form of delayed allergic reaction because the reaction occurs several hours or days after exposure. Tissue specific allergic reaction occurs within 15 to 30 minutes after exposure. Localized reaction occurs within seconds or minutes after exposure. Immune complex reaction occurs within 6 hours of exposure.
Nursing process step: Evaluation
Category of client need: Physiological integrity
Cognitive level: Application
Learning outcome 21-1: Discuss the anatomy and physiology of the pediatric immunological system.
Test-taking tip: Recognize the characteristics of an allergic reaction.

CHAPTER 22

1. The nurse knows the mouth consists of several structures important for intake of food and fluids. When a child has impairment in the papillae, the nurse relates this to the:
1. Taste buds.
2. Openings to the salivary glands.
3. Membranes covering the front of the mouth.
4. A thin membrane attaching the tongue to the floor of the mouth.

Answer: 1
Rationale: The papillae are raised bumps found on the tongue and contain receptors for salty, sour, sweet, and bitter. The salivary glands openings are called ducts. The membrane that covers the front of the mouth and inside the lip is called gingival tissue. The thin membrane attaching the tongue to the floor of the mouth is called the lingual frenulum.
Nursing process step: Assessment
Category of client need: Health promotion and wellness
Cognitive level: Application
Learning outcome 22-1: Describe the basic structures and functioning of the gastrointestinal tract and accessory organs.
Test-taking tip: The correct answer is often the shortest or longest.

2. In caring for a child with gastrointestinal disease realizes absorption of nutrients mostly takes place in the: 1. Cecum. 2. Jejunum. 3. Stomach. 4. Duodenum.	Answer: 2 Rationale: Absorption of nutrients takes place mainly in the jejunum and ileum. The process of chemical digestion is done in the duodenum. Food is mixed with digestive acid and enzymes in the stomach. The cecum propels chime through the large intestine. Nursing process step: Assessment Category of client need: Health promotion and wellness Cognitive level: Application Learning outcome 22-1: Describe the basic structures and functioning of the gastrointestinal tract and accessory organs. Test-taking tip: The key to this question is absorption of nutrients rather than digestion.
3. The nurse is concerned when a child is born with a congenital defect of the gastrointestinal tract. While the parents wait for possible corrective surgery, the parents must watch for (*select all that apply*): 1. Aspiration. 2. Malnutrition. 3. Seizures. 4. Obstruction.	Answer: 1, 2, 4 Rationale: Congenital disorders of the GI tract can lead to aspiration, malnutrition, and obstruction. Seizures would not be directly linked to congenital disorders of the GI tract. Nursing process step: Planning Category of client need: Health promotion and maintenance Cognitive level: Evaluation Learning outcome 22-1: Describe the basic structures and functioning of the gastrointestinal tract and accessory organs. Test-taking tip: Know the function and possible abnormalities of the GI system.
4. The nurse knows chemical digestion is part of the GI tract function. *Number the following in order of occurrence.* 1. Glucose is absorbed into the blood. 2. Peptidase changes peptides into amino acids. 3. Amylase in saliva changes starch into maltose. 4. Pepsin breaks large molecules of protein into smaller molecules.	Answer: 3, 4, 2, 1 Rationale: Amylase found in saliva changes starch into maltose. If swallowing happens too rapidly, this reaction will not take place. When food enters the stomach, hydrochloric acid and pepsin (protease) break up large molecules of protein into smaller molecules. In the small intestine, intestinal juice contains the enzyme peptidase, which changes peptides into amino acids. At the end of chemical digestion, glucose is absorbed into the blood. Nursing process step: Assessment Category of client need: Health promotion and maintenance Cognitive level: Application Learning outcome 22-1: Describe the basic structures and functioning of the gastrointestinal tract and accessory organs. Test-taking tip: Recognize the physiology of digestion.
5. In examining the abdomen of a small child, the nurse knows the order of the examination is (*select all that apply, and place in order of occurrence*): 1. Palpation. 2. Auscultation. 3. Observation. 4. Percussion.	Answer: 3, 2, 1 Rationale: Observation is done first, then auscultation to listen for bowel sounds. Palpation must be last because it can alter bowel sounds. Percussion is not done by the LPN/LVN. Nursing process step: Assessment Category of client need: Safe, effective care environment Cognitive level: Analysis Learning outcome 22-4: Explain appropriate nursing interventions for children with gastrointestinal disorders. Test-taking tip: Recognize techniques of assessment on a child.
6. Postoperatively, after repair of cleft lip, the nurse would expect a 3-month-old to have orders for: 1. Breck feeder. 2. Care of a Logan clamp. 3. Prone position to facilitate drainage. 4. Orogastric tube to low wall suction.	Answer: 2 Rationale: A Logan clamp is used after a cleft lip repair to decrease tension on the suture line. A Breck feeder is a syringe with a rubber hose used to feed infants with a cleft palate. Prone position would allow the child to rub his face on the sheets. An orogastric tube would not be used in this client due to the probability of the tube rubbing on the suture lines. Nursing process step: Planning Category of client need: Physiological integrity Cognitive level: Analysis Learning outcome 22-3: Discuss clinical manifestations, diagnostic procedures, and medical management related to gastrointestinal disorders. Test-taking tip: This question is asking for client safety.

7. Postoperatively, after a cleft palate repair, the nurse knows it is important to (*select all that apply*):
1. Keep the suture line clean.
2. Keep the child medicated for pain.
3. Allow the child to use a straw to keep fluids off the suture line.
4. Use soft elbow restraints to keep the child from putting his fingers in his mouth.

Answer: 1, 2, 4
Rationale: Postoperative care after a cleft palate repair includes keeping the suture line clean, keeping the child comfortable and medicated for pain, and using soft elbow restraints so the child cannot get fingers in his mouth. A straw is never used post-op because it could cause trauma to the suture line or bleeding.
Nursing process step: Implementation
Category of client need: Safe, effective care
Cognitive level: Analysis
Learning outcome 22-4: Explain appropriate nursing interventions for children with gastrointestinal disorders.
Test-taking tip: The priority of postoperative care is to preserve the operative site. Putting something in the client's mouth would not be safe practice.

---

8. A 12-year-old is seen in the physician's office because of lower right quadrant pain. The history is collected by the nurse, and the child states, "All of a sudden my pain went away." The first priority for the nurse is:
1. Inform the doctor.
2. Watch the child for a while longer.
3. Send the child home; he is better.
4. Do nothing, and wait for the physician to exam this child.

Answer: 1
Rationale: If this child was experiencing appendicitis, the sudden relief of pain may mean the appendix has ruptured, and peritonitis can spread rapidly. The child would need immediate surgical intervention.
Nursing process step: Planning
Category of client need: Physiological integrity
Cognitive level: Analysis
Learning outcome 22-4: Explain appropriate nursing interventions for children with gastrointestinal disorders.
Test-taking tip: Refer to Maslow's hierarchy of needs.

---

9. Care for a 14-year-old with a diagnosis of Crohn's disease is based on the knowledge that this adolescent may need:
1. TPN to allow the bowel to rest.
2. Gastrostomy feeding tube for nutrients to allow healing.
3. Surgical removal of affected tissue, which will provide a cure.
4. Corticosteroids, immunosuppressants, and NSAIDs to treat this disease.

Answer: 1
Rationale: TPN is often given during an acute episode to allow the bowel to rest. Gastrostomy tube feedings will not allow bowel rest. Surgical correction would not be curative because ulceration tends to recur in other areas. Corticosteroids and immunosuppressants are used to treat Crohn's disease. NSAIDS would not be used due to the possibility of the side effect of bleeding when utilizing these drugs.
Nursing process step: Planning
Category of client need: Safe, effective care environment
Cognitive level: Application
Learning outcome 22-3: Discuss clinical manifestations, diagnostic procedures, and medical management related to gastrointestinal disorders.
Test-taking tip: Focus on the diagnosis and the associated pathophysiology.

---

10. A 5-year-old is hospitalized with celiac disease. The nurse, in helping the child choose his lunch from the menu, encourages the child to order:
1. Chicken and rice soup.
2. Grilled cheese sandwich on rye.
3. Chicken and rice casserole.
4. Chicken salad on a bed of greens.

Answer: 3
Rationale: Canned soups, rye bread, and mayonnaise all contain gluten, so should not be given to the client.
Nursing process step: Planning
Category of client need: Physiological integrity
Cognitive level: Analysis
Learning outcome 22-4: Explain appropriate nursing interventions for children with gastrointestinal disorders.
Test-taking tip: Read the question carefully, and remember the associations with gluten.

---

11. The pediatric nurse knows that the type of hepatitis that can be seen spreading in day care is:
1. Hepatitis D.
2. Hepatitis C.
3. Hepatitis B.
4. Hepatitis A.

Answer: 4
Rationale: Hepatitis A is also known as infectious hepatitis and is highly contagious. This virus lives on surfaces for 1 month, so diaper changing tables can be a source. Hepatitis D is found in conjunction with hepatitis B. Hepatitis B, called serum hepatitis, is transmitted though blood and body fluids, as in sexual contact or sharing intravenous needles. Most infants have been immunized against hepatitis B. Hepatitis C is transmitted through blood and blood products. This is seen in children who need repeat blood transfusions.
Nursing process step: Assessment
Category of client need: Safe, effective care environment
Cognitive level: Application
Learning outcome 22-2: Describe major gastrointestinal disorders in clear, simple terms.
Test-taking tip: Recognize diseases of the liver.

---

12. The nurse is alerted to the possibility of pyloric stenosis when she observes _____ in the infant. 1. Statorrhea 2. Musty smelling urine 3. Currant-jelly-like stools 4. Peristaltic waves across the abdomen	Answer: 4 Rationale: Pyloric stenosis is characterized by a small round mass felt in the upper right quadrant of the abdomen and peristaltic waves across the abdomen. Statorrhea is seen with cystic fibrosis. Musty smelling urine is indicative of phenylketonuria (PKU). Currant-jelly-like stools are seen in a child with intusseption. Nursing process step: Evaluation Category of client need: Physiological integrity Cognitive level: Analysis Learning outcome 22-2: Describe major gastrointestinal disorders in clear, simple terms. Test-taking tip: Review the pathophysiology of pyloric stenosis.
13. Poisoning is a common cause of injury to a child. When the mother of a 2-year-old calls the pediatrician's office for advice after her child ate some of a poinsettia plant, the nurse should advise the mother: 1. Call the local poison control center. 2. Give the child syrup of ipecac immediately. 3. Take the child to the nearest emergency room. 4. Do nothing; poinsettias are not poisonous.	Answer: 1 Rationale: The mother must call the local poison control center and follow the advice given. Syrup of ipecac is no longer used because it can be harmful in some situations and may not remove all of the poison. Taking the child immediately to the emergency room can delay treatment. Nursing process step: Evaluation Category of client need: Health promotion and maintenance Cognitive level: Analysis Learning outcome 22-4: Explain appropriate nursing interventions for children with gastrointestinal disorders. Test-taking tip: Recognize emergency measures appropriate to children.
14. A 2-year-old has been treated with two rounds of antibiotics for otitis media. The mother calls the pediatrician's office because her child still has five days to go on her second antibiotic and is having six diarrhea stools a day. The recommendation for this child would most likely be: 1. Stop the antibiotics. 2. Give the child robotic supplements. 3. Give the child a diet high in sugar and starch. 4. Six stools/day is not unusual; call if stools increase to 10 or more a day.	Answer: 2 Rationale: Robotic supplements help to replace normal flora in the GI tract after antibiotic use. A diet high in sugar and starch may prevent normal flora from flourishing. Six diarrhea stools/day can be problematic for the child, depending on size and amount of fluid lost. Antibiotics would not be stopped unless the diarrhea could not be stopped any other way. Nursing process step: Evaluation Category of client need: Health promotion and maintenance Cognitive level: Analysis Learning outcome 22-1: Describe the basic structures and functioning of the gastrointestinal tract and accessory organs. Test-taking tip: Know key terms.
15. An overdose of acetaminophen (Tylenol) can be serious in a small child. The nurse knows a safe dose for a small child is 10–15 mg/kg/dose. In a 13-kg child, the safe range of Tylenol is: 1. 80–130 mg/dose. 2. 130–195 mg/dose. 3. 130–260 mg/dose. 4. 195–260 mg/dose.	Answer: 2 Rationale: 10 mg $\times$ 13 kg $=$ 130 mg. 15 mg $\times$ 13 kg $=$ 195 mg, so this is the safe range for this child. Nursing process step: Implementation Category of client need: Physiological integrity Cognitive level: Application Learning outcome 22-4: Explain appropriate nursing interventions for children with gastrointestinal disorders. Test-taking tip: Need to know formula for figuring pediatric medications.

CHAPTER 23

1. In calculating fluid output for a small child, the nurse should expect this client's hourly output to equal: 1. 30 mL/hr. 2. 10–30 mL/hr. 3. 0.5–2 mL/kg/hr. 4. 2–4.5 mL/kg/hr.	Answer: 3 Rationale: An infant is expected to have 2 mL/kg/hr output, and a child should have 0.5–1 mL/kg/hr, thus a small child could have an output of 0.5–2 mL/kg/hr. Nursing process step: Implementation Category of client need: Safe, effective care environment Cognitive level: Application Learning outcome 23-1: Describe the anatomy and physiology of the pediatric urinary and reproductive system. Test-taking tip: Know formula to calculate normal output in a child.

2. A 10-month-old is admitted to the outpatient surgical department for repair of a hypospadias. The nurse recognizes the child will have a (an):
1. Dorsal urethral opening.
2. Ventral urethral opening.
3. Ventral curvature of the penis.
4. Absence of part of the abdominal wall.

Answer: 2
Rationale: Hypospadias occurs with a ventral urethra opening in the penile shaft. A dorsal urethral opening is indicative of an epispadias. A ventral curve of the penis is called a chordee. An absence of the abdominal wall is seen with bladder exstrophy.
Nursing process step: Assessment
Category of client need: Physiological integrity
Cognitive level: Application
Learning outcome 23-2: Describe urinary and reproductive disorders, including urinary tract infections, acute and chronic renal failure, Wilms' tumor, hypospadias, phimosis, cryptorchidism, ambiguous genitalia, and menstrual disorders.
Test-taking tip: Know abnormalities of the genitourinary system.

3. The nurse caring for a child post-hypospadias repair expects to see the client manifest (select all that apply):
1. Pain.
2. Dysuria.
3. Bladder spasms.
4. Hematuria for a few days.

Answer: 1, 3, 4
Rationale: The client with a hypospadias repair may have bladder spasms, will experience pain, and is expected to have bloody urine for a few days. The client should not have difficulty with urination due to the stent that is placed in the new urethral opening.
Nursing process step: Planning
Category of client need: Physiological integrity
Cognitive level: Analysis
Learning outcome 23-3: Discuss clinical manifestations, diagnostic procedures, medical management, and nursing interventions related to urinary and reproductive disorders.
Test-taking tip: Recognize symptoms related to the genitourinary system.

4. In the infant, the pediatric office nurse knows urinary tract infections (UTI) should be suspected if the infant presents with:
1. Diarrhea.
2. Unexplained illness.
3. Sweet-smelling urine.
4. Hydronephrosis.

Answer: 2
Rationale: Signs of a UTI are less specific in an infant than in an older child. Anytime an infant presents with an unexplained illness, the possibility of UTI should be suspected. Diarrhea is not seen commonly with UTI. Strong-smelling urine can be a symptom of a UTI in an infant. Hydronephrosis is the distension of the renal pelvis caused by increased pressure due to urine backup.
Nursing process step: Evaluation
Category of client need: Physiological integrity
Cognitive level: Analysis
Learning outcome 23-3: Discuss clinical manifestations, diagnostic procedures, medical management, and nursing interventions related to urinary and reproductive disorders.
Test-taking tip: Know the symptoms of urinary tract infections in the child.

5. The mother of a 3-year-old boy who is being treated for a urinary tract infection needs to know how to avoid urinary tract infections in her child for the future. The nurse reinforces the following teaching (select all that apply):
1. Give the child cranberry juice daily.
2. Retract the foreskin daily.
3. Use bubble baths no more than once a day.
4. Give the child plenty of fiber to avoid constipation.

Answer: 1, 2, 4
Rationale: Cranberry juice may change the acidity of the urine and cause it to be less likely to become infected. Constipation distends the rectum and distorts the bladder, which hinders complete emptying of the bladder. Retraction of the foreskin is necessary for an uncircumcised male. Bubble baths are not recommended at all because bubble baths are a skin irritant and provide a medium for growth of harmful bacteria.
Nursing process step: Implementation
Category of client need: Safe, effective care environment
Cognitive level: Analysis
Learning outcome 23-4: Explain appropriate nursing interventions for children with urinary and reproductive disorders.
Test-taking tip: Recognize ways to avoid urinary tract infections in children.

6. A 5-year-old is admitted to the hospital with a diagnosis of primary nephrotic syndrome. The nurse knows the following symptoms may be present:
1. Proteinuria and hypoalbuminemia.
2. Proteinuria and hyperalbuminemia.
3. Hypoalbuminemia and hypolipidemia.
4. Hyperlipidemia and hyperalbuminemia.

Answer: 1
Rationale: Proteinuria, hypoalbuminemia, hyperlipidemia, and altered immunity are seen with nephrotic syndrome. The glomerular permeability is altered, allowing albumin to move from the blood to the urine. A low osmotic pressure stimulates the liver to make lipoproteins, leading to hyperlipidemia.
Nursing process step: Assessment
Category of client need: Physiological integrity
Cognitive level: Analysis

Learning outcome 23-2: Describe urinary and reproductive disorders, including urinary tract infections, acute and chronic renal failure, Wilms' tumor, hypospadias, phimosis, cryptorchidism, ambiguous genitalia, and menstrual disorders.
Test-taking tip: Recognize symptoms of nephrotic syndrome.

7. Treatment of the child with nephrotic syndrome is multifaceted. Dietary management is achieved through a diet of: 1. High protein. 2. Low protein. 3. High sodium. 4. Low sodium.	Answer: 4 Rationale: A low-sodium diet is recommended to prevent further protein loss by the kidneys and to allow return of normal blood protein levels. Nursing process step: Planning Category of client need: Safe, effective care environment Cognitive level: Application Learning outcome 23-3: Discuss clinical manifestations, diagnostic procedures, medical management, and nursing interventions related to urinary and reproductive disorders. Test-taking tip: Recognize care of the child with nephrotic syndrome.
8. Demineralization of the bone is seen in children with chronic renal failure (CRF). This symptom is exacerbated in children by (*select all that apply*): 1. Anemia. 2. Fractures. 3. Weakness. 4. Growth retardation.	Answer: 1, 4 Rationale: Growth retardation and anemia are seen in children with CRF due to demineralization of the bone. Nursing process step: Assessment Category of client need: Physiological integrity Cognitive level: Application Learning outcome 23-2: Describe urinary and reproductive disorders, including urinary tract infections, acute and chronic renal failure, Wilms' tumor, hypospadias, phimosis, cryptorchidism, ambiguous genitalia, and menstrual disorders. Test-taking tip: Know the pathophysiology of renal failure in children.
9. A 4-year-old is admitted to the pediatric intensive care unit with a diagnosis of acute renal failure (ARF). As the admitting nurse is assessing the client, the LPN is setting up the equipment to get intravenous (IV) fluids started. The IV fluids that are appropriate in this situation are: 1. Lactated Ringers. 2. D5W. 3. D5lactated Ringers. 4. Plasmalyte.	Answer: 1 Rationale: Isotonic fluids such as Ringer's lactate or normal saline are used for fluid replacement in a child with ARF. If the fluid deficit is caused by blood loss, albumin is given. Nursing process step: Implementation Category of client need: Safe, effective care environment Cognitive level: Analysis Learning outcome 23-3: Discuss clinical manifestations, diagnostic procedures, medical management, and nursing interventions related to urinary and reproductive disorders. Test-taking tip: Know the pathophysiology of renal failure in children.
10. In monitoring a child who is undergoing peritoneal dialysis, the nurse knows symptoms of peritonitis must be watched for. Symptoms to alert the nurse of this include: 1. Fever and constipation. 2. Vomiting and diarrhea. 3. Abdominal tenderness and headache. 4. Abdominal pain and constipation.	Answer: 2 Rationale: The child with peritonitis may have cloudy dialysate, fever, vomiting, diarrhea, abdominal tenderness, and/or pain. Nursing process step: Assessment Category of client need: Safe, effective care environment Cognitive level: Analysis Learning outcome 23-3: Discuss clinical manifestations, diagnostic procedures, medical management, and nursing interventions related to urinary and reproductive disorders. Test-taking tip: Recognize the symptoms of peritonitis.
11. A 5-year-old is seen in the pediatric office for a yearly checkup. The mother reports noticing an abdominal mass while bathing the child last week. If a Wilm's tumor is suspected, the nurse knows to post signs at the bedside of this client that remind caregivers to: 1. Weigh the client daily. 2. Follow strict intake and output. 3. Avoid palpating this client's abdomen. 4. Give pain medication around the clock.	Answer: 3 Rationale: Never palpate the abdomen of a child with potential Wilm's tumor. These tumors are fragile. Palpation could cause the tumor to rupture, dispersing cancerous cells throughout the abdomen. Nursing process step: Assessment Category of client need: Safe, effective care environment Cognitive level: Application Learning outcome 23-4: Explain appropriate nursing interventions for children with urinary and reproductive disorders. Test-taking tip: Recognize safe care for a child with a Wilm's tumor.

12. In children with enuresis, a diagnostic test that may be ordered is bladder capacity. The pediatric nurse knows the approximate bladder capacity for an 8-year-old child is:
1. 100 mL.
2. 200 mL.
3. 300 mL.
4. 500 mL.

Answer: 3
Rationale: An estimate of a child's bladder capacity can be made by adding 2 to the child's age in years. This approximates the ounces of bladder capacity in the child. The bladder of an 8-year-old can hold approximately 10 ounces, which is 300 mL.
Nursing process step: Evaluation
Category of client need: Health promotion and maintenance
Cognitive level: Application
Learning outcome 23-1: Describe the anatomy and physiology of the pediatric urinary and reproductive systems.
Test-taking tip: Know the calculation for bladder capacity in children.

13. A 15-year-old is seen at the pediatrician's office for a yearly screening. The nurse recognizes the client may be feeling some anxiety about her exam. In responding to this possible anxiety, the nurse should:
1. Allow the mother to stay in the exam room.
2. Ask the mother to stay in the waiting room.
3. Ask the mother where she would like to be.
4. Ask the client if she wants her mother with her in the exam room.

Answer: 4
Rationale: The nurse must realize physical exams are embarrassing to a client at this age. The nurse must maintain a professional manner and communicate respect to the client verbally and nonverbally.
Nursing process step: Evaluation
Category of client need: Health promotion and maintenance
Cognitive level: Analysis
Learning outcome 23-4: Explain appropriate nursing interventions for children with urinary and reproductive disorders.
Test-taking tip: Recognize normal development in an adolescent.

14. Testicular self-examination is important for all males, starting at the age of 15. The nurse recommends to her 16-year-old client this examination be done:
1. Weekly.
2. Daily.
3. Monthly.
4. Yearly.

Answer: 3
Rationale: Young men should choose a day of the month, perhaps their birthday, and examine the testicles every month.
Nursing process step: Assessment
Category of client need: Health promotion and maintenance
Cognitive level: Application
Learning outcome 23-3: Discuss clinical manifestations, diagnostic procedures, medical management, and nursing interventions related to urinary and reproductive disorders.
Test-taking tip: Recognize health promotion for the adolescent.

15. A woman should have her first Pap smear within three years of becoming sexually active or by the age of 21. Research has shown that the most common cause of cervical cancer is:
1. *Streptococcus*.
2. *Staphylococcus*.
3. Epstein Barr virus.
4. Human papillomavirus.

Answer: 4
Rationale: Human papillomavirus infection is the most common cause of cervical cancer.
Nursing process step: Implementation
Category of client need: Health promotion and maintenance
Cognitive level: Application
Learning outcome 23-2: Describe urinary and reproductive disorders, including urinary tract infections, acute and chronic renal failure, Wilms' tumor, hypospadias, phimosis, cryptorchidism, ambiguous genitalia, and menstrual disorders.
Test-taking tip: Recognize health promotion for the adolescent.

16. In a 4-year-old with a Wilms' tumor, a diagnostic procedure shows the cancer has spread beyond the kidney to soft tissue and blood vessels. The nurse knows the stage of this Wilms' tumor is:
1. Stage I.
2. Stage II.
3. Stage III.
4. Stage IV.

Answer: 2
Rationale: Stage II is when the tumor has spread beyond the kidney to fat or soft tissue or blood vessels. Stage I cancer is found only in the kidney. In stage III, the cancer has spread within the abdomen and may have spread to lymph nodes, blood vessels, or peritoneum. In stage IV, the cancer has spread to the lungs, liver, bone, or brain.
Nursing process step: Assessment
Category of client need: Physiological integrity
Cognitive level: Application
Learning outcome 23-3: Discuss clinical manifestations, diagnostic procedures, medical management, and nursing interventions related to urinary and reproductive disorders.
Test-taking tip: Recognize the signs found in Wilms' tumors.

17. Ditropan is often used to treat enuresis in children. In a 6-year-old child who weighs 27 kg, the physician has ordered 0.2 mg/kg/day to be given by mouth three times a day. The nurse knows the safe dose of this drug is:
1. 1.8 mg/dose.
2. 1.8 mg/day.
3. 5.4 mg/dose.
4. 1.35 mg/dose.

Answer: 1
Rationale: The order is 0.2 mg/kg/day, to be given three times a day. 0.2 mg $\times$ 27 kg = 5.4 mg/day, divided by 3 = 1.8 mg/dose.
Nursing process step: Planning
Category of client need: Safe, effective care environment
Cognitive level: Application
Learning outcome 23-3: Explain appropriate nursing interventions for children with urinary and reproductive disorders.
Test-taking tip: Know drug calculations in children.

CHAPTER 24

1. The skin is the largest organ system of the body. The purpose of the dermis is to (*select all that apply*):
1. Secrete melanin.
2. Allow cells to multiply and grow.
3. Provide nourishment to the epidermis.
4. Produce collagen.

Answer: 3, 4
Rationale: The dermal layer is highly vascular and provides nourishment to the dermis. Collagen is produced by fibroblast cells, which are the primary cells in the dermis. Melanin is secreted in the epidermis. The epidermis is where cells multiply, grow, and move toward the skin's surface, causing the surface layer to be replaced about every four weeks.
Nursing process step: Assessment
Client category of need: Health promotion and maintenance
Cognitive level: Application
Learning outcome 24-1: Review the basic structure and function of the skin and describe the differences between the skin of a child and an adult.
Test-taking tip: Know the function of the layers of the skin.

2. Sudoriferous glands are also known as:
1. Sweat glands.
2. Sebaceous glands.
3. Stratum germinativum.
4. Keratinized epidermal cells.

Answer: 1
Rationale: Sweat glands are also called sudoriferous glands. Stratum germinativum is the skin's basal cell layer where cells multiply, grow, and move toward the skin's surface. Keratinized epidermal cells are nails.
Nursing process step: Assessment
Category of client need: Health promotion and maintenance
Cognitive level: Application
Learning outcome 24-1: Review the basic structure and function of the skin and describe the differences between the skin of a child and an adult.
Test-taking tip: Know the function of the layers of the skin.

3. In a newborn, body temperature is regulated by the:
1. Epidermis.
2. Subcutaneous fat.
3. Exocrine sweat glands.
4. Apocrine sweat glands.

Answer: 3
Rationale: The newborn's body regulates temperature through the exocrine sweat glands. The apocrine glands do not function in a newborn. Newborns have little subcutaneous fat, so lose heat rapidly. The epidermis does not have a function in temperature regulation of the newborn.
Nursing process step: Assessment
Category of client need: Health promotion and maintenance
Cognitive level: Application
Learning outcome 24-1: Review the basic structure and function of the skin and describe differences between the skin of a child and an adult.
Test-taking tip: Know the skin's regulatory system.

4. Suspicious or malignant lesions should be inspected using the acronym ABCDE. This stands for (*select all that apply*):
1. Asymmetry of shape.
2. Border irregularity.
3. Contour of edges.
4. Elevation of lesion.

Answer: 1, 2, 4
Rationale: The acronym ABCDE stands for asymmetry of shape, border irregularity, color variation, diameter larger than 6 mm, and elevation of the lesion.
Nursing process step: Assessment
Client category of need: Health promotion and maintenance
Cognitive level: Application
Learning outcome 24-1: Review the basic structure and function of the skin and describe differences between the skin of a child and an adult.
Test-taking tip: Recognize abnormal growths of the skin.

5. A small child with a port-wine stain is seen in the pediatrician's office for an evaluation. The nurse knows a port-wine stain can be related to:
1. Glaucoma.
2. Tumors of the neck.
3. Congenital cataracts.
4. Feeding difficulties.

Answer: 1
Rationale: Port-wine stains are permanent vascular stains that may be associated with other structural malformations, such as glaucoma or tumors of the blood or lymph vessels in the pia mater and arachnoid layers of the meninges.
Nursing process step: Evaluation
Client category of need: Physiological integrity
Cognitive level: Analysis
Learning outcome 24-2: Discuss common congenital disorders of the skin, their treatment, and nursing care.
Test-taking tip: Recognize abnormal growths of the skin.

6. Excessive heat and moisture can cause irritation to the skin. This is known as:
1. Eczema.
2. Prickly heat.
3. Intertrigo.
4. Dermatitis.

Answer: 3
Rationale: Intertrigo is skin irritation caused when opposing skin creates friction. Prickly heat is caused from exocrine glands becoming blocked when a child is exposed to high temperatures. Dermatitis is a general term meaning inflammation of the skin. Eczema is a chronic inflammatory skin disorder.
Nursing process step: Assessment
Client category of need: Physiological integrity
Cognitive level: Application
Learning outcome 24-3: Discuss common infections and infestations of the skin in children.
Test-taking tip: Know the definition of key words relating to the skin.

7. A 7-month-old is brought to the pediatrician due to a diaper rash. The infant has been well, has just started eating more solid foods, and is on a commercial dairy-based formula. The nurse explains to the mother:
1. She is not changing the baby's diaper often enough.
2. Introduction of solid foods can change the pH level of urine.
3. Diaper rash is commonly caused from this formula; the mother should change the infant's formula to a commercial soy-based formula.
4. Diarrhea commonly causes diaper rash and as the diarrhea improves, so will the diaper rash.

Answer: 2
Rationale: Diaper dermatitis is caused by irritation of stool and/or urine. Introduction of solid foods changes the pH level, leaving the infant more prone to diaper dermatitis. Diarrhea can cause diaper rash, but this infant has been well. It would not be necessary to change the baby's formula at this time.
Nursing process step: Evaluation
Category of client need: Safe, effective care environment
Cognitive level: Analysis
Learning outcome 24-4: Discuss various types of skin trauma in children as well as treatment and nursing care.
Test-taking tip: Recognize common forms of skin irritation in infants.

8. Nursing considerations in a 4-year-old child with eczema are:
1. Keep the environment warm.
2. Give Benadryl three times a day.
3. Wear clothing with natural fibers, such as wool.
4. Apply wet compresses soaked in aluminum acetate.

Answer: 4
Rationale: Wet compresses soaked in aluminum acetate solution help to remove the crusts of eczema and decrease inflammation. The environment should be cool. Benadryl can be given, but only at bedtime, due to its sedating properties. Wool can be an irritant to eczema.
Nursing process step: Implementation
Category of client need: Physiological integrity
Cognitive level: Application
Learning outcome 24-3: Discuss common infections and infestations of skin in children as well as treatment and nursing care.
Test-taking tip: Recognize nursing care related to skin conditions.

9. A 7-year-old in the second grade has been diagnosed with pediculus capitis. The nurse instructs the mother to:
1. Use Elimite (premethrin cream) prescribed by the physician.
2. Seal all items that cannot be washed in a plastic bag for 2 weeks.
3. Treat the whole family, even if they do not have symptoms.

Answer: 2
Rationale: Placing items that cannot be washed in a plastic bag for 2 weeks will break the cycle of infestation by preventing the lice that hatch from finding a new host. Elimite is used to treat scabies. Only family members who actually have head lice or nits should be treated. Hair is combed with a comb dipped in vinegar to remove stubborn nits.
Nursing process step: Planning
Category of client need: Health promotion and maintenance

4. Comb hair with a fine-tooth comb dipped in olive oil so the nits slide off the hair.	Cognitive level: Application Learning outcome 24-3: Discuss common infections and infestations of skin in children as well as treatment and nursing care. Test-taking tip: Recognize nursing care related to conditions of the skin.
10. A 4-year-old is admitted to the pediatric unit with a diagnosis of cellulitis of the face, extending from the cheekbone to the jaw line on the left side of the face. Nursing care for this client includes (*select all that apply*): 1. Frequent vital signs. 2. Give all antibiotics on time. 3. Cool compresses to the affected area. 4. Have the mother cut the child's fingernails short, so the child cannot scratch.	Answer: 1, 2 Rationale: Frequent vital signs are needed to watch for fever, which could indicate septicemia. Strict adherence to antibiotics administration is necessary to achieve therapeutic levels of the drug(s) and prevent sepsis. Warm, rather than cool, compresses are used to improve circulation and promote healing. Cellulitis may have been caused from a bug bite that itched and the child scratched. Cellulitis, though, does not itch and can actually be painful and/or tender. Nursing process step: Planning Category of client need: Physiological integrity Cognitive level: Analysis Learning outcome 24-3: Discuss common infections and infestations of skin in children as well as treatment and nursing care. Test-taking tip: Recognize nursing care related to conditions of the skin.
11. A breastfed 3-month-old is diagnosed with oral candidiasis. She has just finished a round of antibiotics for otitis media. The mother asks how her baby has gotten the candidiasis. The nurse replies: 1. It probably came from day care. 2. Oral candidiasis can be spread from breast milk. 3. Oral candidiasis can be a suprainfection, sometimes experienced after the treatment of antibiotics. 4. This baby needs to be switched to a commercial formula.	Answer: 3 Rationale: This can be common after treatment of antibiotics. Antibiotics can kill some of the normal flora that maintains a balance in the mouth. Oral candidiasis is not spread in breast milk. It is not necessary to switch to formula, and it is not spread in day care. Nursing process step: Evaluation Category of client need: Health promotion and maintenance Cognitive level: Analysis Learning outcome 24-3: Discuss common infections and infestations of skin in children as well as treatment and nursing care. Test-taking tip: Know the skin's regulatory system.
12. The office nurse is speaking to a mother of a 7-year-old who had a bicycle accident three days ago. The mother is calling because the scrapes and cuts on the left knee "don't look right." The nurse needs which of the following information (*select all that apply*): 1. Presence of swelling. 2. Body temperature. 3. Drainage from wound. 4. Color of skin around wound.	Answer: 1, 2, 3, 4 Rationale: The nurse would want to know the presence of swelling, fever, drainage, and a description of the skin around the wound. Nursing process step: Evaluation Category of client need: Physiological integrity Cognitive level: Analysis Learning outcome 24-4: Discuss various types of skin trauma in children as well as treatment and nursing care. Test-taking tip: Recognize the data necessary for the nurse to assess the injured area.
13. A 5-year-old was playing with matches and started a fire in the woods. The child received burns to hands, face, and chest when trying to put this fire out. Immediate treatment for this client involves: 1. Pain relief. 2. Monitor airway. 3. Replace fluid loss. 4. Prevent infection.	Answer: 2 Rationale: Pain relief, replacing fluid loss, and preventing infection are all important in the care of a child with a burn. The first priority, however, is airway maintenance. Nursing process step: Evaluation Category of client need: Physiological integrity Cognitive level: Analysis Learning outcome 24-4: Discuss various types of skin trauma in children as well as treatment and nursing care. Test-taking tip: Know that airway, breathing, and circulation (ABCs) are always the priority.
14. The LPN knows a secondary lesion, lichenification, is seen with chronic dermatitis in children. A lichenification can be described as: 1. Leathery hardening and thickening of the skin. 2. Fibrous tissue that replaces normal tissue after injury.	Answer: 1 Rationale: Leathery hardening and thickening of the skin is known as lichenification. Fibrous tissue that replaces normal tissue after an injury is scar tissue. Hypoplastic scar tissue with irregular bands of collagen is a keloid, and the wearing away of superficial epidermis by friction or pressure is erosion. Nursing process step: Assessment Category of client need: Health promotion and maintenance Cognitive level: Application

3. Hyperplastic scar tissue with irregular bands of collagen. 4. A wearing away of the superficial epidermis by friction or pressure.	Learning outcome 24-1: Review the basic structure and function of skin and describe differences between the skin of a child and an adult. Test-taking tip: Know the definition of key words relating to the skin.
15. A mother of a 21-month-old calls the pediatrician's office for advice. The family is going camping over the weekend, and the mother wants to know how to protect her child from bug bites. The nurse advises the mother to: 1. Avoid sweet-smelling baby lotion, as it may attract insects. 2. Use DEET, which is safe due to the thickness of the baby's epidermis. 3. Apply insect repellent with DEET to all exposed areas of the baby's skin. 4. Use insect repellants that have at least 10% DEET to be effective.	Answer: 1 Rationale: Sweet-smelling lotion or cream may attract insects. DEET must be used with caution in children, due to the thinness of the epidermis. Many manufacturers recommend applying DEET to a child's clothing rather than to their skin. Avoid repellents containing more than 10% DEET. Nursing process step: Planning Category of client need: Health promotion and maintenance Cognitive level: Analysis Learning outcome 24-1: Review the basic structure and function of the skin and describe differences between the skin of a child and an adult. Test-taking tip: When three of the answers are similar, the correct answer is most likely the answer that is different.

CHAPTER 25

1. Which of the following statements correctly describes a negative feedback mechanism? 1. When insulin levels rise, glucose levels drop. 2. Melatonin levels increase during darkness. 3. A deficit of growth hormone will restrict a child's growth. 4. Oxytocin production stops after delivery of the baby.	Answer: 1 Rationale: In a negative feedback system, an increase in one substance causes a decrease in the other. Melatonin production stops when light enters the eye but is not a negative feedback system since there is no limit to the amount of melatonin that can be produced. The two are not dependent on one another. The relationship between a deficit of growth hormone and a child's growth represents a positive relationship since the absence of growth hormone restricts growth and an increase of growth hormone will increase growth. Oxytocin production increases during labor but stops after delivery; this represents a positive feedback system. Nursing process step: Diagnosis Category of client need: Physiological integrity Cognitive level: Application Learning outcome 25-2: Discuss the interrelationship of the normally functioning endocrine system. Test-taking tip: Look for the answer that is different from the others. Three choices describe situations where changes occur in the same direction. Only the correct answer describes a system where an increase of one substance produces a decrease in another.
2. Increased levels of growth hormone will: 1. Promote the deposit of fat in subcutaneous tissues. 2. Slow the production of insulin by the pancreas. 3. Stimulate the passage of amino acids into the cells. 4. Increase glucose storage by the liver.	Answer: 3 Rationale: Growth hormone stimulates growth by enhancing amino acid utilization. Growth hormone will increase fat breakdown. Growth hormone will indirectly cause increased insulin levels since glucose levels rise with hormone production. Glucose levels will rise and storage will decrease with increased levels of growth hormone. Nursing process step: Diagnosis Category of client need: Physiological integrity Cognitive level: Analysis Learning outcome 25-1: Identify the location of each endocrine gland, the hormones produced, and the function of each. Test-taking tip: Look for the answer that would represent an effect of the change described in the question.
3. If a client's diet is deficient in iodine, production of which of the following hormones will decrease? 1. Thyroid-stimulating hormone 2. Calcitonin	Answer: 2 Rationale: Calcitonin is a thyroid hormone. Iodine is necessary for thyroid hormone production. Thyroid-stimulating hormones will rise with low iodine levels. Insulin level is not dependent on iodine in the diet. Aldosterone is secreted by the adrenal cortex and is not affected by iodine levels in the diet. Nursing process step: Diagnosis

3. Insulin 4. Aldosterone	Category of client need: Physiological integrity Cognitive level: Analysis Learning outcome 25-3: Discuss disorders of each endocrine gland, including pathology, diagnostic procedures, and medical treatment. Test-taking tip: Must know that thyroid hormone production will decrease with low iodine intake. Calcitonin is the only hormone produced in the thyroid.
4. Glucocorticoid production may result in which of the following? *Select all that apply.* 1. Muscle breakdown 2. Glucose regulation 3. Lowering blood pressure 4. Increasing urine production 5. Increasing the sex drive	Answer: 1, 2 Rationale: Glucocorticoid production will stimulate muscle breakdown and glucose production. Glucocorticoids tend to increase blood pressure. Glucocorticoids have no role in urine production or in promoting the sex drive. Nursing process step: Diagnosis Category of client need: Physiological integrity Cognitive level: Application Learning outcome 25-1: Identify the location of each endocrine gland, the hormones produced, and the function of each. Test-taking tip: Look for physiological similarities that could be caused by the same stimulus.
5. You are caring for a hospitalized infant newly diagnosed with galactosemia. Which of the following is expected to be a priority in the plan of care? 1. Give lactose-free formula 1–2 ounces every 2–4 hours 2. Check specific gravity of each voiding 3. Check blood glucose levels every 6 hours 4. Check direct bilirubin levels each morning	Answer: 1 Rationale: Galactosemia is a disease that prevents the breakdown of milk sugars and requires a lactose-free formula to prevent liver damage. Urine specific gravity is unaffected by galactosemia. Blood glucose levels may fall, but with a lactose-free diet, glucose levels should be unaffected. Liver enlargement may result from galactosemia, but by following the prescribed diet, the bilirubin levels should remain within the normal range. Nursing process step: Implementation Category of client need: Safe, effective care environment Cognitive level: Analysis Learning outcome 25-3: Discuss disorders of each endocrine gland, including pathology, diagnostic procedures, and medical treatment. Test-taking tip: When prioritizing care, look for the most critical element.
6. Teaching for the parent of a child with growth hormone deficiency should include which of the following? 1. The child will not be permitted to participate in sports 2. The child will have lifelong replacement injections 3. The child may have a delayed onset of puberty 4. The child may always look small and thin	Answer: 3 Rationale: The child may have a delayed onset of puberty to allow for more growth. Sports are not contraindicated for this child. The child may have injections until normal height is reached. Obesity may be a problem for children with growth hormone deficiency. Nursing process step: Planning Category of client need: Health promotion and maintenance Cognitive level: Application Learning outcome 25-3: Discuss disorders of each endocrine gland, including pathology, diagnostic procedures, and medical treatment. Test-taking tip: Eliminate choices that describe absolutes, using phrases such as "will have" and "will not have," and choose a more general answer.
7. The child with diabetes insipidus is expected to: 1. Produce large amounts of dilute urine. 2. Require insulin to maintain normal blood glucose levels. 3. Have low serum sodium and high serum potassium. 4. Follow a high-protein, low-carbohydrate diet.	Answer: 1 Rationale: Diabetes insipidus results from a decreased production of ADH; without adequate ADH, the renal tubules will not reabsorb water. Diabetes insipidus is unrelated to diabetes mellitus and glucose metabolism. Clients with diabetes insipidus tend to have high sodium levels and low potassium levels. Clients with diabetes insipidus should be on a protein-restricted diet. Nursing process step: Assessment Category of client need: Physiological integrity Cognitive level: Analysis Learning outcome 25-3: Discuss disorders of each endocrine gland, including pathology, diagnostic procedures, and medical treatment. Test-taking tip: Look for an answer that is physiologically possible given the disease in question. The student should know that diabetes insipidus is a fluid balance problem, not a glucose management problem.

8. Which of the following meals would be best for a client with diabetes insipidus? 1. Chicken nuggets and chocolate pudding 2. Vegetable soup and oatmeal cookie 3. A taco and milk shake 4. Tuna salad sandwich and carrot sticks	Answer: 2 Rationale: Clients with diabetes insipidus should follow a low-protein diet. Vegetable soup and oatmeal cookie are the lowest choice in protein. Chicken nuggets and pudding are high in protein. A taco and milk shake would have too much protein. Tuna would be a good second choice for the selections, but still has a high level of protein. Nursing process step: Implementation Category of client need: Health promotion and maintenance Cognitive level: Analysis Learning outcome 25-5: Discuss teaching topics for children with diabetes and their parents. Test-taking tip: Look for the answer that is different from the others. Three of the choices are high protein and only one is a low-protein option.
9. The parent of a child with hypothyroidism should be alert to the signs of too much levothyroxin (Synthroid), which would include: 1. Weight gain. 2. Heart palpitations. 3. Cold intolerance. 4. Constipation.	Answer: 2 Rationale: Tachycardia, restlessness, heat intolerance, diarrhea, weight loss, and exophthalmos are all signs of too much thyroid hormone replacement. Weight gain is a sign of too little thyroid hormone. Cold intolerance is a sign of ineffective therapy and too little hormone. Digestive problems of hyperthyroidism include diarrhea, not constipation. Nursing process step: Evaluation Category of client need: Health promotion and maintenance Cognitive level: Analysis Learning outcome 25-5: Discuss teaching topics for children with diabetes and their parents. Test-taking tip: Know that the side effects of too much medication represent a excess of the desired therapeutic effect of the medication.
10. Which of the following assessment findings would concern the nurse caring for a 5-year-old child immediately following thyroid surgery? 1. The child cries and refuses to let the nurse obtain vital signs 2. The child has a blood pressure of 96/54 3. The nurse sees 1–2 cm of serous drainage on the surgical dressing 4. The child speaks with a hoarse sounding voice	Answer: 4 Rationale: A hoarse voice might be a sign that the airway is swelling and could be an early sign of respiratory distress. A child being shy of strangers might be regressive behavior, which would be normal following surgery. A blood pressure reading of 96/54 would be normal for a 5-year-old. The thyroid is very vascular, so a small amount of drainage would be expected. Nursing process tip: Assessment Category of client need: Physiological integrity Cognitive level: Analysis Learning outcome 25-4: Explain appropriate nursing interventions for children with endocrine disorders. Test-taking tip: Prioritize care to detect the most serious problems, airway being the most important.
11. You are providing care for an 8-year-old hospitalized child with Cushing's syndrome. Which of the following would be an expected finding during your assessment? 1. Gradual weight loss over the past 6 months 2. Breast development indicative of precocious puberty 3. Height and weight in the 95th percentile 4. The face is very round, with full cheeks	Answer: 4 Rationale: Children with Cushing's syndrome tend to be small for their age. Cushing's syndrome often results in weight gain. Physical maturity is likely to be delayed. A "moon" face is a common characteristic for a child with Cushing's syndrome. Nursing process step: Assessment Category of client need: Physiological integrity Cognitive level: Application Learning outcome 25-3: Discuss disorders of each endocrine gland, including pathology, diagnostic procedures, and medical treatment. Test-taking tip: Choose an answer that is physiologically possible when dealing with a specific disease assessment.
12. Hypofunction of the adrenal gland may produce which of the following assessment findings in the newborn? 1. A deposit of fat between the shoulder blades 2. A heart rate of 150 beats per minute 3. An enlarged malformed clitoris 4. A blood sugar level of 62	Answer: 3 Rationale: Hypofunction of the adrenal gland may result in an over production of androgens that will cause a malformation of genitalia development of precocious puberty. Newborns often have a fat deposit between the shoulder blades. A heart rate of 150 beats per minute is a normal finding in the newborn. A blood sugar of 62 is normal for the newborn. Nursing process step: Assessment Category of client need: Physiological integrity

Cognitive level: Analysis
Learning outcome 25-3: Discuss disorders of each endocrine gland, including pathology, diagnostic procedures, and medical treatment.
Test-taking tip: Look for the answer that is different from the others.

13. Your client is learning to prepare and self-administer a mixture of regular and NPH insulin. Which of the following is most appropriate in this situation? *Select all that apply.*
1. Have the client's meal tray available and watch the client prepare the injection before eating breakfast.
2. Tell the client to administer injections in the same area of the body (abdomen, thigh, etc.) each day.
3. Remind the client that each type of insulin requires a separate syringe for injection.
4. Show the client how to inject air first into the NPH insulin and then into the regular insulin.
5. Have the client verbalize that exercise or acute illness may require an adjustment in the insulin dosage.

Answer: 1, 2, 5
Rationale: Regular and NPH insulin should be given before meals. Air should first be injected into the regular insulin and then into the NPH insulin. Exercise can decrease insulin needs, and acute illness may increase insulin needs. Insulin absorption can be affected by rotating injections from one area of the body to another. Regular and NPH insulins may be mixed in the same syringe.
Nursing process step: Intervention
Category of client need: Health promotion and maintenance
Cognitive level: Analysis
Learning outcome 25-5: Discuss teaching topics for children with diabetes and their parents.
Test-taking tip: Eliminate choices that sound too complicated or impractical.

14. Which of the following is a true statement regarding type I, insulin-dependent diabetes?
1. The client's pancreas will produce some insulin, except when the client experiences stress.
2. Oral antidiabetic agents will usually be prescribed with good glucose control obtained.
3. Most clients will receive an initial diagnosis of the disease between the ages of 2 and 8.
4. There is an autoimmune component to the disease, and onset often follows an acute viral illness.

Answer: 4
Rationale: There is an autoimmune link to type I diabetes, and the onset often follows an acute viral illness. One of the factors that differentiates type I diabetes from type II diabetes is the complete lack of insulin production in type I diabetes. Insulin injections are used for management of type I diabetes. Most children are diagnosed between the ages of 10 and 14.
Nursing process step: Diagnosis
Category of client need: Physiological integrity
Cognitive level: Analysis
Learning outcome 25-1: Identify the location of each endocrine gland, the hormones produced, and the function of each.
Test-taking tip: Look for an answer that represents a physiological possibility, not something that is too complicated or detailed

15. Which of the following diabetic children is demonstrating signs of hypoglycemia?
1. A 10-year-old who complains of frequent urination
2. A 4-year-old who has a slow weak pulse
3. An 8-year-old with a distinctly fruity breath
4. A 12-year-old who is shaking and reporting dizziness

Answer: 4
Rationale: Shakiness and dizziness are signs of hypoglycemia. Signs of hyperglycemia include polyuria, polydipsia, and polyphagia. The child with excess ketones will have a fruity breath.
Nursing process step: Implementation
Category of client need: Safe, effective care environment
Cognitive level: Assessment
Learning outcome 25-3: Discuss disorders of each endocrine gland, including pathology, diagnostic procedures, and medical treatment.
Test-taking tip: Look for the answer that is different from the others.

CHAPTER 26

1. Which of the following is considered a communicable disease? *Select all that apply.*
1. Diabetes mellitus
2. Varicella
3. Cystic fibrosis

Answer: 2, 4, 5
Rationale: Varicella, rotavirus, and poliomyelitis are all diseases that are spread directly from one person to another. Diabetes mellitus may have an autoimmune or lifestyle origin. Cystic fibrosis is a genetic disease that is inherited from the affected individual's parents.
Nursing process step: Assessment

4. Rotavirus 5. Poliomyelitis	Category of client need: Physiological integrity Cognitive level: Analysis Learning outcome 26-1: Discuss the chain of infection. Test-taking tip: Look for diseases that fit the questions: Which diseases can cause general outbreaks in the population? Are there vaccines for any of the choices? Those diseases would likely be spread from person to person.
2. Children, in general, are more susceptible to or have a poorer prognosis for some diseases than adults because: 1. Children come in contact with more people in a day than most adults. 2. Most children are not tall enough or coordinated enough to wash their hands. 3. Children have a higher metabolic rate than adults. 4. Adults have a more mature immune system than children.	Answer: 4 Rationale: Children have an immature immune system and have fewer neutrophils than an adult and so are more at risk for acquiring disease from the many organisms they encounter. While some children may contact more people than an adult, many adults encounter active disease-causing organisms and transmit them to children. Children can be taught to wash their hands and should be supervised and encouraged to do so. Metabolic rate has no affect on disease susceptibility. Nursing process step: Diagnosis Category of client need: Health promotion and maintenance Cognitive level: Analysis Learning outcome 26-2: Explain the specific risk factors for communicable diseases in children. Test-taking tip: Look for answers that are both physiologically possible and make sense when comparing two groups such as adults and children.
3. Careful and frequent cleaning of toys in a pediatric office waiting room will break the "chain of infection" by eliminating the: 1. Disease reservoir. 2. Portal of exit. 3. Mode of transmission. 4. Portal of entry.	Answer: 3 Rationale: Toys can serve as a fomite for transmitting disease organisms from one person to another. Careful cleaning can remove the organisms and prevent transmission. The disease reservoir is where the organisms grow and multiply. An example might be a person or animal. The portal of exit represents how an organism leaves the reservoir; it might be a sneeze or cough. The portal of entry is how the disease enters a new individual, such as through the respiratory or digestive tract. Nursing process step: Implementation Category of client need: Health promotion and maintenance Cognitive level: Application Learning outcome 26-1: Discuss the chain of infection. Test-taking tip: By knowing the definitions of key terms, you can apply the terms to a real-life situation.
4. Which of the following behaviors could increase the spread of disease by direct transmission? The nurse who: 1. Does not wear gloves when changing an infant's diaper. 2. Does not wear a face mask when caring for a child on reverse isolation precautions. 3. Allows the child to take a favorite toy when the child leaves the floor for an x-ray. 4. Sneezes into a tissue and discards the tissue in the client's trash container.	Answer: 1 Rationale: The nurse's hands may become contaminated while changing a diaper, so gloves should always be worn and the hands cleansed between clients. A child on reverse isolation precautions should wear the face mask, not the nurse. The child may spread disease if the toy is given to another child, but this would be indirect transmission. Sneezing would not increase the risk for direct transmission, but would spread disease by indirect transmission. Nursing process step: Implementation Category of client need: Safe, effective care environment Cognitive level: Application Learning outcome 26-2: Explain the specific risk factors for communicable diseases in children Test-taking tip: Look for answers that relate directly to the question asked. Only one answer is an example of direct transmission.
5. Which of the following children is in the incubation stage of the infectious process? 1. The 3-year-old exposed to chickenpox who remains active and healthy. 2. The 2-month-old who is not feeding well after exposure to rotovirus. 3. The 16-year-old sexually active male complaining of dysuria. 4. The 9-year-old who remains weak and fatigued following an *E. coli* infection.	Answer: 1 Rationale: The incubation period is the period between exposure and the appearance of symptoms, so the child who appears healthy would fit this category. Vague symptoms such as poor feeding in an infant would represent the prodromal period and a time when the child is contagious. The illness phase would be characterized by the symptoms of the infectious disease, and a child in the convalescent period would remain weak following recovery. Nursing process step: Assessment Category of client need: Physiological integrity Cognitive level: Analysis Learning outcome 26-1: Discuss the chain of infection. Test-taking tip: The correct answer is often the one that meets the definition of key terms used in the question.

6. An example of active immunity is when:

1. Antibodies present in breast milk protect the breastfeeding newborn.
2. Maternal antibodies cross the placenta and protect the fetus from infections for a short time after birth.
3. A child plays with a pet that becomes sick, but the child remains healthy.
4. A fully immunized child does not become ill despite close contact with infected individuals.

Answer: 4

Rationale: Active immunity results when the child's immune system produces antibodies following infection or immunizations. Breast milk and placental transfer of antibodies are examples of passive immunity; and when a child does not prove susceptible to a disease that an animal gets, the child will not need immunity.

Nursing process step: Evaluation

Category of client need: Physiological integrity

Cognitive level: Application

Learning outcome 26-3: Describe methods of communicable disease prevention in children.

Test-taking tip: The correct answer is often the one that meets the definition of key terms used in the question.

---

7. Which of the following clients is most at risk for acquiring a nosocomial infection?

1. The 6-year-old leukemia client being cared for at home by attentive parents.
2. The 9-year-old cystic fibrosis client hospitalized for 2 weeks with pneumonia.
3. The 18-month-old hospitalized overnight following a motor vehicle accident.
4. The 3-year-old whose tonsils were removed at a same-day surgery center.

Answer: 2

Rationale: The longer a child is hospitalized, the greater the risk of a nosocomial, or hospitalized, infection; thus the cystic fibrosis client in the hospital would be most at risk. A child at home, hospitalized for a short time, or an outpatient surgery client is at lower risk for a nosocomial infection.

Nursing process step: Planning

Category of client need: Physiological integrity

Cognitive level: Analysis

Learning outcome 26-2: Explain the specific risk factors for communicable diseases in children.

Test-taking tip: The correct answer is often the one that meets the definition of key terms used in the question. By knowing what a nosocomial infection is, the question can be answered.

---

8. A nurse following standard precautions would:

1. Wear gloves while obtaining blood pressure, pulse, and respirations and tympanic temperature.
2. Always keep the door to the client's room closed.
3. Designate equipment such as thermometers for single client use for those with infectious diseases.
4. Instruct parents and visitors to wear gown and mask each time they enter the room.

Answer: 3

Rationale: Standard precautions include not transferring equipment from room to room when a client has an infectious disease. A nurse should wear gloves when there is a chance of contacting body fluids, not likely in obtaining simple noninvasive vital signs. Closing a door and wearing gowns and masks routinely are not part of standard precautions.

Nursing process step: Implementation

Category of client need: Safe, effective care environment

Cognitive level: Application

Learning outcome 26-5: Explain appropriate nursing interventions for children with childhood communicable diseases.

Test-taking tip: By knowing the different types of infection control procedures, the student can choose the answer that describes only standard precautions.

---

9. Select all of the following that are included in droplet precautions:

1. The client must be in a private room.
2. The door to the room must be closed at all times.
3. The nurse should wash hands before and after any procedures.
4. Caregivers must wear a high-efficiency respirator when in contact with the client.
5. Everyone must wear a mask when within 3 feet of the client.

Answer: 1, 3, 5

Rationale: Droplet precautions are implemented to prevent transmission of diseases that may be spread by droplets along with full standard precautions. This would include a private room, hand washing, and wearing a mask within 3 feet of the client. The room door may remain open and respirators are not part of this infection control policy.

Nursing process step: Implementation

Category of client need: Safe, effective care environment

Cognitive level: Application

Learning outcome 26-5: Explain appropriate nursing interventions for children with childhood communicable diseases.

Test-taking tip: By knowing the different types of infection control procedures, the student can choose the answer that describes droplet precautions.

---

10. Reverse isolation precautions would be most effective for:

1. The 6-year-old with a suspected case of tuberculosis.
2. The 2-year-old following a heart transplant.

Answer: 2

Rationale: Reverse isolation is to protect an immunocompromised child, such as a child following a heart transplant taking anti-rejection drugs. The child with tuberculosis or hepatitis A should be on transmission-based precautions, and the immigrant may not need to be on any precautions if not acutely ill.

Nursing process step: Implementation

<table>
<tr>
<td>

3. A 16-year-old recent immigrant from China with no immunization history.

4. A 10-year-old with hepatitis A.

</td>
<td>

Category of client need: Safe, effective care environment

Cognitive level: Application

Learning outcome 26-5: Explain appropriate nursing interventions for children with childhood communicable diseases.

Test-taking tip: By knowing the different types of infection control procedures, the student can choose the answer that describes applicable precautions.

</td>
</tr>
<tr>
<td>

11. A vaccine that uses a weakened or attenuated form of a microorganism to stimulate antibody production is a _____ vaccine.

1. Conjugated
2. Recombinant
3. Toxoid
4. Live virus

</td>
<td>

Answer: 4

Rationale: A live virus vaccine can stimulate the immune system through exposure to a weakened form of the organism. Conjugated and recombinant vaccines are genetically altered, and the toxoid is only part of the organism and not an organism itself.

Nursing process step: Diagnosis

Category of client need: Physiological integrity

Cognitive level: Application

Learning outcome 26-3: Describe methods of communicable disease prevention in children.

Test-taking tip: If you know the definitions of key terms, you are able to correctly identify which of the given answers are possible.

</td>
</tr>
<tr>
<td>

12. Before administering the fifth dose of a Diphtheria, Tetanus, and acellular Pertussis (DTaP) vaccination, the nurse should notify the physician if the parent reports:

1. The client is allergic to eggs.
2. The client has a temperature of 99.6°F axillary.
3. The client had a red swollen spot on the thigh after the first dose.
4. The client had an unexplained seizure the previous week.

</td>
<td>

Answer: 4

Rationale: A client receiving the DTaP vaccine should be observed and given Tylenol if there is a history of seizures; therefore, the physician should be notified. An allergy to eggs and a slight temperature elevation are not contraindications to the DTaP vaccine. A local reaction is not uncommon with the fourth or fifth dose of the DTaP vaccine.

Nursing process step: Planning

Category of client need: Health promotion and maintenance

Cognitive level: Analysis

Learning outcome 26-4: Discuss clinical manifestations, diagnostic procedures, and medical management related to childhood communicable diseases.

Test-taking tip: By looking for the most serious implication of an adverse reaction, you will often identify the correct answer.

</td>
</tr>
<tr>
<td>

13. A child with diphtheria may have:

1. Rhinorrhea and a dark membrane on the pharynx.
2. Muscle spasms and jaw stiffness.
3. Joint inflammation and chest pain.
4. Tremors and hyperactive reflexes.

</td>
<td>

Answer: 1

Rationale: Rhinorrhea and a membrane that may obstruct the pharynx are signs of diphtheria. Muscle spasms and jaw stiffness are signs of tetanus. Joint inflammation and chest pain may occur after flu infection, and tremors and hyperactive reflexes may be signs of early polio infection.

Nursing process step: Diagnosis

Category of client need: Physiological integrity

Cognitive level: Analysis

Learning outcome 26-4: Discuss clinical manifestations, diagnostic procedures, and medical management related to childhood communicable diseases.

</td>
</tr>
<tr>
<td>

14. The parents of a child with hepatitis B should know that:

1. The client may become a lifetime carrier of the disease.
2. The client may develop a rash that spreads from the face to the trunk.
3. The incubation period may be from 14 to 21 days.
4. The administration of aspirin may promote Reye's syndrome.

</td>
<td>

Answer: 1

Rationale: Hepatitis B can be transmitted even after recovery from the acute phase of the disease. Measles may cause a rash that spreads from the face to the trunk. The incubation period for hepatitis B can be up to 6 months, and aspirin has been associated with Reye's syndrome during a varicella outbreak.

Nursing process step: Intervention

Category of client need: Physiological integrity

Cognitive level: Application

Learning outcome 26-5: Explain appropriate nursing interventions for children with childhood communicable diseases

Test-taking tip: Look for the answer that is physiologically possible from the given choices.

</td>
</tr>
<tr>
<td>

15. A pregnant woman should avoid contact with an infected child if the woman is not immune to:

1. Varicella.
2. Tetanus.

</td>
<td>

Answer: 1

Rationale: The varicella virus can cause great harm to the unborn fetus if the pregnant woman contracts the virus. Tetanus, pertussis, and roseola are not transmitted through the placenta, and the fetus would not be at risk from maternal exposure.

</td>
</tr>
</table>

3 Pertussis. 4. Roseola.	Nursing process step: Planning Category of client need: Physiological integrity Cognitive level: Analysis Learning outcome 26-4: Discuss clinical manifestations, diagnostic procedures, and medical management related to childhood communicable diseases. Test-taking tip: By knowing how the disease is transmitted, the correct answer is the only one that is possible

CHAPTER 27

1. Holistic health, when applied to the realm of pediatric nursing, encompasses: 1. Physical and mental health. 2. Physical and emotional health. 3. Physical, mental, spiritual, and emotional health. 4. Physical and mental health, plus growth and development.	Answer: 3 Rationale: Holistic health is a concept that approaches an individual's health as an integrated system, and includes physical, emotional, intellectual, and spiritual health. Though growth and development are vital parts of health in the pediatric client, these fall under the physical, emotional, and intellectual health. Nursing process step: Evaluation Category of client need: Health promotion and maintenance Cognitive level: Application Learning outcome 27-1: Describe an appropriate psychosocial assessment of the child. Test-taking tip: Know definitions of key terms.
2. Observation by the nurse is important in caring for the pediatric client. As the nurse begins to establish a relationship with the pediatric client, the nurse is observing the child's (*select all that apply*): 1. Lung sounds. 2. Speech pattern. 3. General appearance. 4. Body posture and gait.	Answer: 2, 3, 4 Rationale: Speech pattern, general appearance, body posture, and gait can all be observed. Lung sounds can only be heard accurately with a stethoscope. Nursing process step: Assessment Category of client need: Health promotion and maintenance Cognitive level: Application Learning outcome 27-1: Describe an appropriate psychosocial assessment of the child. Test-taking tip: Recognize the components of an assessment of the child.
3. A 9-year-old is admitted to the pediatric unit with a diagnosis of pneumonia. His physician orders antibiotics and Adderall (amphetamine sulfate). The nurse knows the Adderall is to treat: 1. Depression. 2. Anxiety disorders. 3. Bipolar disorder. 4. Attention deficit disorder.	Answer: 4 Rationale: Adderall is used in children to treat attention deficit disorder. Nursing process step: Evaluation Category of client need: Safe, effective care environment Cognitive level: Application Learning outcome 27-4: Discuss clinical manifestations, diagnostic procedures, medical management, and nursing interventions related to psychosocial disorders. Test-taking tip: Recognize the medications used to treat children with psychosocial disorders.
4. A 7-year-old is seen at the pediatrician's office for his yearly exam. The mother tells the nurse her child does not complete his homework and is not doing well in school. The nurse advises the mother to develop: 1. A system of rewards. 2. A system of punishments. 3. A record of each behavior, to be more specific. 4. Time for her child to stay after school for additional help.	Answer: 1 Rationale: Establishing a system of rewards for appropriate behavior can help the child learn and foster a positive self-image. The expected behavior must be realistically achievable. Nursing process step: Planning Category of client need: Psychosocial integrity Cognitive level: Analysis Learning outcome 27-2: Describe psychosocial disorders, including autism, Asperger's syndrome, attention deficit disorder, Giles de la Tourette syndrome, anxiety, depression, anorexia nervosa and bulimia, child abuse (physical and emotional), and substance abuse. Test-taking tip: Know the symptoms and care for a child with attention deficit disorder.
5. Children with attention deficit disorder (ADD) are often prescribed stimulants to help treat this disorder. The nurse knows the mother understands	Answer: 2 Rationale: Drug holidays can be implemented during vacation periods and summer months when academic performance is not necessary. Giving a stimulant at night can cause a child with ADD to be unable to sleep. It takes 10 to 14 days

how the stimulants work when she says to the nurse:
1. "I will give this medication to my child at night."
2. "My child may not need this drug during his summer vacation."
3. "My child will start showing improved behavior after taking this medication for 1 week."
4. "I will bring my child back to the pediatrician next year for his checkup."

before effects of the medication will be recognized. The child with ADD should be evaluated on a regular basis, sooner than a yearly checkup.
Nursing process step: Evaluation
Category of client need: Safe, effective care environment
Cognitive level: Application
Learning outcome 27-2: Describe psychosocial disorders, including autism, Asperger's syndrome, attention deficit disorder, Giles de la Tourette syndrome, anxiety, depression, anorexia nervosa and bulimia, child abuse (physical and emotional), and substance abuse.
Test-taking tip: Know medications and side effects in the treatment of ADD.

---

6. An 8-year-old child has been complaining of a "stomachache" for the last several school mornings, saying she did not want to go to school. This morning the child has a stomachache, headache, and a temperature of 99°F orally. The best advice for this mother is:
1. Call the school.
2. Call the pediatrician.
3. Send the child to school.
4. Make a counseling appointment for this child.

Answer: 2
Rationale: The mother should make sure there is not something physically wrong with her child. If the pediatrician does not find something physiologically wrong, then the mother perhaps should call school and see if something has happened to cause this child to have school phobia.
Nursing process step: Planning
Category of client need: Psychosocial integrity
Cognitive level: Analysis
Learning outcome 27-4: Discuss clinical manifestations, diagnostic procedures, medical management, and nursing interventions related to psychosocial disorders.
Test-taking tip: Rule out physical problem first.

---

7. A 5-year-old has been diagnosed with attention deficit/hyperactivity disorder (ADHD) and is prescribed Strattera (atomoxetine hydrochloride). The safe dose for this 27 kg child ranges from 0.5 mg–1.2 mg/day. In milligrams, the child's dosage should be:
1. Between 10.8 mg and 15.2 mg.
2. Between 15.4 mg and 33.0 mg.
3. Between 12.8 mg and 28.7 mg.
4. Between 13.5 mg and 32.4 mg.

Answer: 4
Rationale: The safe dose range for this child is 13.5 mg to 32.4 mg daily. The formula for this calculation is 0.5 mg $\times$ 27 kg = 13.5 mg
1.2 mg $\times$ 27 kg = 32.4 mg
Nursing process step: Evaluation
Category of client need: Safe, effective care environment
Cognitive level: Analysis
Learning outcome 27-5: Explain appropriate nursing interventions for children with psychosocial disorders.
Test-taking tip: Know the formula to calculate pediatric drug doses.

---

8. A 13-year-old is seen at the physician's office for complaints of headaches, irritability, and sleeping "all of the time," according to her mother. Upon weighing and measuring this child, the nurse finds her BMI to be in the 98th percentile. Other tests the physician may order are (*select all that apply*):
1. Chest x-ray.
2. Triglycerides.
3. Hemoglobin A1c.
4. Bariatric surgery consult.

Answer: 2, 3
Rationale: This child is at risk for diabetes, orthopedic problems, and cardiovascular problems. A baseline must be established and goals set to help this teenager make good choices. This child would not be a candidate for bariatric surgery at this time. A chest x-ray would not be necessary unless the child has some pulmonary symptoms.
Nursing process step: Planning
Category of client need: Health promotion and maintenance
Cognitive level: Analysis
Learning outcome 27-3: Describe associated manifestations of psychological disorders, including overeating and obesity and suicide.
Test-taking tip: Know the laboratory tests needed to diagnose children with an eating disorder.

---

9. The mother of a 15-year-old has brought her to the pediatrician for a check-up. The expected weight for this 5 ft 6 in. teenager is 130 pounds. In assessing this teenager, the nurse finds she weighs 107 pounds. The nurse knows this weight:
1. Is within normal limits.
2. Is no reason for concern.
3. May mean an eating disorder.
4. Means the child is in good physical shape.

Answer: 3
Rationale: One hundred seven pounds is lower than 85% of the expected weight for this teenager. This leads a person to consider the possibility of an eating disorder.
Nursing process step: Assessment
Category of client need: Health promotion and maintenance
Cognitive level: Analysis
Learning outcome 27-4: Discuss clinical manifestations, diagnostic procedures, medical management, and nursing interventions related to psychosocial disorders.
Test-taking tip: If three of the answers are similar, the correct answer is most likely the one that is different.

10. In times of great stress, like with a terrorist attack, children can be easily influenced by what they see and hear. The parents of a 5-year-old who is beginning to have difficulty concentrating need to (*choose all that apply*):
1. Talk to the child honestly.
2. Allow the child time to draw and color.
3. Give the child physical contact, as in hugging.
4. Let her watch as much television as she wants.

Answer: 1, 2, 3
Rationale: Talking to the child honestly in an appropriate developmental level is important. The child may need the close contact of the parent, and drawing and coloring may be a way for the child to express feelings. The parent must be careful and protect the child from too much television and media coverage.
Nursing process step: Planning
Category of client need: Psychosocial integrity
Cognitive level: Analysis
Learning outcome 27-6: Discuss the impact to children of traumatic events and natural disasters.
Test-taking tip: Recognize psychosocial needs of a child after a traumatic event.

---

11. In assessing a child with possible fetal alcohol syndrome (FAS), the nurse knows to look for characteristics of:
1. Microcephaly and small eyes.
2. Halitosis and drowsiness.
3. Enuresis and encopresis.
4. Tachycardia and diaphoresis.

Answer: 1
Rationale: Craniofacial abnormalities like microcephaly and small eyes are seen in a child who was born with fetal alcohol syndrome. Enuresis and encopresis can be seen in children who have been sexually abused. Tachycardia and diaphoresis can be seen in children with anxiety disorders. Halitosis and drowsiness can be seen in children who are substance abusers.
Nursing process step: Assessment
Category of client need: Physiological integrity
Cognitive level: Application
Learning outcome 27-4: Discuss clinical manifestations, diagnostic procedures, medical management, and nursing interventions related to psychosocial disorders.
Test-taking tip: Three of the answers are symptoms, and one lists characteristics. Read the question carefully to see what is asked.

---

12. Therapy is important in treating children with psychosocial disorders. In a teenager with an eating disorder the therapy most effective at this age is:
1. Pet therapy.
2. Play therapy.
3. Family therapy.
4. Group therapy.

Answer: 4
Rationale: Teenagers are especially receptive to group therapy because teens are more responsive to their peers than to an authority figure. Appropriate suggestions from peers can be accepted more readily than from a therapist or parent.
Nursing process step: Evaluation
Category of client need: Psychosocial integrity
Cognitive level: Analysis
Learning outcome 27-5: Explain appropriate nursing interventions for children with psychosocial disorders.
Test-taking tip: Recognize appropriate development of teenagers.

---

13. A priority nursing consideration in caring for a child with autism is:
1. Play.
2. Safety.
3. Nutrition.
4. Communication.

Answer: 2
Rationale: A priority in nursing care of the child with autism is safety. These children have no fear of dangerous situations and may have repeated behaviors, such as head banging. Nutrition, communication, and play all are important with a child with autism, but not the priority.
Nursing process step: Planning
Category of client need: Safe, effective care environment
Cognitive level: Analysis
Learning outcome 27-5: Explain appropriate nursing interventions for children with psychosocial disorders.
Test-taking tip: Use Maslow's hierarchy as a guide for the correct answer.

---

14. A physician is seeing a 6-year-old with a fracture of the humerus. Last year the same child had a fracture in her radius. The physician talks with the parents to find out how this fracture occurred. The mother states this child was riding her bike, going down a hill, and when she fell, she hit the handlebars. The physician at this point should:
1. Not do anything, accidents happen.
2. Consider this child abuse and report it immediately.

Answer: 4
Rationale: Though the physician has a responsibility to report child abuse, he first has a responsibility to make sure this child does not have a physiological origin to these fractures. Certainly children do have accidents, so having 2 fractures in a year may not have much significance, and may be a normal part of development of a 6-year-old girl.
Nursing process step: Evaluation
Category of client need: Safe, effective care environment
Cognitive level: Analysis
Learning outcome 27-2: Describe psychosocial disorders, including autism, Asperger's syndrome, attention deficit disorder, Giles de la Tourette syndrome,

---

3. Send the parents and child for family counseling
4. See if there is a physiological reason for these fractures.

anxiety, depression, anorexia nervosa and bulimia, child abuse (physical and emotional), and substance abuse.

Test-taking tip: Use Maslow's hierarchy as a guide for the correct answer.

---

15. The nurse is administering Zoloft (sertraline hydrochloride) to an 8-year-old child for depression. This drug comes in a solution of 20 mg/mL. The dose that is ordered for this child is 32 mg once a day. The correct amount of Zoloft to administer is:
1. 1.0 ml.
2. 1.6 ml.
3. 1.8 ml.
4. 2.2 ml.

Answer: 2
Rationale: The correct dose is 1.6 ml. The formula to find this dose is: dose divided by what is on hand, then multiplied by the quantity. The dose is 32 mg/ 20 mg × 1 = 1.6 mL.
Nursing process step: Implementation
Category of client need: Safe, effective care environment
Cognitive level: Analysis
Learning outcome 27-5: Explain appropriate nursing interventions for children with psychosocial disorders.
Test-taking tip: Know formulas for drug calculations.

CHAPTER 28

1. A 16-year-old who had been in a motor vehicle accident dies while in the intensive care unit. The father, who has just been told the news, replies "This is a bad dream, and I will wake up soon." This parent is in which state of grief?
1. Anger
2. Bargaining
3. Depression
4. Shock and disbelief

Answer: 4
Rationale: This parent is in the shock and disbelief stage of grief. The intense shock is the initial stage of grief and usually passes in 24 hours. Anger is the second stage, bargaining the third, and depression is the fourth stage.
Nursing process step: Implementation
Category of client need: Psychosocial integrity
Cognitive level: Analysis
Learning outcome 28-2: Describe the stages of grief.
Test-taking tip: Recognize the stages of grief.

---

2. In the last stages of life for a 14-year-old with cystic fibrosis, the mother tells the physician that she wants her child to be resuscitated if he stops breathing so that she can have one more day with her child. The nurse knows this parent is experiencing grief and is probably in what stage?
1. Anger
2. Bargaining
3. Depression
4. Shock and disbelief

Answer: 2
Rationale: The mother is experiencing bargaining, and the parent is bargaining with the physician to try to prolong her child's life. Shock and disbelief are the first stage of grief, in which a parent may feel like "things are not real." Anger is the second stage, in which a parent may direct anger to themselves or to the health care providers. Depression is a state of persistent sadness.
Nursing process step: Evaluation
Category of client need: Psychosocial integrity
Cognitive level: Analysis
Learning outcome 28-2: Describe the stages of grief.
Test-taking tip: Recognize the stages of grief.

---

3. The mother of a child is talking to the nurse about the behavior of this child who is dying of cancer. This child has been behaving aggressively—throwing things, hitting, and so on—and is afraid to go to sleep at night. This child has also been asking lots of questions about death. The nurse knows this child is most likely in which age group?
1. Toddler
2. Preschooler
3. School-age
4. Prepuberty

Answer: 2
Rationale: The preschooler shows aggression, throws things, hits, and may be hyperactive. This age has a fear of going to sleep because of nightmares and asks lots of questions about death. The toddler who has separation anxiety may hit and bite and refuse to eat or sleep. The toddler may fear bodily mutilation and pain. A school-age child may keep his fears to himself. A child in prepuberty is old enough to understand death and what is happening.
Nursing process step: Analysis
Category of client need: Psychosocial integrity
Cognitive level: Analysis
Learning outcome 28-4: Describe the role of the LPN/LVN in caring for dying children and their families.
Test-taking tip: Recognize the stages of grief.

---

4. The biggest fear in a 5-year-old who has leukemia and is aware that his body is deteriorating is: 1. Fear of body mutilation. 2. Fear of acceptance. 3. Fear of rejection. 4. Fear of loneliness.	Answer: 1 Rationale: Five-year-olds can tell the seriousness of an illness. They may realize they are dying based on their own body image, and they express fear of body mutilation. This age child does not realize the permanence of death and commonly does not experience loneliness, rejection or acceptance. Nursing process step: Analysis Category of client need: Psychological integrity Cognitive level: Analysis Learning outcome 28-4: Describe the role of the LPN/LVN in caring for dying children and their families. Test-taking tip: Recognize normal growth and development in a child.
5. If the death of a child is impending, the focus of the LVN/LPN changes. The focus now becomes (*select all that apply*): 1. Beginning the grief process. 2. Keeping the child comfortable. 3. Identifying resources available to the family. 4. Attending professional support groups.	Answer: 2, 3, 4 Rationale: The client focus is placed on keeping the child comfortable, the family focus on helping them find resources for additional support, and it is vital for the LVN/LPN to attend professional groups so he or she will have the personal resources to deal with difficult situations, such as the death of a child. Nursing process step: Assessment Category of client need: Safe, effective care environment Cognitive level: Evaluation Learning outcome 28-4: Describe the role of the LPN/LVN in caring for dying children and their families. Test-taking tip: Recognize the role of the nurse in supporting clients and families through difficult times.
6. In working with parents of a dying child, it is many times helpful and supportive to the parents for the nurse to: 1. Cheer them up. 2. Sit quietly with the parents. 3. Send the parents home and sit with the child. 4. Find a volunteer to sit with the child so the parents can leave.	Answer: 2 Rationale: The most important aspect of care for the child and family is to provide care with compassion and understanding of the extreme stress the family is undergoing. Many times sitting quietly with the family is the best intervention at the time. Nursing process step: Implementation Category of client need: Psychosocial integrity Cognitive level: Analysis Learning outcome 28-4: Describe the role of the LPN/LVN in caring for dying children and their families. Test-taking tip: Recognize the role of the nurse in supporting families through difficult times.
7. The death of a child is among the most painful experiences a parent will have to endure. At times, parents may experience dysfunctional grief after this death. Signs of dysfunctional grief are (*select all that apply*): 1. Sleep disturbances. 2. Continuous crying. 3. No emotional response. 4. Unable to work within 2 months of the death.	Answer: 1, 2, 3 Rationale: Parents who experience dysfunctional grief may have sleep disturbances, continuous crying, and no emotional response. Usually dysfunctional grieving is seen in those who are unable to work within 3 to 6 months of the death. Nursing process step: Evaluation Category of client need: Psychosocial integrity Cognitive level: Analysis Learning outcome 28-1: Define key terms. Test-taking tip: Be familiar with key terms to select the correct answer.
8. After a closed head injury in a 3-year-old, the child is unable to gain consciousness and is dying in the intensive care unit. The LPN is sitting with the family at the child's bedside when the charge nurse comes to talk with the family about organ donation. The parents have many questions about this process, and though they have not given consent yet, it is important to give them all the information so they can make a decision. The nurse informs the parents	Answer: 1, 2 Rationale: Organ donation is not a financial responsibility of the family, and it should not change the funeral plans. There is a specialty team of surgeons, anesthesiologists, nurses, and technicians who must be flown in to retrieve the organs, plus the child who is to receive the organ must be notified and brought to a hospital where the transplants can be performed. All of these people must be in place before the child will be removed from life support. Nursing process step: Implementation Category of client need: Psychosocial integrity Cognitive level: Analysis Learning outcome 28-5: Discuss the process of organ donation. Test-taking tip: Know the procedure for harvesting organs.

the following related to organ donation (*select all that apply*):
1. Organ donation will not alter the funeral ceremony.
2. The cost of organ donation is not the responsibility of the family.
3. The child's primary physician will be the one to harvest the organs.
4. The child will be taken off the ventilator as soon as a recipient is found.

---

9. A 5-year-old has been in pain since surgery and radiation for a Wilms' tumor. The nurse knows skin stimulation can be useful in enhancing the effects from pain medications. This is done by:
1. Rubbing the area of radiation.
2. Exerting firm pressure near the pain.
3. Never using vibration over the area of pain.
4. Exerting firm pressure to the area for 5 minutes.

Answer: 2
Rationale: Exerting pressure near or on the area of pain for about 10 seconds to 1 minute can help to lessen pain. Areas of radiation should not have skin stimulation because it could increase trauma to the skin.
Nursing process step: Planning
Category of client need: Physiological integrity
Cognitive level: Analysis
Learning outcome 28-4: Describe the role of the LPN/LVN in caring for dying children and their families.
Test-taking tips: Recognize alternatives and enhancements to control pain in children.

---

10. A 10-year-old with terminal leukemia is in the process of dying. One of the first signs that this may be happening is:
1. Increased respirations.
2. Increased heart rate.
3. Decreased heart rate.
4. Decreased respirations.

Answer: 2
Rationale: As the heart becomes less proficient at pumping blood, the rate increases to compensate. Changes in respiratory status follow increased heart rate.
Nursing process step: Assessment
Category of client need: Physiological integrity
Cognitive level: Evaluation
Learning outcome 28-3: Describe the signs of impending death.
Test-taking tip: Recognize the signs of impending death in a child.

---

11. As the child progresses in the process of dying, the child will become mottled in appearance. This mottling usually begins:
1. On the face.
2. On the trunk.
3. In the hands and feet.
4. In mucous membranes.

Answer: 3
Rationale: Mottling usually begins in the extremities, the farthest areas from the heart. As the heart pump is failing, it is difficult to get oxygenated blood to the extremities, and the blood is shunted to the vital organs.
Nursing process step: Assessment
Category of client need: Physiological integrity
Cognitive level: Application
Learning outcome 28-3: Describe the signs of impending death.

---

12. A 6-year-old who is in the process of dying has Cheyne–Stokes respirations. The nurse would classify this type of respiration as:
1. Fast and deep.
2. Slow and deep.
3. Shallow and slow.
4. Deep breaths, followed by periods of apnea.

Answer: 4
Rationale: Cheyne–Stokes respirations are characterized by a progressive depth of breathing, followed by a period of apnea.
Nursing process step: Assessment
Category of client need: Physiological integrity
Cognitive level: Application
Learning outcome 28-1: Define key terms.
Test-taking tip: Know definitions of key terms to select correct answer.

---

13. The family of a 4-year-old spent an hour with their child after death before they felt they could leave the hospital. The nurse, in doing postmortem care, notes the child has algor mortis. This means the body has:
1. Stiffening of the joints.
2. Decrease in body temperature.
3. Stiffening of the involuntary muscles.
4. A deep discoloration in the dependent areas of the body.

Answer: 2
Rationale: Algor mortis is the gradual decrease of body temperature, due to termination of circulation and cessation of hypothalamus function. Stiffening of the joints and stiffening of the involuntary muscles is called rigor mortis. The deep discoloration in the dependent areas of the body is known as liver mortis.
Nursing process step: Assessment
Category of client need: Physiological integrity
Cognitive level: Application
Learning outcome 28-1: Define key terms
Test-taking tip: Know definitions of key terms to select correct answer.

---

14. The hospice nurse is caring for an 8-year-old who is in the final stages of life with a tumor of the brain. The nurse has an order for morphine sulfate to be given intravenously (IV) as needed for pain. The nurse notes the child's blood pressure is 82/44 and respiratory rate is 10. The child is moaning but otherwise not responding to the nurse or his family. When the family asks the nurse about more pain medication for this child, the nurse replies:

1. "Yes, I agree, he needs more medicine."
2. "Let's wait and see if he wakes up and asks for pain medication."
3. "He is probably dreaming, let's watch him for awhile and see what he does."
4. "He already has had too much pain medication; that is why he is breathing so slowly."

Answer: 1

Rationale: It is important for the nurse to recognize a dying child must be kept comfortable to decrease suffering. Respirations can decrease with the use of pain medication; this is expected during the dying process.

Nursing process step: Assessment

Category of client need: Safe, effective care environment

Cognitive level: Analysis

Learning outcome 28-4: Describe the role of the LPN/LVN in caring for dying children and their families.

Test-taking tip: When three of the answers are similar, choose the answer that is different.

---

15. The nurse who is providing postmortem care needs to handle the body of the child with respect. Rough handling of the child during this care may result in:

1. Tears of the skin.
2. Fecal incontinence.
3. Urine incontinence.
4. Opening of the eyelids.

Answer: 1

Rationale: After death, skin loses its elasticity and can easily be broken. Fecal and urine incontinence are the result of sphincters relaxing and are not affected by handling. Opening of the eyelids would be unrelated to handling of the child, though eyelids may not remain closed even if they were closed by the nurse.

Nursing process step: Implementation

Category of client need: Safe, effective care environment

Cognitive level: Analysis

Learning outcome 28-4: Describe the role of the LPN/LVN in caring for dying children and their families.

Test-taking tip: Recognize the effects of death on the body of a child.